Nanostructured Materials: Synthesis, Functionalization and Applications in Biomedicine

Nanostructured Materials: Synthesis, Functionalization and Applications in Biomedicine

Guest Editors

Ying-Jie Zhu
Heng Li

MDPI

Basel • Beijing • Wuhan • Barcelona • Belgrade • Novi Sad • Cluj • Manchester

Guest Editors

Ying-Jie Zhu
Biomaterials and Tissue Engineering Research Center
Shanghai Institute of Ceramics (SICCAS), CAS
Shanghai
China

Heng Li
Biomaterials and Tissue Engineering Research Center
Shanghai Institute of Ceramics (SICCAS), CAS
Shanghai
China

Editorial Office
MDPI AG
Grosspeteranlage 5
4052 Basel, Switzerland

This is a reprint of the Special Issue, published open access by the journal *Molecules* (ISSN 1420-3049), freely accessible at: https://www.mdpi.com/journal/molecules/special_issues/Nanostructured_Materials.

For citation purposes, cite each article independently as indicated on the article page online and as indicated below:

Lastname, A.A.; Lastname, B.B. Article Title. *Journal Name* **Year**, *Volume Number*, Page Range.

ISBN 978-3-7258-8045-4 (Hbk)
ISBN 978-3-7258-8046-1 (PDF)
https://doi.org/10.3390/books978-3-7258-8046-1

Contents

About the Editors

Ying-Jie Zhu

Ying-Jie Zhu received his Master's degree and Ph.D. from the University of Science and Technology of China in 1992 and 1994, respectively. He served as an assistant professor and associate professor at the University of Science and Technology of China from 1994 to 1997. From 1998 to 1999, he was an Alexander von Humboldt Research Fellow at the Fritz-Haber Institute of the Max Planck Society, Germany. He subsequently worked as a postdoctoral fellow at the University of Utah and the University of Delaware, USA, from 1999 to 2002. In 2002, he was recruited by the Chinese Academy of Sciences through the Program for Recruiting Overseas Outstanding Talents and began his tenure as a full professor and research group leader at the Shanghai Institute of Ceramics, Chinese Academy of Sciences. He has received many honors, including being selected as a "Person of Scientific Chinese" in 2006, recognition as an Outstanding Leader of the Shanghai Subject Chief Scientist Program in 2007, being awarded the ZhuLiYueHua Excellent Teacher Prize of the Chinese Academy of Sciences in 2008, and receiving the First-Class Prize of Natural Sciences from the Shanghai Municipality in 2009 (shared with colleagues). He has published more than 400 peer-reviewed journal papers, including in many ESI highly cited papers, 1 monograph, and 7 book chapters, with his research being cited approximately 25,000 times. From 2014 to 2025, he was listed 12 times among Elsevier's Annual List of Most Cited Chinese Researchers. He also holds 72 authorized patents. His research interests include nanostructured materials and biomaterials.

Heng Li

Heng Li received his Ph.D. from the Shanghai Institute of Ceramics, Chinese Academy of Sciences, in 2019, and he subsequently worked at the Center of Super-Diamond and Advanced Films, the City University of Hong Kong. He is currently an associate professor at the Chinese Academy of Sciences. In 2021, he became a faculty member at the Chinese Academy of Sciences. His research interest focuses on high-safety and biocompatible battery materials.

molecules

MDPI

Article

Microwave-Heating-Assisted Synthesis of Ultrathin and Ultralong Hydroxyapatite Nanowires Using Biogenic Creatine Phosphate and Their Derived Flexible Bio-Paper with Drug Delivery Function

Yu Zhang [1,2], Ying-Jie Zhu [1,2,*], Si-Yi Li [1,2], Li-Ying Dong [1] and Han-Ping Yu [1,*]

[1] State Key Laboratory of High Performance Ceramics and Superfine Microstructure, Shanghai Institute of Ceramics, Chinese Academy of Sciences, Shanghai 200050, China; zgzyaizg@163.com (Y.Z.); lain9221@163.com (S.-Y.L.); lydong@mail.sic.ac.cn (L.-Y.D.)

[2] Center of Materials Science and Optoelectronics Engineering, University of Chinese Academy of Sciences, Beijing 100049, China

* Correspondence: y.j.zhu@mail.sic.ac.cn (Y.-J.Z.); yuhanping@mail.sic.ac.cn (H.-P.Y.)

Abstract: With an ultrahigh aspect ratio and a similar chemical composition to the biomineral in bone and tooth, ultralong hydroxyapatite nanowires (UHAPNWs) exhibit a meritorious combination of high flexibility, excellent mechanical performance, high biocompatibility, and bioactivity. Despite these exciting merits, the rapid and green synthesis of UHAPNWs remains challenging. In this work, we have developed an environment-friendly, rapid, and highly efficient synthesis of ultrathin UHAPNWs by the microwave-assisted calcium oleate precursor hydrothermal method using biogenic creatine phosphate as the bio-phosphorus source. Owing to the controllable hydrolysis of bio-phosphorus-containing creatine phosphate and the highly efficient heating of microwave irradiation, ultrathin UHAPNWs with a homogeneous morphology of several nanometers in diameter (single nanowire), several hundred micrometers in length, and ultrahigh aspect ratios (>10,000) can be rapidly synthesized within 60 min. This effectively shortens the synthesis time by about two orders of magnitude compared with the traditional hydrothermal method. Furthermore, ultrathin UHAPNWs are decorated in situ with bioactive creatine and self-assembled into nanowire bundles along their longitudinal direction at the nanoscale. In addition, ultrathin UHAPNWs exhibit a relatively high specific surface area of 84.30 m^2 g^{-1} and high ibuprofen drug loading capacity. The flexible bio-paper constructed from interwoven ibuprofen-loaded ultrathin UHAPNWs can sustainably deliver ibuprofen in phosphate-buffered saline, which is promising for various biomedical applications such as tissue regeneration with anti-inflammatory and analgesic functions.

Keywords: hydroxyapatite; nanowire; microwave; hydrothermal; creatine phosphate

1. Introduction

With the rapid and energetic development of nanotechnology in recent decades, various kinds of nanomaterials have been created for widespread applications [1–4]. Nanowires, in particular, with their merits of anisotropy, superior mechanical properties, weaving ability, and high surface-to-volume ratio, have attracted tremendous attention in recent years [5,6]. Nanowires and their assembled materials usually exhibit very different physical and chemical properties from their monolithic bulk analogues [7,8]. For example, many ceramic nanowires have been found to be more flexible than traditional ceramic pieces [9–12], and they can be woven into a variety of porous scaffolds for tissue regeneration [13–16]. Moreover, nanowires can provide abundant surface-active points for high drug loading capacity and controlled drug release [17,18].

Hydroxyapatite (HAP, $Ca_{10}(PO_4)_6(OH)_2$) is a popular inorganic biomaterial for bone tissue engineering, tooth repair, and drug delivery [19–21]. HAP nanowires (HAPNWs) show outstanding properties, such as high mechanical properties, biocompatibility, bioactivity, osteo-conductivity, and osteo-induction, owing to their compositional similarity to the inorganic mineral in human bones and teeth [22,23]. It is well-accepted that high aspect ratio HAP nanostructures encourage rich functions [24]. In recent years, the authors' research group has developed a kind of ultralong HAP nanowire (UHAPNW) with ultrahigh aspect ratios (>10,000), about 10 nm in diameter, and several hundred micrometers in length [25–27]. In contrast to the traditional brittle HAP ceramic materials, UHAPNWs exhibit high flexibility. UHAPNWs can be twisted and interwoven owing to their extremely high aspect ratios, and they can assemble into various flexible functional materials with the networked structure [26,27]. Moreover, UHAPNWs show a high surface-to-volume ratio and significant interface phenomena, providing abundant sites for the attachment of drug molecules, metal ions, and functional groups [25–28].

The traditional synthesis of HAP materials is still facing the challenges of uncontrollable formation of calcium phosphate nuclei and lengthy reaction times [29–31]. In our previous work, we developed a microwave-assisted calcium oleate precursor–biophosphorus hydrothermal method, which is promising for the preparation of UHAPNWs with uniform morphology, high mechanical flexibility, and high bioactivity [32]. Moreover, owing to the controlled hydrolysis of phosphorus-containing biomolecules as well as the rapid and uniform heating by microwaves [33,34], the nucleation and growth of crystals can be regulated, resulting in HAP nanowires with small diameters and high aspect ratios. Unfortunately, until now, only adenosine triphosphate (ATP) has been explored for the synthesis of UHAPNWs. The chemical structure of ATP is shown in Scheme 1. More potential phosphorus-containing biomolecules need to be explored, yet this is challenging. Unlike the case of inorganic phosphates as the phosphorus source, the complexity of the structure and hydrolysis process of phosphorus-containing biomolecules may prohibit the satisfactory preparation of high-quality UHAPNWs.

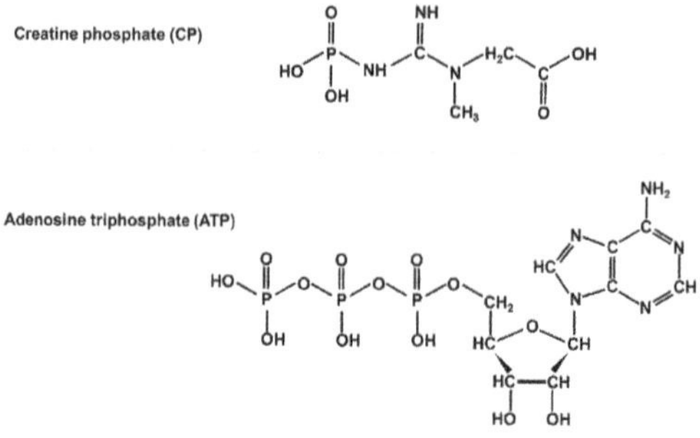

Scheme 1. The chemical structures of creatine phosphate and adenosine triphosphate (ATP).

Creatine phosphate (phosphocreatine) is a high-energy phosphate compound commonly found in muscle or other excitable tissues [35,36]. The chemical structure of creatine phosphate is shown in Scheme 1. It is a storage form of high-energy phosphate groups. When organisms consume ATP and produce adenosine diphosphate, creatine phosphate can rapidly release high-energy phosphate groups into adenosine diphosphate under enzymatic action, so that ATP can be rapidly restored to the normal high supply levels [37]. In the past, studies focused on the in vitro hydrolysis of creatine phosphate and its mechanisms of interconversion with ATP and creatine in order to understand its role in influencing the body during exercise [38]. Because of its close association with high-energy phosphate compounds, creatine phosphate is often used as a reference for testing the metabolic performance of muscle [39–41]. In recent years, creatine phosphate has been explored for the synthesis of nanostructured materials. For instance, Cao et al. reported a microwave solvothermal method for the preparation of hollow hierarchical mesoporous structured hydroxyapatite microflowers with a high drug loading capacity using creatine phosphate as the phosphorus source and template [42]. Qi et al. used creatine phosphate to synthesize magnesium phosphate pentahydrate nanosheets with pH-responsive solubility, which is promising for use as pH-responsive nanocarriers for drug and gene delivery [43]. However, neither of them successfully prepared UHAPNWs using creatine phosphate as the bio-phosphorus source. We speculate that creatine phosphate may be used as the bio-phosphorus source to synthesize UHAPNWs like ATP.

In this work, we successfully prepared UHAPNWs with ultrathin diameters (only several nanometers for a single nanowire) using creatine phosphate as the bio-phosphorus source and calcium oleate as the precursor by the microwave-assisted calcium oleate precursor hydrothermal method. The optimized parameters for the synthesis of ultrathin UHAPNWs were investigated. The as-prepared ultrathin UHAPNWs have ultrasmall diameters (only several nanometers for a single nanowire), ultralong lengths (hundreds of micrometers), and ultrahigh aspect ratios (>10,000), and can self-assemble along their longitudinal direction to form nanowire bundles with a high BET specific surface area (84.30 m^2 g^{-1}). Moreover, the as-prepared ultrathin UHAPNWs show a high ibuprofen loading capacity (0.33 g drug per gram of nanocarrier). After loading ibuprofen, ultrathin UHAPNWs still exhibit a high specific surface area of 79.21 m^2 g^{-1}. The ibuprofen-loaded ultrathin UHAPNWs can be further interwoven into flexible and porous bio-paper, and it can continuously release the drug in phosphate-buffered saline (PBS), which is promising for various biomedical applications such as inflammatory treatment and promoting tissue regeneration.

2. Results and Discussion

2.1. Characterization of Ultrathin UHAPNWs

In this work, we chose sodium creatine phosphate tetrahydrate as the bio-phosphorus source and calcium oleate as the precursor, and used microwave-assisted hydrothermal heating to rapidly synthesize ultrathin UHAPNWs. The synthetic process of ultrathin UHAPNWs is demonstrated in Figure 1. As shown in the schematic diagram, calcium ions are combined with oleate groups to form calcium oleate precursor. It is known that the phosphate groups are fixed within creatine phosphate biomolecules [44,45]. In the initial reaction system, there are no free PO_4^{3-} ions because creatine phosphate molecules are not hydrolyzed to release free PO_4^{3-} ions, which can prevent the premature formation of calcium phosphate nuclei and uncontrollable crystal growth. During microwave heating, the temperature of the reaction system rises rapidly, and creatine phosphate molecules hydrolyze and release free PO_4^{3-} ions to supply the phosphorus source for the formation of ultrathin UHAPNWs. Moreover, microwave-assisted heating shows the advantages of rapid volumetric heating, higher efficiency and reaction rates, shorter reaction times, and lower energy consumption compared with the conventional heating methods [34,46–48], which is beneficial for controlling the hydrolysis of creatine phosphate molecules as well as for the environmentally friendly rapid synthesis of homogeneous and well-crystallized ultrathin UHAPNWs. In our previous review article [34], we discussed the comparison of energy consumption between microwave heating and conventional heating, confirming that the energy consumption of microwave heating is reduced significantly compared with conventional heating methods.

In addition, in our previous studies, the microwave heating time needed for the synthesis of UHAPNWs was much shorter (less than 1 h) than the conventional heating methods (usually about 24 h or longer), and the microwave heating time needed for the synthesis of UHAPNWs decreased by about two orders of magnitude, further verifying that the energy consumption by microwave heating can be reduced significantly compared with conventional heating methods [25,28,32,47]. Microwave heating can significantly enhance the chemical reaction rate, selectivity, and yield of the product, and microwave heating synthesis can exhibit order-of-magnitude enhancements in the reaction rate as compared with the conventional heating synthesis. Due to the merits of microwave dielectric volumetric heating for rapid temperature ramping of the reaction system, the conventional heating system needs more than six times the energy consumption for the synthesis of cubic $BaTiO_3$ nanoparticles compared with that of the microwave heating system [34,49]. As a result, the microwave heating calcium oleate precursor hydrothermal method provides a promising pathway to significantly enhance the efficiency and reduce the energy consumption for the rapid synthesis of UHAPNWs.

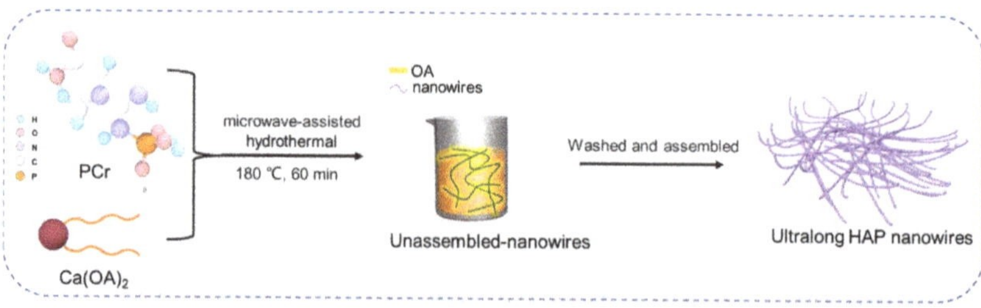

Figure 1. Schematic diagram of the rapid synthesis of ultrathin UHAPNWs by the microwave-assisted calcium oleate precursor hydrothermal method using sodium creatine phosphate as the bio-phosphorus source, and the self-assembly of ultrathin UHAPNWs into ultralong nanowire bundles.

Figure 2 shows the SEM images of the ultrathin UHAPNWs synthesized by the microwave-assisted calcium oleate precursor hydrothermal method using creatine phosphate as the bio-phosphorus source, and the reaction time and temperature are 60 min and 180 °C, respectively. As expected, ultrathin UHAPNWs can be successfully prepared by the microwave-assisted calcium oleate precursor hydrothermal method using creatine phosphate as the bio-phosphorus source. The as-prepared ultrathin UHAPNWs are morphologically homogeneous, and their diameters are dozens of nanometers, and their lengths can reach hundreds of micrometers. In addition, ultrathin UHAPNWs can self-assemble along their longitudinal direction to form nanowire bundles with larger diameters. Ultrathin UHAPNWs are highly flexible and can be bent at large angles without fracture. Due to the high aspect ratios and high flexibility of ultrathin UHAPNWs, they tend to interweave into a porous nanowire network.

Energy dispersive spectroscopy (EDS) elemental mapping results (Figure 3) indicate that the as-prepared ultrathin UHAPNWs contain Ca, P, O, N, and C elements. The Ca, P, and O elements originate from ultrathin UHAPNWs. Both the N and C elements are from the components of creatine phosphate, suggesting the presence of creatine phosphate molecules adsorbed on the surface of ultrathin UHAPNWs.

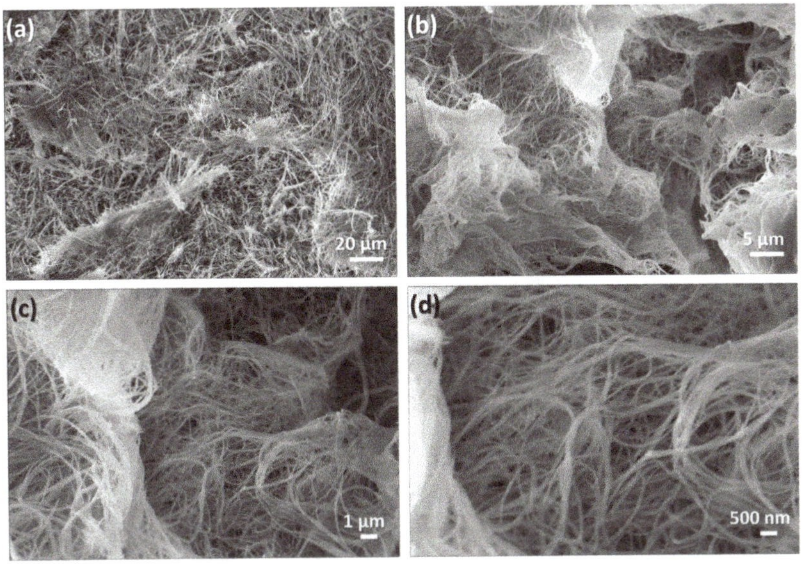

Figure 2. SEM images with different magnifications (**a–d**) of UHAPNWs prepared by the microwave-assisted calcium oleate precursor hydrothermal method using creatine phosphate as the bio-phosphorus source at 180 °C for 60 min.

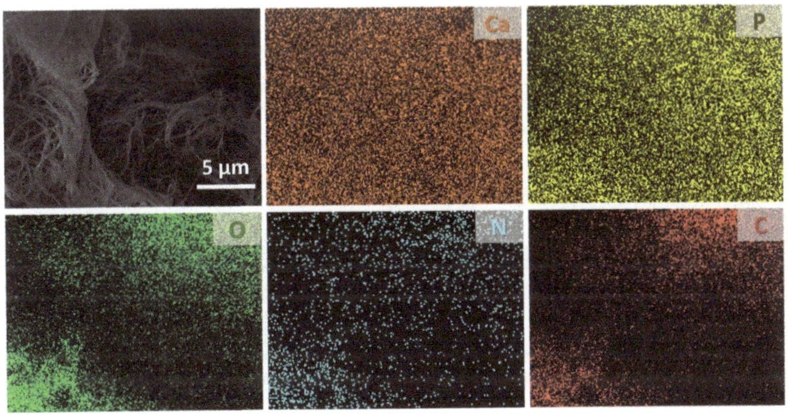

Figure 3. EDS elemental mapping of the ultrathin UHAPNWs prepared by the microwave-assisted calcium oleate precursor hydrothermal method using creatine phosphate as the bio-phosphorus source at 180 °C for 60 min.

Higher-resolution structural analysis of the as-prepared ultrathin UHAPNWs was performed by TEM, and the results are shown in Figure 4. One can see that ultrathin UHAPNWs are self-assembled along their longitudinal direction to form nanowire bundles with diameters of 10 to ~100 nanometers (Figure 4a). The diameter of a single ultralong HAP nanowire is only ~6 nm (Figure 4b), which is lower than those of UHAPNWs prepared using inorganic phosphate salts as the phosphorus source, and consistent with those of UHAPNWs synthesized using ATP as the bio-phosphorus source in our previous work [32]. This suggests that the combination of rapid microwave heating and the use of phosphorus-containing biomolecules as the bio-phosphorus source can rapidly synthesize UHAPNWs with ultrasmall diameters compared with those prepared by the conventional heating methods using inorganic phosphates. It is calculated that the aspect ratios of the as-prepared ultrathin UHAPNWs are more than 10,000. The TEM image of the nanowire bundles clearly reveals that ultrathin UHAPNWs self-align along their longitudinal direction at the nanoscale (Figure 4c). Such nanoscale ordered structures are beneficial to the superior microscopic flexibility of the ultralong HAP nanowire bundles [50].

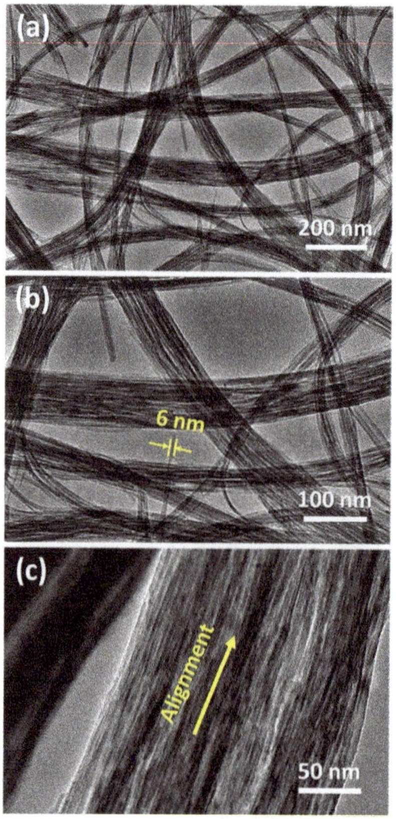

Figure 4. TEM images of ultrathin UHAPNWs and nanowire bundles with high flexibility (**a**), ultrasmall nanowire diameter (**b**), and nanoscale self-alignment (**c**) prepared by the microwave-assisted calcium oleate precursor hydrothermal method using creatine phosphate as the bio-phosphorus source at 180 °C for 60 min.

2.2. Effects of Experimental Parameters on the Formation of Ultrathin UHAPNWs

We explored the influence of the reaction time on the formation of ultrathin UHAPNWs prepared by the microwave-assisted calcium oleate precursor hydrothermal method using creatine phosphate as the bio-phosphorus source at 180 °C. As shown in Figure 5, one-dimensional (1-D) wire-like structures are formed for a reaction time of 15 min, accompanying many irregular-shaped particles (Figure 5a,b). When the microwave heating time increases to 30 min, the particles disappear and HAP nanowires are obtained. However, the as-prepared HAP nanowires show significantly heterogeneous sizes, and some microfibers with diameters of several micrometers can be observed (Figure 5c,d). As discussed above, when the microwave heating time further increases to 60 min, well-defined ultrathin UHAPNWs with a uniform morphology, ultrasmall diameters, ultralong lengths, ultrahigh aspect ratios, and high flexibility are obtained (Figure 2). In contrast to the traditional hydrothermal method that requires tens of hours to synthesize UHAPNWs, the microwave heating in this work can produce high-quality ultrathin UHAPNWs within 60 min, which can greatly enhance the reaction rate and efficiency, and shorten the reaction time.

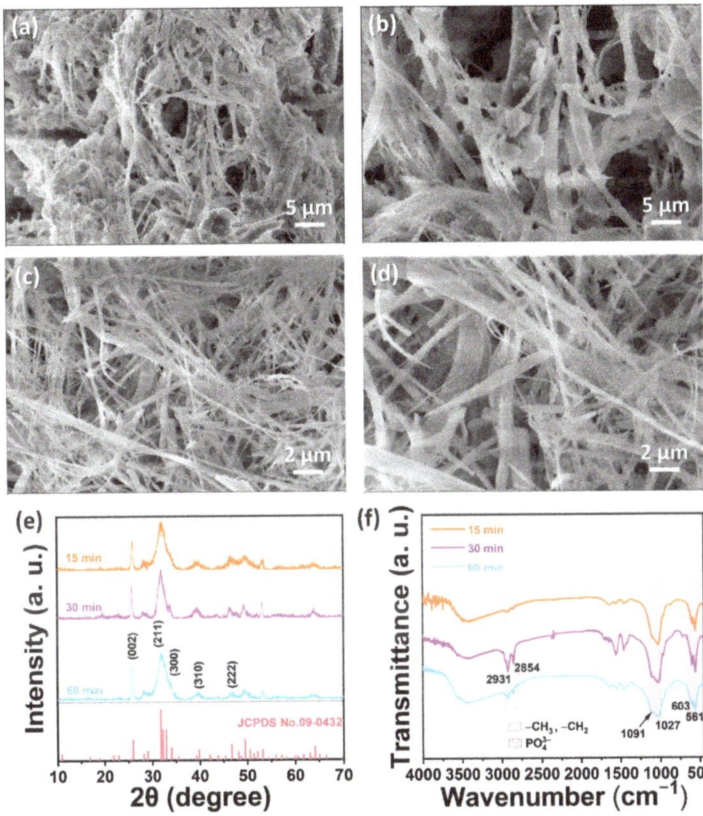

Figure 5. Evaluation of the influence of the reaction time on the formation of the product prepared by the microwave-assisted calcium oleate precursor hydrothermal method using creatine phosphate as the bio-phosphorus source at 180 °C. (**a**–**d**) SEM images of the products prepared for different reaction times: (**a**,**b**) 15 min; (**c**,**d**) 30 min. (**e**) XRD patterns. (**f**) FTIR spectra.

Figure 5e shows the XRD patterns of the products synthesized by the microwave-assisted calcium oleate precursor hydrothermal method using creatine phosphate as the bio-phosphorus source at 180 °C for different times. The XRD patterns indicate that the as-prepared samples are composed of a single crystal phase of hexagonal hydroxyapatite (JCPDS No. 09-0432). This experimental result indicates that a single crystal phase of hydroxyapatite is formed in a short period of the microwave-assisted hydrothermal time (<15 min). With an increase in the reaction time, the crystallinity of the product is enhanced. Therefore, well-crystalline HAP nanowires have already formed within 30 min.

The experimental results show the microwave heating time has a great impact on the morphology and size of the product. It usually takes about 24 h or longer for the synthesis of UHAPNWs and other one-dimensional (1-D) hydroxyapatite nanomaterials by traditional heating methods [25,28,51–59], indicating the high efficiency and energy-saving advantage of the microwave heating method. The FTIR spectra (Figure 5f) show absorption peaks at 2931 cm^{-1} and 2854 cm^{-1}, corresponding to the $-CH_3$ and $-CH_2$ groups, and absorption peaks at 1091 cm^{-1}, 1027 cm^{-1}, 603 cm^{-1}, and 561 cm^{-1}, belonging to the ${PO_4}^{3-}$ group [28,56], suggesting the formation of ultrathin UHAPNWs and the presence of organic components (oleate and creatine phosphate) on their surface. Ultrathin UHAPNWs with a uniform morphology, ultrasmall diameters, ultralong lengths, ultrahigh aspect ratios, and high crystallinity can be obtained when microwave hydrothermal heating is performed for a sufficient time, and 60 min is preferred.

On this basis, we investigated the effect of microwave hydrothermal temperature on the formation of the product. As shown in Figure 6a, when the microwave hydrothermal temperature is 120 °C, the XRD pattern of the product shows a low crystallinity of hydroxyapatite and a broad diffraction peak from ~20° to ~40°, corresponding to amorphous calcium phosphate. That is, the product obtained by the microwave-assisted hydrothermal treatment at 120 °C for 60 min consists of a mixture of low-crystallinity hydroxyapatite and amorphous calcium phosphate. When the microwave hydrothermal temperature increases to 140 °C, the amount of the amorphous phase decreases significantly. When the microwave hydrothermal temperature is elevated to 160 °C or above, the product is composed of a single-phase crystalline hydroxyapatite with a hexagonal structure. The FTIR spectra of the products prepared by the microwave-assisted calcium oleate precursor hydrothermal method using creatine phosphate as the bio-phosphorus source at different temperatures for 60 min are shown in Figure 6b. The absorption peak at ~3569 cm^{-1} is ascribed to the –OH group of hydroxyapatite. The absorption peaks at 1027 cm^{-1} and 1091 cm^{-1} correspond to the stretching mode of the PO_4^{3-} group, and the absorption peaks located at 603 cm^{-1} and 561 cm^{-1} correspond to the bending mode of the O–P–O of the PO_4^{3-} group. Furthermore, the absorption peaks from 1300 to 1700 cm^{-1} originate from the presence of the groups from phosphocreatine, indicating that the phosphocreatine molecules are adsorbed on the surface of the products.

The experimental results indicate that the microwave hydrothermal temperature has a great effect on the morphology of the product (Figure 6c–h). When the microwave hydrothermal temperature is 120 °C or 140 °C, irregular structures are obtained, although their XRD patterns show the formation of the crystal phase of hexagonal hydroxyapatite. Thus, UHAPNWs cannot be prepared at low reaction temperatures by this method. From the crystallographic perspective, the oriented growth of hydroxyapatite into ultralong nanowires along its *c*-axis direction requires sufficiently high temperatures and pressures. As expected, when the reaction temperature is enhanced to 160 °C, UHAPNWs are formed without irregular structures, and the UHAPNWs become longer and thinner when the reaction temperature further increases to 180 °C. Therefore, an adequately high reaction temperature is essential for the formation of ultrathin UHAPNWs. In order to obtain ultrathin UHAPNWs, the minimum reaction temperature should be 180 °C.

Furthermore, we investigated the influence of the Ca/P molar ratio of the reactants on the structure of the product (Figure 7). For the samples discussed above, we fixed the Ca/P molar ratio of the reactants at 1:2. Here, we modulated this ratio to 1:1.5 and 1:1 by varying the amount of creatine phosphate but fixing the amount of $CaCl_2$. As shown in Figure 7a), the modulation of the Ca/P molar ratio of the reactants does not change the crystalline phase of the product, and all samples can be indexed to a single crystalline phase of hexagonal hydroxyapatite (JCPDS No. 09-0432). The FTIR spectra of the samples prepared at different Ca/P molar ratios of the reactants are shown in Figure 7b. The characteristic absorption peaks at 2927 cm^{-1} and 2854 cm^{-1}, corresponding to the $–CH_3$ and $–CH_2$ groups, are observed in all FTIR spectra of the products. In addition, the characteristic absorption peaks at 1650 cm^{-1} and 1558 cm^{-1} are ascribed to the bending vibrations of $–NH_2$ and C–N–H. These results suggest the presence of characteristic groups from phosphocreatine in the product.

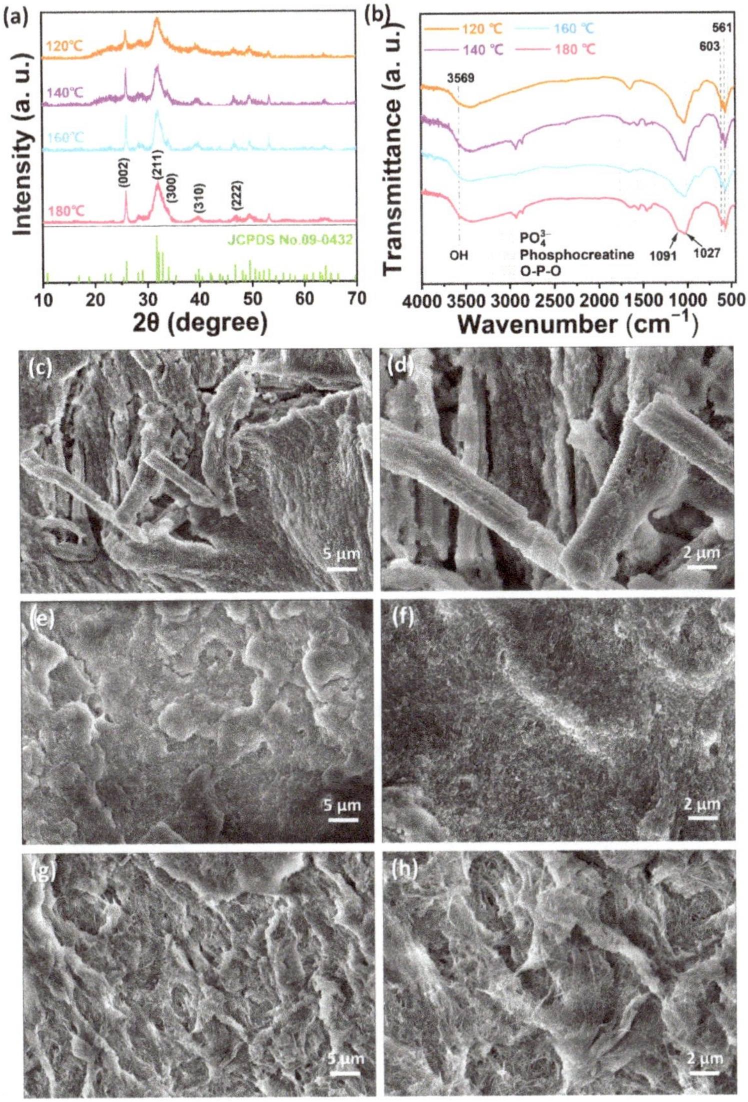

Figure 6. Characterization of the products obtained by the microwave-assisted calcium oleate precursor hydrothermal method using creatine phosphate as the bio-phosphorus source at different temperatures for 60 min. (**a**) XRD patterns; (**b**) FTIR spectra; (**c**–**h**) SEM images: (**c**,**d**) 120 °C, (**e**,**f**) 140 °C, and (**g**,**h**) 160 °C.

The SEM investigation results reveal that the Ca/P molar ratio of the reactants also influences the morphology of the product. Although ultrathin UHAPNWs can be prepared by the modulation of Ca/P molar ratios ranging from 1:1 to 1:2, they exhibit a distinct size and uniformity. When the Ca/P molar ratio is 1:1, the as-prepared UHAPNWs show uneven diameters and lengths, and some thick HAP microfibers can be observed (Figure 7c,d). When the Ca/P molar ratio decreases to 1:1.5, the HAP nanowire bundles become thicker, with some particles. As discussed above, when the Ca/P molar ratio is 1:2, relatively uniform ultrathin UHAPNWs are synthesized. Therefore, hexagonal structured UHAPNWs can be obtained at different molar ratios of calcium and phosphorus sources of reactants, but ultrathin UHAPNWs with uniform sizes and higher aspect ratios are obtained when the Ca/P molar ratio is 1:2.

Therefore, the reaction time, reaction temperature, and Ca/P molar ratio of the reactants are important parameters to modulate the size and morphology of the product. We can conclude that the optimized parameters for the preparation of ultrathin UHAPNWs are as follows: adopting the microwave-assisted calcium oleate precursor hydrothermal method using creatine phosphate as the bio-phosphorus source heated at 180 °C for 60 min with the Ca/P molar ratio of the reactants being 1:2.

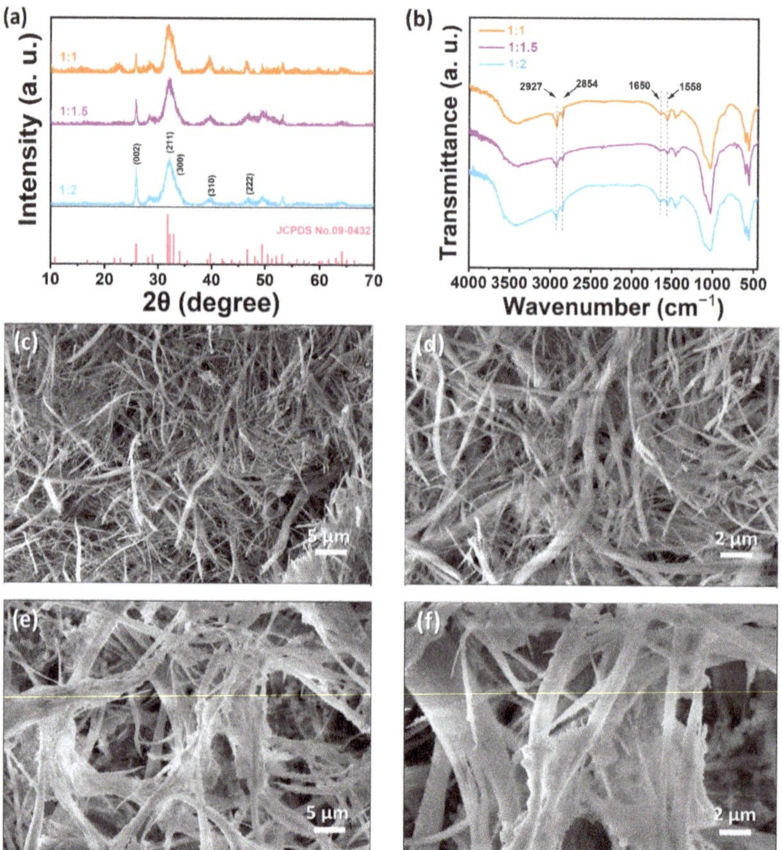

Figure 7. Characterization of the products prepared by the microwave-assisted calcium oleate precursor hydrothermal method using creatine phosphate as the bio-phosphorus source at different Ca/P molar ratios at 180 °C for 60 min. (**a**) XRD patterns; (**b**) FTIR spectra; (**c**–**f**) SEM images of the samples prepared at different Ca/P molar ratios: (**c**,**d**) 1:1 and (**e**,**f**) 1:1.5.

2.3. The Formation Mechanism of Ultrathin UHAPNWs

The oleate plays an important role in the formation of ultrathin UHAPNWs. As shown in Figure 8a, although sodium oleate is absent from the reaction system, the XRD pattern of the obtained product is also indexed to a single crystal phase of hexagonal hydroxyapatite (JCPDS No. 09-0432). This is consistent with the results obtained with the synthetic system using sodium oleate. Therefore, sodium oleate does not alter the crystal phase of the product in this method. It is noted that the product obtained without sodium oleate shows a higher degree of crystallinity than ultrathin UHAPNWs prepared in the presence of sodium oleate. This may be attributed to the fact that ultrathin UHAPNWs possess ultrasmall diameters but extraordinarily long lengths, leading to the significant disarrangement of surface atoms. Similarly, as shown in Figure 8b, the FTIR spectra of the products obtained by the microwave-assisted hydrothermal method using creatine phosphate as the bio-phosphorus source both with and without sodium oleate exhibit the characteristic absorption peaks of PO_4^{3-} located at 1091 cm^{-1}, 1027 cm^{-1}, 603 cm^{-1}, and 561 cm^{-1}, suggesting the formation of hydroxyapatite. However, the FTIR spectra of the ultrathin UHAPNWs prepared in the presence of sodium oleate show more pronounced C–N–H and $-CH_3$ absorption peaks at 1558 cm^{-1} and 1457 cm^{-1}, respectively, compared with those of the product prepared without sodium oleate. These peaks originate from creatine phosphate, suggesting that the interaction between oleate and creatine phosphate can better facilitate the in situ modification of the surface of ultrathin UHAPNWs with creatine phosphate molecules.

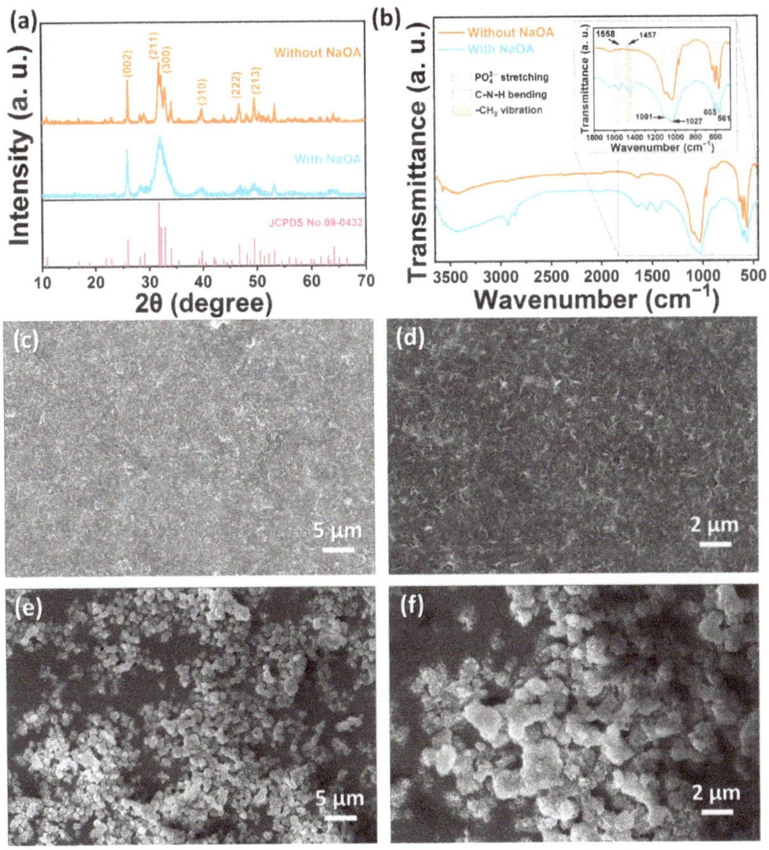

Figure 8. (**a**,**b**) XRD patterns (**a**) and FTIR spectra (**b**) of the products prepared by the microwave-assisted hydrothermal method using creatine phosphate as the bio-phosphorus source with or without sodium oleate at 180 °C for 60 min (Ca/P molar ratio 1:2). (**c**,**d**) SEM images of calcium oleate obtained by the reaction between sodium oleate and $CaCl_2$ in an aqueous solution. (**e**,**f**) SEM images of the product synthesized by the microwave-assisted hydrothermal method using creatine phosphate as the bio-phosphorus source in the absence of sodium oleate at 180 °C for 60 min (Ca/P molar ratio 1:2).

As shown in Figure 8c,d, the calcium oleate precursor formed by the reaction between oleate groups and calcium ions consists of irregular particles. During the microwave heating process, the hydrolysis of creatine phosphate results in the release of PO_4^{3-} ions, and PO_4^{3-} ions react with calcium oleate to gradually form ultrathin UHAPNWs. However, without the addition of sodium oleate to the reaction system, no calcium oleate precursor is formed, lacking structural guidance for the growth of ultrathin UHAPNWs. Therefore, only severely aggregated HAP particles are obtained in the reaction system in the absence of the calcium oleate precursor, and their diameters range from hundreds of nanometers to several micrometers (Figure 8e,f). The chemical reactions associated with the formation of ultrathin UHAPNWs using the calcium oleate precursor and creatine phosphate as the bio-phosphorus source is described below.

$$Ca^{2+} + 2R\text{-}COO^{-} \rightarrow Ca(R\text{-}COO)_2$$

$$\text{Phosphocreatine} + H_2O \rightarrow \text{Creatine} + H_3PO_4$$

$$10Ca(R\text{-}COO)_2 + 6H_3PO_4 + 2H_2O \rightarrow Ca_{10}(PO_4)_6(OH)_2 + 20R\text{-}COOH$$

where $R = CH_3(CH_2)_7CH = CH(CH_2)_7$.

Phosphocreatine is unable to hydrolyze in an aqueous solution at room temperature without creatine kinase, and can only hydrolyze at high temperatures without creatine kinase. Thus, unlike the case of inorganic phosphates as the phosphorus source, phosphocreatine can prevent undesired premature chemical reactions between calcium oleate precursor and PO_4^{3-} ions before the microwave-assisted hydrothermal treatment.

As shown in Figure 9, the FTIR spectrum of the dried product obtained by mixing the calcium oleate precursor and sodium creatine phosphate in aqueous solution (labelled as $Ca(OA)_2$-CP) is consistent with that of the pure calcium oleate precursor (labelled as $Ca(OA)_2$), indicating that the premature chemical reactions between calcium oleate precursor and sodium creatine phosphate did not occur. This can avoid the uncontrolled chemical reaction, nucleation, and crystal growth of the product.

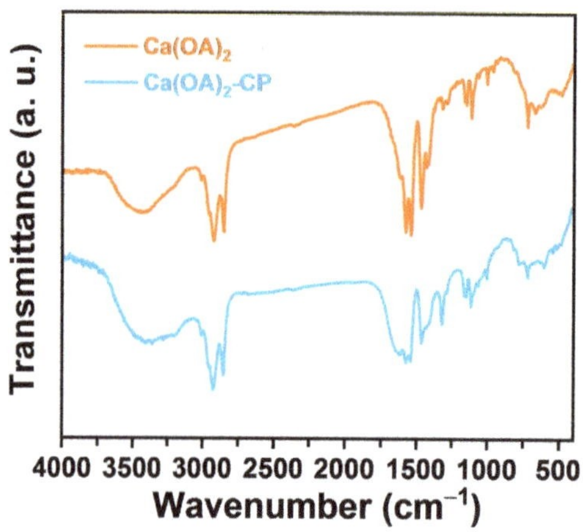

Figure 9. FTIR spectra of the calcium oleate ($Ca(OA)_2$) precursor and the dried product ($Ca(OA)_2$-CP) obtained by mixing the calcium oleate precursor with sodium creatine phosphate tetrahydrate in an aqueous solution at room temperature.

In addition, microwave heating shows competitive superiorities such as environmental friendliness, high efficiency, and energy savings. Therefore, during the microwave-assisted hydrothermal treatment, the temperature of the reaction system is rapidly and uniformly elevated to the hydrolysis temperature of phosphocreatine, and the hydrolysis of phosphocreatine releases free PO_4^{3-} ions in an aqueous solution to participate in the formation of ultrathin UHAPNWs. This can avoid the problem that calcium phosphate nuclei prematurely form and subsequently grow into byproducts during the lengthy heating process of the conventional hydrothermal treatment using inorganic phosphates as the phosphorus source, which results in an inhomogeneous morphology and size.

As expected, the experimental results verify our speculation that creatine phosphate is a rational phosphorus-containing biomolecule to control the formation of ultrathin UHAPNWs through the microwave-assisted calcium oleate precursor hydrothermal method. The advantages of creatine phosphate as a bio-phosphorus source for the synthesis of UHAPNWs are summarized as follows: (1) creatine phosphate is a biogenic and small biomolecule containing only one phosphate group in each molecule with the same breaking energy, which can provide PO_4^{3-} ions for the formation of UHAPNWs by hydrolysis in an aqueous solution under hydrothermal conditions; (2) since the hydrolysis of creatine phosphate requires creatine kinase at room temperature, and can only hydrolyze at high temperatures in the absence of creatine kinase, this can prevent the undesired premature chemical reactions between calcium oleate precursor and PO_4^{3-} ions before the microwave-assisted hydrothermal treatment; (3) the hydrolysis conditions for creatine phosphate to release PO_4^{3-} ions are consistent with the hydrothermal treatment required for the formation of UHAPNWs; (4) creatine phosphate and its hydrolyzed product show high biocompatibility.

In our previous work, we chose ATP as the bio-phosphorus source for synthesizing UHAPNWs [32]. The chemical structure of creatine phosphate is very different from that of ATP, and thus their hydrolysis processes are different. Creatine phosphate and ATP cannot hydrolyze without enzymes at room temperature, and they can only hydrolyze at high temperatures in the absence of enzymes, but their hydrolysis behaviors are different at high temperatures under hydrothermal conditions. One ATP molecule contains three phosphate groups with different breaking energies, which gradually hydrolyze to form adenosine diphosphate, adenosine monophosphate, and adenosine under hydrothermal conditions, and the phosphate ions are released in an aqueous solution. In comparison, one creatine phosphate molecule contains only one phosphate group, and the same activated energy is needed for its hydrolysis. Therefore, creatine phosphate can hydrolyze to provide phosphate ions for the formation of UHAPNWs in a short period of time, which is beneficial for obtaining ultrathin UHAPNWs with a uniform morphology. Moreover, creatine phosphate, as a common drug for the treatment of hypertension and cardiovascular disease [60,61], is cheaper than ATP and thus is more promising to be used as the bio-phosphorus source for the synthesis of UHAPNWs with a reduced cost.

2.4. Ultrathin UHAPNWs as Drug Nanocarriers for Drug Delivery

Owing to their ultrasmall diameter, ultralong length, and ultrahigh aspect ratio, the as-prepared ultrathin UHAPNWs are the ideal nanocarrier for drug delivery. Herein, we investigated the drug loading performance of ultrathin UHAPNWs as the drug carrier using ibuprofen, a typical anti-inflammatory drug, as the model drug. The TG-DSC analysis was applied to calculate the drug loading capacity of ultrathin UHAPNWs. As shown in Figure 10a, the pure ultrathin UHAPNWs without ibuprofen loading exhibit a weight loss of about 12.08 wt.% from room temperature to 800 °C. This weight loss is ascribed to the evaporation of adsorbed water (5.32 wt.%), as well as the oxidative decomposition of creatine phosphate and residual oleate (6.76 wt.%). Thus, the organic content of UHAPNWs is calculated to be approximately 7.14%. The weight loss of ultrathin UHAPNWs loaded with ibuprofen is only 0.5 wt.% when it is heated from room temperature to 150 °C, mainly due to the evaporation of the adsorbed water. Compared with the TG curve of pure ultrathin UHAPNWs, the adsorbed water of ibuprofen-loaded UHAPNWs obviously decreases, which may be ascribed to the solvent exchange (water and hexane) during the ibuprofen loading process. When the temperature is further enhanced to 800 °C, the weight loss of ultrathin UHAPNWs loaded with ibuprofen reaches 29.88 wt.%. The increased weight loss results from the oxidative decomposition of ibuprofen. As evidence, there is a clear exothermic peak at 352.8 °C in the DSC curve of ibuprofen-loaded ultrathin UHAPNWs, whereas there is no obvious peak in the DSC curve of unloaded ultrathin UHAPNWs in the same temperature range (Figure 10b).

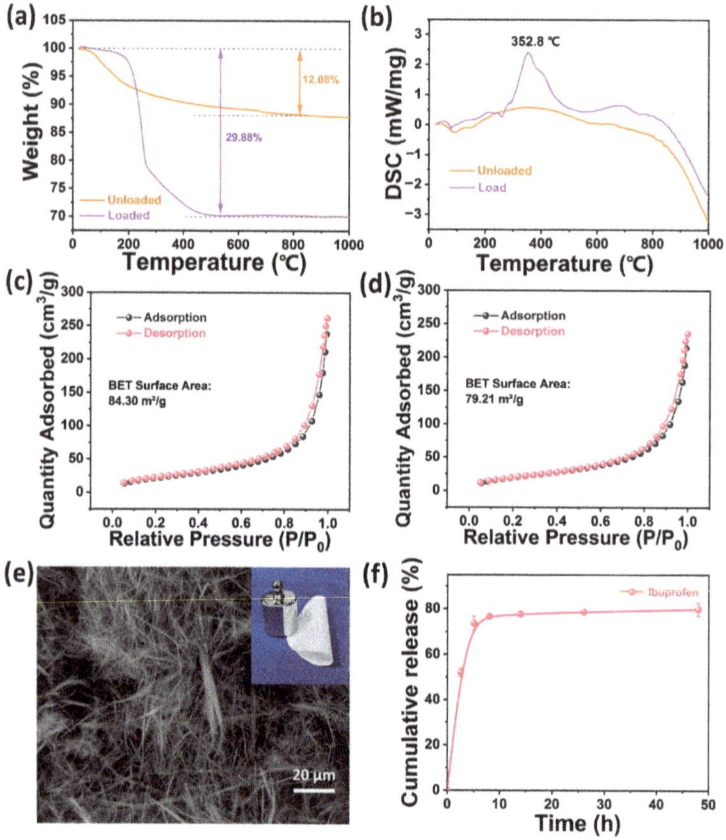

Figure 10. (**a**,**b**) Thermal analysis of the ultrathin UHAPNWs prepared by the microwave-assisted calcium oleate precursor hydrothermal method using creatine phosphate as the bio-phosphorus source at 180 °C for 60 min (Ca/P molar ratio 1:2) before and after loading ibuprofen: (**a**) TG curve; (**b**) DSC curve. (**c**,**d**) Nitrogen absorption/desorption curves of ultrathin UHAPNWs before (**c**) and after (**d**) ibuprofen loading. (**e**) SEM image of the ibuprofen-loaded ultrathin UHAPNW bio-paper. The inset is a digital image showing the high flexibility of the bio-paper. (**f**) Cumulative ibuprofen drug release profile of the ibuprofen-loaded ultrathin UHAPNW bio-paper in PBS (pH = 7.4, 37 °C).

As the TG curve shows significant stepwise weight loss, it can be used to evaluate the ibuprofen loading. According to the thermogravimetric analysis results, the ibuprofen loading capacity (drug (g)/carrier (g)) in ultrathin UHAPNWs can be calculated using the following equation:

$$\text{content}\ (\%) = 1 - \frac{m_2}{m_1} = \frac{m_1 - m_2}{m_1} \times 100\%$$

$$\text{Loading capacity}\ (g/g) = \frac{(1 - \frac{m_2}{m_1})}{\frac{m_2}{m_1}} = \frac{m_1 - m_2}{m_2}$$

In the above equation, m_1 and m_2 are the percentages of the remaining weights of unloaded ultrathin UHAPNWs and ibuprofen-loaded ultrathin UHAPNWs, respectively, after being heated at a high temperature of 900 °C in the TG curves. According to this equation, the drug loading of ibuprofen in the ultrathin UHAPNW carrier is calculated as 0.33 g g^{-1}, i.e., 0.33 g of ibuprofen can be loaded per gram of the ultrathin UHAPNW carrier, indicating the good drug loading capacity of the as-prepared ultrathin UHAPNWs.

In order to investigate the change in the ultrathin UHAPNWs before and after ibuprofen loading, the Brunauer–Emmett–Teller (BET) specific surface areas of the samples were measured. As shown in Figure 10c, the BET specific surface area of the pure ultrathin UHAPNWs without ibuprofen loading is measured to be about 84.30 $m^2\ g^{-1}$, while after loading ibuprofen, the specific surface area is slightly reduced to 79.21 $m^2\ g^{-1}$ (Figure 10d). In comparison with our previously reported ultralong UHAPNWs prepared by the calcium oleate precursor traditional hydrothermal/solvothermal method using the inorganic phosphate as the phosphorus source, the BET specific surface area of ultrathin UHAPNWs in this work is much higher because of the ultrasmall diameter, ultralong length, and ultrahigh aspect ratio. The high specific surface area of ultrathin UHAPNWs can provide plenty of active sites for drug loading, leading to a high drug loading capacity.

Furthermore, the ibuprofen-loaded ultrathin UHAPNWs can be interwoven into flexible and porous bio-paper. As shown in Figure 10e, the SEM image of the as-prepared bio-paper shows a continuous networked porous structure randomly interwoven with ibuprofen-loaded ultrathin UHAPNWs. This structure endows the bio-paper with high flexibility, which can be bent at large angles without noticeable damage (Figure 10e). The porous network structure provides a suitable microenvironment for cell adhesion, proliferation, and differentiation, and thus favors tissue regeneration [62–64]. In addition, the ibuprofen-loaded ultrathin UHAPNW bio-paper can sustainably release ibuprofen. As shown in Figure 10f, the ibuprofen drug is released at a suitable rate from the bio-paper in the first 12 h, which is beneficial for rapid anti-inflammatory pain relief. Then, the drug release rate decreases gradually.

The drug release kinetics of ibuprofen from the ibuprofen-loaded ultrathin UHAPNW bio-paper can be described well by the Higuchi model, with a high coefficient of determination (R^2) of 0.99 (Figure 11). According to this model, the cumulative amount of the released drug has a linear relationship with the square root of the release time

$$Q_t = k \cdot t^{1/2}$$

where Q_t is the amount of the drug released at time t, and k is the release rate constant for the Higuchi model [65,66]. This model is the common description for the diffusion-controlled release of a drug from insoluble carriers [67]. Therefore, as the ultrathin UHAPNWs exhibit a slow biodegradation rate in PBS, the drug release kinetics of ibuprofen from ultrathin UHAPNW bio-paper can be described as a process governed by the diffusion of drug molecules. It is expected that the as-prepared drug-loaded ultrathin UHAPNW bio-paper is promising for various biomedical applications such as anti-inflammatory, analgesic, wound healing, and bone defect repair.

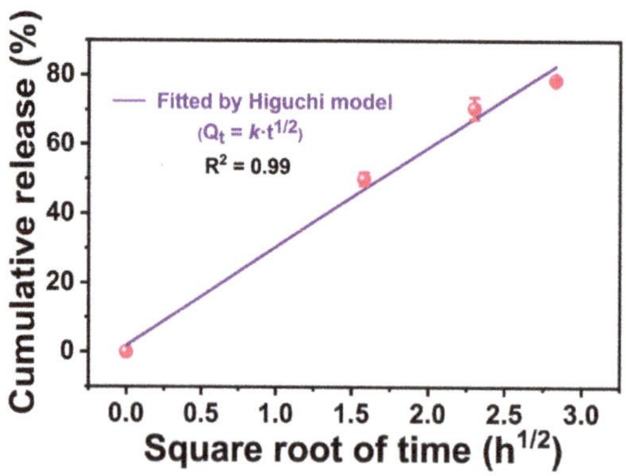

Figure 11. The linear relationship between the cumulative drug release percentage and the square root of the release time, which is consistent with the Higuchi model.

3. Experimental

3.1. Materials and Chemicals

Calcium chloride ($CaCl_2$) and hexane were purchased from Sinopharm Chemical Reagent Co., Ltd. (Shanghai, China). Sodium oleate and sodium creatine phosphate tetrahydrate were purchased from Aladdin Industrial Corporation. Ethanol was obtained from Shanghai Lingfeng Chemical Reagent Co., Ltd. (Shanghai, China). All chemicals were used as received without further purification. Deionized water was used in the related experiments.

3.2. Synthesis of Ultralong HAP Nanowires with Ultrathin Diameters

Ultralong HAP nanowires (UHAPNWs) with ultrathin diameters were synthesized by the microwave-assisted calcium oleate precursor hydrothermal method. Typically, $CaCl_2$ (0.110 g) was dissolved in 5 mL deionized water. 2.634 g sodium oleate was dissolved in 15 mL hot deionized water, cooled, and then slowly added into the $CaCl_2$ aqueous solution under magnetic stirring at room temperature. After 15 min of stirring, 5 mL of the aqueous solution containing 0.667 g sodium creatine phosphate tetrahydrate was added dropwise to the above mixture under magnetic stirring at room temperature. After that, the obtained aqueous suspension was transferred into an autoclave, sealed, and heated in a microwave oven (MDS-6, Sineo, Shanghai, China) for 60 min. The autoclave in this work was a modified polytetrafluoroethylene (TFM) cylindrical autoclave (total volume = 60 mL). Its inner diameter, outer diameter, and inner height were 3.0 cm, 3.8 cm, and 9.3 cm, respectively. It was fixed in a high-strength outer vessel. The microwave oven was a microwave hydrothermal/solvothermal synthesis system with a continuous heating mode, and the autoclave was continuously rotated during the microwave irradiation to ensure relatively uniform heating. After microwave heating, the autoclave was cooled down to room temperature, and the product was washed with ethanol and deionized water 3 times each. All samples were dried at 60 °C for 24 h before further use. Other samples were prepared by a similar procedures but with varying experimental parameters.

3.3. Material Characterization

X-ray powder diffraction (XRD) patterns were recorded by an X-ray diffractometer (D/max 2550 V, Rigaku, Tokyo, Japan) with Cu Kα radiation (λ = 1.54178 Å). Fourier transform infrared (FTIR) spectra were obtained with a FTIR spectrometer (FTIR-7600, Lambda Scientific, Edwardstown, Australia). Morphological observations of the samples were performed using scanning electron microscopy (SEM, Gemini 450, Zeiss, Oberkochen,

Germany, and TM-3000, Hitachi, Tokyo, Japan) and transmission electron microscopy (TEM, JEM-2100F, JEOL, Tokyo, Japan). The elemental mapping of UHAPNWs was performed by SEM energy-dispersive X-ray spectroscopy (EDS, Ultim Extreme, Oxford Instrument, Oxford, UK) and SEM (Gemini 450, Zeiss, Oberkochen, Germany) at 10 kV. The samples were sputtered with gold for 15 s. The thermal properties of samples were tested by thermogravimetric (TG) analysis and differential scanning calorimetry (DSC) (STA 409/PC, Netzsch, Selb, Germany) at a heating rate of 10 °C·min^{-1} in flowing air. The Brunauer–Emmett–Teller (BET) specific surface area of the samples was measured by analyzing N_2 adsorption/desorption using a surface area and pore size analyzer (Tristar II 3020, Micromeritics, Norcross, GA, USA). Before the measurement, the samples were outgassed at 80 °C for at least 4 h. The cumulative release of ibuprofen from the bio-paper of ibuprofen-loaded ultrathin UHAPNWs was assessed by soaking it in PBS at 37 °C under constant shaking (160 rpm) in a temperature-controlled shaker (HZQ-X 160, Peiying, Suzhou, China). At various intervals, 1 mL of the supernatant was withdrawn and analyzed by ultraviolet–visible (UV–vis) absorption spectroscopy (UV-2300II, Techcomp Instrument, Shanghai, China) to analyze its absorbance at a wavelength of 263 nm. Meanwhile, fresh PBS was added to replace the withdrawn volume to maintain a constant volume throughout the experiment.

3.4. Ibuprofen Loading

In a typical procedure of ibuprofen drug loading, ibuprofen was dissolved into hexane to form a solution with a concentration of 50 mg mL^{-1}. Then, 50 mg of the as-prepared powder of ultrathin UHAPNWs was added into 20 mL of the above ibuprofen solution under magnetic stirring. It should be noted that the container was covered with a lid to avoid the evaporation of hexane. After being soaked for 4 h, the supernatant was removed, and the ibuprofen-loaded ultrathin UHAPNWs were collected, washed with clean hexane, and dried to obtain the ibuprofen-loaded ultrathin UHAPNW drug delivery system.

4. Conclusions

To sum up, we have developed the microwave-assisted calcium oleate precursor hydrothermal method for the rapid synthesis of ultrathin UHAPNWs using creatine phosphate as the bio-phosphorus source. This method has the advantages of environmental friendliness, efficient heating, a short reaction time, high efficiency, and energy savings. The controllable hydrolysis of phosphocreatine prevents the undesired premature formation of calcium phosphate nuclei, and microwave heating rapidly and uniformly elevates the temperature for phosphocreatine hydrolysis, which releases free PO_4^{3-} ions for the formation of homogeneous ultrathin UHAPNWs. Ultrathin UHAPNWs with ultrathin diameters (only ~6 nm for a single nanowire), ultralong lengths (several hundred micrometers), and ultrahigh aspect ratios (>10,000) can be rapidly prepared within 60 min, shortening the synthesis time by about two orders of magnitude compared with the traditional hydrothermal method. Ultrathin UHAPNWs can self-assemble along their longitudinal direction to form nanowire bundles with a high BET specific surface area (84.30 m^2 g^{-1}). Moreover, the as-prepared ultrathin UHAPNWs show a high ibuprofen loading capacity (0.33 g drug per gram of nanocarrier). After loading ibuprofen, ultrathin UHAPNWs still exhibit a high specific surface area of 79.21 m^2 g^{-1}. The ibuprofen-loaded ultrathin UHAPNWs can be further interwoven into flexible and porous bio-paper, and it can continuously release the drug in phosphate-buffered saline, which is promising for various biomedical applications such as inflammatory treatment and accelerated tissue regeneration. In future research, the in vitro/in vivo biocompatibility of the as-prepared ultrathin UHAPNWs as drug nanocarriers should be investigated. Moreover, experiments can be performed to load other drugs in the ultrathin UHAPNWs drug nanocarriers for a variety of biomedical applications.

Author Contributions: Y.Z.: methodology, formal analysis, data curation, and writing—original draft; Y.-J.Z.: conceptualization, funding acquisition, methodology, project administration, supervision, and writing—review and editing; S.-Y.L.: investigation; L.-Y.D.: funding acquisition, investigation; H.-P.Y.: conceptualization, funding acquisition, investigation, project administration, writing—original draft, and writing—review and editing. All authors have read and agreed to the published version of the manuscript.

Funding: This research was funded by the National Natural Science Foundation of China (Nos 52302358, 52072395, and 52372099).

Institutional Review Board Statement: Not applicable.

Informed Consent Statement: Not applicable.

Data Availability Statement: The data presented in this study are available on reasonable request from the corresponding authors.

Conflicts of Interest: The authors declare no conflicts of interest.

References

1. Baig, N.; Kammakakam, I.; Falath, W. Nanomaterials: A review of synthesis methods, properties, recent progress, and challenges. *Mater. Adv.* **2021**, *2*, 1821–1871. [CrossRef]
2. Mitchell, M.J.; Billingsley, M.M.; Haley, R.M.; Wechsler, M.E.; Peppas, N.A.; Langer, R. Engineering precision nanoparticles for drug delivery. *Nat. Rev. Drug Discov.* **2021**, *20*, 101–124. [CrossRef] [PubMed]
3. Harish, V.; Tewari, D.; Gaur, M.; Yadav, A.B.; Swaroop, S.; Bechelany, M.; Barhoum, A. Review on Nanoparticles and Nanostructured Materials: Bioimaging, Biosensing, Drug Delivery, Tissue Engineering, Antimicrobial, and Agro-Food Applications. *Nanomaterials* **2022**, *12*, 457. [CrossRef] [PubMed]
4. Cho, N.H.; Guerrero-Martínez, A.; Ma, J.; Bals, S.; Kotov, N.A.; Liz-Marzán, L.M.; Nam, K.T. Bioinspired chiral inorganic nanomaterials. *Nat. Rev. Bioeng.* **2023**, *1*, 88–106. [CrossRef]
5. Liu, H.; Haider, B.; Fried, H.R.; Ju, J.; Bolonduro, O.; Raghuram, V.; Timko, B.P. Nanobiotechnology: 1D nanomaterial building blocks for cellular interfaces and hybrid tissues. *Nano Res.* **2018**, *11*, 5372–5399. [CrossRef]
6. Garnett, E.; Mai, L.; Yang, P. Introduction: 1D Nanomaterials/Nanowires. *Chem. Rev.* **2019**, *119*, 8955–8957. [CrossRef]
7. Wang, S.; Shan, Z.; Huang, H. The Mechanical Properties of Nanowires. *Adv. Sci.* **2017**, *4*, 1600332. [CrossRef]
8. He, Z.; Wang, J.L.; Chen, S.M.; Liu, J.W.; Yu, S.H. Self-Assembly of Nanowires: From Dynamic Monitoring to Precision Control. *Acc. Chem. Res.* **2022**, *55*, 1480–1491. [CrossRef]
9. Wu, F.; Qiang, S.; Zhang, X.; Wang, F.; Yin, X.; Liu, L.; Yu, J.; Liu, Y.T.; Ding, B. The Rising of Flexible and Elastic Ceramic Fiber Materials: Fundamental Concept, Design Principle, and Toughening Mechanism. *Adv. Funct. Mater.* **2022**, *32*, 2207130. [CrossRef]
10. Jia, C.; Xu, Z.; Luo, D.; Xiang, H.; Zhu, M. Flexible Ceramic Fibers: Recent Development in Preparation and Application. *Adv. Fiber Mater.* **2022**, *4*, 573–603. [CrossRef]
11. Si, Y.; Wang, X.; Dou, L.; Yu, J.; Ding, B. Ultralight and fire-resistant ceramic nanofibrous aerogels with temperature-invariant superelasticity. *Sci. Adv.* **2018**, *4*, eaas8925. [CrossRef] [PubMed]
12. Su, L.; Jia, S.; Ren, J.; Lu, X.; Guo, S.W.; Guo, P.; Cai, Z.; Lu, D.; Niu, M.; Zhuang, L.; et al. Strong yet flexible ceramic aerogel. *Nat. Commun.* **2023**, *14*, 7057. [CrossRef]
13. Zhang, Y.; Li, J.; Soleimani, M.; Giacomini, F.; Friedrich, H.; Truckenmüller, R.; Habibovic, P. Biodegradable Elastic Sponge from Nanofibrous Biphasic Calcium Phosphate Ceramic as an Advanced Material for Regenerative Medicine. *Adv. Funct. Mater.* **2021**, *31*, 2102911. [CrossRef]
14. Zhang, Y.; Li, J.; Mouser, V.H.M.; Roumans, N.; Moroni, L.; Habibovic, P. Biomimetic Mechanically Strong One-Dimensional Hydroxyapatite/Poly(D,L-lactide) Composite Inducing Formation of Anisotropic Collagen Matrix. *ACS Nano* **2021**, *15*, 17480–17498. [CrossRef] [PubMed]
15. Zheng, Y.; Ma, W.; Yang, Z.; Zhang, H.; Ma, J.; Li, T.; Niu, H.; Zhou, Y.; Yao, Q.; Chang, J.; et al. An ultralong hydroxyapatite nanowire aerogel for rapid hemostasis and wound healing. *Chem. Eng. J.* **2022**, *430*, 132912. [CrossRef]
16. Hao, L.; Liang, S.; Han, Q.; Jing, Y.; Li, J.; Li, Q.; Wang, A.; Bai, S.; Yin, J. Ultralong hydroxyapatite nanowires-incorporated dipeptide hydrogel with enhanced mechanical strength and superior in vivo osteogenesis activity. *Colloids Surf. A Physicochem. Eng. Asp.* **2023**, *664*, 131153. [CrossRef]

17. Peng, F.; Su, Y.; Ji, X.; Zhong, Y.; Wei, X.; He, Y. Doxorubicin-loaded silicon nanowires for the treatment of drug-resistant cancer cells. *Biomaterials* **2014**, *35*, 5188–5195. [CrossRef]
18. Martinez-Banderas, A.I.; Aires, A.; Quintanilla, M.; Holguin-Lerma, J.A.; Lozano-Pedraza, C.; Teran, F.J.; Moreno, J.A.; Perez, J.E.; Ooi, B.S.; Ravasi, T.; et al. Iron-Based Core-Shell Nanowires for Combinatorial Drug Delivery and Photothermal and Magnetic Therapy. *ACS Appl. Mater. Interfaces* **2019**, *11*, 43976–43988. [CrossRef]
19. Filip, D.G.; Surdu, V.A.; Paduraru, A.V.; Andronescu, E. Current Development in Biomaterials—Hydroxyapatite and Bioglass for Applications in Biomedical Field: A Review. *J. Funct. Biomater.* **2022**, *13*, 248. [CrossRef]
20. Mondal, S.; Park, S.; Choi, J.; Vu, T.T.H.; Doan, V.H.M.; Vo, T.T.; Lee, B.; Oh, J. Hydroxyapatite: A journey from biomaterials to advanced functional materials. *Adv. Colloid Interface Sci.* **2023**, *321*, 103013. [CrossRef]
21. Liu, C.; Xu, M.; Wang, Y.; Yin, Q.; Hu, J.; Chen, H.; Sun, Z.; Liu, C.; Li, X.; Zhou, W.; et al. Exploring the potential of hydroxyapatite-based materials in biomedicine: A comprehensive review. *Mater. Sci. Eng. R Rep.* **2024**, *161*, 100870. [CrossRef]
22. Du, M.; Chen, J.; Liu, K.; Xing, H.; Song, C. Recent advances in biomedical engineering of nano-hydroxyapatite including dentistry, cancer treatment and bone repair. *Compos. Part B Eng.* **2021**, *215*, 108790. [CrossRef]
23. Zhao, H.; Liu, S.; Lu, J.; Yang, X.; Yang, Z.; Li, F.; Guo, L. Natural tooth enamel and its analogs. *Cell Rep. Phys. Sci.* **2022**, *3*, 100945. [CrossRef]
24. Diez-Escudero, A.; Espanol, M.; Ginebra, M.P. High-aspect-ratio nanostructured hydroxyapatite: Towards new functionalities for a classical material. *Chem. Sci.* **2023**, *15*, 55–76. [CrossRef] [PubMed]
25. Lu, B.Q.; Zhu, Y.J.; Chen, F. Highly flexible and nonflammable inorganic hydroxyapatite paper. *Chem.-A Eur. J.* **2014**, *20*, 1242–1246. [CrossRef]
26. Zhu, Y.J. Multifunctional Fire-Resistant Paper Based on Ultralong Hydroxyapatite Nanowires. *Chin. J. Chem.* **2021**, *39*, 2296–2314. [CrossRef]
27. Zhu, Y.-J. *Fire-Resistant Paper: Materials, Technologies, and Applications*; CRC Press: Boca Raton, FL, USA, 2021.
28. Yu, H.-P.; Zhu, Y.-J. Bioinspired flexible, high-strength, and versatile hydrogel with the fiberboard-and-mortar hierarchically ordered structure. *Nano Res.* **2021**, *14*, 3643–3652. [CrossRef]
29. Wang, L.; Nancollas, G.H. Calcium Orthophosphates: Crystallization and Dissolution. *Chem. Rev.* **2008**, *108*, 4628–4669. [CrossRef]
30. Lin, K.; Wu, C.; Chang, J. Advances in synthesis of calcium phosphate crystals with controlled size and shape. *Acta Biomater.* **2014**, *10*, 4071–4102. [CrossRef]
31. Mohd Pu'ad, N.A.S.; Abdul Haq, R.H.; Mohd Noh, H.; Abdullah, H.Z.; Idris, M.I.; Lee, T.C. Synthesis method of hydroxyapatite: A review. *Mater. Today Proc.* **2019**, *29*, 233–239. [CrossRef]
32. Zhang, Y.; Zhu, Y.-J.; Yu, H.-P. Microwave-Assisted Hydrothermal Rapid Synthesis of Ultralong Hydroxyapatite Nanowires Using Adenosine 5′-Triphosphate. *Molecules* **2022**, *27*, 5020. [CrossRef] [PubMed]
33. Qi, C.; Musetti, S.; Fu, L.H.; Zhu, Y.J.; Huang, L. Biomolecule-assisted green synthesis of nanostructured calcium phosphates and their biomedical applications. *Chem. Soc. Rev.* **2019**, *48*, 2698–2737. [CrossRef] [PubMed]
34. Zhu, Y.-J.; Chen, F. Microwave-assisted preparation of inorganic nanostructures in liquid phase. *Chem. Rev.* **2014**, *114*, 6462–6555. [CrossRef] [PubMed]
35. Gaddi, A.V.; Galuppo, P.; Yang, J. Creatine phosphate administration in cell energy impairment conditions: A summary of past and present research. *Heart Lung Circ.* **2017**, *26*, 1026–1035. [CrossRef] [PubMed]
36. Wu, S.H.; Chen, K.L.; Hsu, C.; Chen, H.C.; Chen, J.Y.; Yu, S.Y.; Shiu, Y.J. Creatine Supplementation for Muscle Growth: A Scoping Review of Randomized Clinical Trials from 2012 to 2021. *Nutrients* **2022**, *14*, 1255. [CrossRef]
37. Yquel, R.J.; Arsac, L.M.; Thiaudiere, E.; Canioni, P.; Manier, G. Effect of creatine supplementation on phosphocreatine resynthesis, inorganic phosphate accumulation and pH during intermittent maximal exercise. *J. Sports Sci.* **2002**, *20*, 427–437. [CrossRef]
38. Bessman, S.P.; Carpenter, C.L. The Creatine-Creatine Phosphate Energy Shuttle. *Annu. Rev. Biochem.* **1985**, *54*, 831–862. [CrossRef]
39. Andres, R.H.; Ducray, A.D.; Schlattner, U.; Wallimann, T.; Widmer, H.R. Functions and effects of creatine in the central nervous system. *Brain Res. Bull.* **2008**, *76*, 329–343. [CrossRef]
40. Williams, C.; Rollo, I. Carbohydrate Nutrition and Team Sport Performance. *Sports Med.* **2015**, *45* (Suppl. 1), S13–S22. [CrossRef]
41. Hargreaves, M.; Spriet, L.L. Skeletal muscle energy metabolism during exercise. *Nat. Metab.* **2020**, *2*, 817–828. [CrossRef]
42. Cao, X.; Wang, G.; Yang, Y.; Cao, X. Biomolecules induce the synthesis of hollow hierarchical mesoporous structured hydroxyapatite microflowers: Application in macromolecule drug delivery. *J. Mater. Sci.* **2021**, *56*, 7034–7049. [CrossRef]
43. Qi, C.; Zhu, Y.-J.; Wu, C.-T.; Sun, T.-W.; Chen, F.; Wu, J. Magnesium phosphate pentahydrate nanosheets: Microwave-hydrothermal rapid synthesis using creatine phosphate as an organic phosphorus source and application in protein adsorption. *J. Colloid Interface Sci.* **2016**, *462*, 297–306. [CrossRef] [PubMed]
44. Du, T.-m.; Yang, H.-s.; Niu, X.-f. Phosphorus-containing compounds regulate mineralization. *Mater. Today Chem.* **2021**, *22*, 100579. [CrossRef]
45. Balestrino, M. Role of Creatine in the Heart: Health and Disease. *Nutrients* **2021**, *13*, 1215. [CrossRef]

46. Gawande, M.B.; Shelke, S.N.; Zboril, R.; Varma, R.S. Microwave-Assisted Chemistry: Synthetic Applications for Rapid Assembly of Nanomaterials and Organics. *Chem. Rev.* **2014**, *47*, 1338–1348. [CrossRef]
47. Yu, H.-P.; Zhu, Y.-J.; Lu, B.-Q. Highly efficient and environmentally friendly microwave-assisted hydrothermal rapid synthesis of ultralong hydroxyapatite nanowires. *Ceram. Int.* **2018**, *44*, 12352–12356. [CrossRef]
48. Kumar, A.; Kuang, Y.; Liang, Z.; Sun, X. Microwave chemistry, recent advancements, and eco-friendly microwave-assisted synthesis of nanoarchitectures and their applications: A review. *Mater. Today Nano* **2020**, *11*, 100076. [CrossRef]
49. Katsuki, H.; Furuta, S.; Komarneni, S. Semi-continuous and fast synthesis of nanophase cubic $BaTiO_3$ using a single-mode home-built microwave reactor. *Mater. Lett.* **2012**, *83*, 8–10. [CrossRef]
50. Yu, H.P.; Zhu, Y.J. Guidelines derived from biomineralized tissues for design and construction of high-performance biomimetic materials: From weak to strong. *Chem. Soc. Rev.* **2024**, *53*, 4490–4606. [CrossRef]
51. Zhang, H.; Darvell, B.W. Synthesis and characterization of hydroxyapatite whiskers by hydrothermal homogeneous precipitation using acetamide. *Acta Biomater.* **2010**, *6*, 3216–3222. [CrossRef]
52. Lee, J.-H.; Kim, Y.-J. Hydroxyapatite nanofibers fabricated through electrospinning and sol–gel process. *Ceram. Int.* **2014**, *40*, 3361–3369. [CrossRef]
53. Stojanović, Z.S.; Ignjatović, N.; Wu, V.; Žunič, V.; Veselinović, L.; Škapin, S.; Miljković, M.; Uskoković, V.; Uskoković, D. Hydrothermally processed 1D hydroxyapatite: Mechanism of formation and biocompatibility studies. *Mater. Sci. Eng. C* **2016**, *68*, 746–757. [CrossRef] [PubMed]
54. Ko, H.-S.; Lee, S.; Jho, J.Y. Synthesis and Modification of Hydroxyapatite Nanofiber for Poly(Lactic Acid) Composites with Enhanced Mechanical Strength and Bioactivity. *Nanomaterials* **2021**, *11*, 213. [CrossRef] [PubMed]
55. Jeong, E.J.; Kim, J.H.; Park, J.; Kang, H.C. Synthesis and characterization of hydroxyapatite nanowires on tricalcium phosphate bone discs using a hydrothermal reaction. *Ceram. Int.* **2024**, *50*, 55609–55616. [CrossRef]
56. Yu, H.-P.; Zhu, Y.-J.; Xiong, Z.-C.; Lu, B.-Q. Bioinspired fiberboard-and-mortar structural nanocomposite based on ultralong hydroxyapatite nanowires with high mechanical performance. *Chem. Eng. J.* **2020**, *399*, 125666. [CrossRef]
57. Nakayama, M.; Kajiyama, S.; Kumamoto, A.; Nishimura, T.; Ikuhara, Y.; Yamato, M.; Kato, T. Stimuli-responsive hydroxyapatite liquid crystal with macroscopically controllable ordering and magneto-optical functions. *Nat. Commun.* **2018**, *9*, 568. [CrossRef]
58. Sebastian, T.; Preisker, T.R.; Gorjan, L.; Graule, T.; Aneziris, C.G.; Clemens, F.J. Synthesis of hydroxyapatite fibers using electrospinning: A study of phase evolution based on polymer matrix. *J. Eur. Ceram. Soc.* **2020**, *40*, 2489–2496. [CrossRef]
59. Das, P.; Jana, N.R. Length-Controlled Synthesis of Calcium Phosphate Nanorod and Nanowire and Application in Intracellular Protein Delivery. *ACS Appl. Mater. Interfaces* **2016**, *8*, 8710–8720. [CrossRef]
60. Horjus, D.L.; Oudman, I.; van Montfrans, G.A.; Brewster, L.M. Creatine and creatine analogues in hypertension and cardiovascular disease. *Cochrane Database Syst. Rev.* **2011**, *11*, CD005184. [CrossRef]
61. Clarke, H.; Hickner, R.C.; Ormsbee, M.J. The Potential Role of Creatine in Vascular Health. *Nutrients* **2021**, *13*, 857. [CrossRef]
62. Meng, C.; Liu, X.; Li, R.; Malekmohammadi, S.; Feng, Y.; Song, J.; Gong, R.H.; Li, J. 3D Poly (L-lactic acid) fibrous sponge with interconnected porous structure for bone tissue scaffold. *Int. J. Biol. Macromol.* **2024**, *268*, 131688. [CrossRef] [PubMed]
63. Meng, C.; Song, J.; Malekmohammadi, S.; Meng, J.; Wei, W.; Li, R.; Feng, J.; Gong, R.H.; Li, J. Hierarchical porous poly (L-lactic acid) fibrous vascular graft with controllable architectures and stable structure. *Mater. Des.* **2024**, *240*, 112829. [CrossRef]
64. Yu, H.; Chen, X.; Cai, J.; Ye, D.; Wu, Y.; Fan, L.; Liu, P. Novel porous three-dimensional nanofibrous scaffolds for accelerating wound healing. *Chem. Eng. J.* **2019**, *369*, 253–262. [CrossRef]
65. Higuchi, T. Rate of Release of Medicaments from Ointment Bases Containing Drugs in Suspension. *J. Pharm. Sci.* **1961**, *50*, 874–875. [CrossRef]
66. Higuchi, T. Mechanism of sustained-action medication. Theoretical analysis of rate of release of solid drugs dispersed in solid matrices. *J. Pharm. Sci.* **1963**, *52*, 1145–1149. [CrossRef]
67. Andersson, J.; Rosenholm, J.; Areva, S.; Lindén, M. Influences of Material Characteristics on Ibuprofen Drug Loading and Release Profiles from Ordered Micro- and Mesoporous Silica Matrices. *Chem. Mater.* **2004**, *16*, 4160–4167. [CrossRef]

molecules

MDPI

Article

Multifunctional Biocomposites: Synthesis, Characterization, and Prospects for Regenerative Medicine and Controlled Drug Delivery

Mohamed Aaddouz [1], Ridouan El Yousfi [1], Rachid Sabbahi [2,3,*], Khalil Azzaoui [3,4], Meryem Idrissi Yahyaoui [5], Abdeslam Asehraou [5] Belkheir Hammouti [3], Fouad Laoutid [6] Mohammed M. Alanazi [7] and Elmiloud Mejdoubi [1]

1 Laboratory of Applied Chemistry and Environment, Department of Chemistry, Faculty of Sciences. Mohammed First University, Oujda 60000, Morocco; aaddouzmed@gmail.com (M.A.); red1elyousfi@gmail.com (R.E.Y.); ee.mejdoubi@gmail.com (E.M.)

2 Research Team in Science and Technology, Higher School of Technology, Ibn Zohr University, Quartier 25 Mars, Laayoune 70000, Morocco

3 Euromed Research Center, Euromed Polytechnic School, Euromed University of Fes, UEMF, Fes 30030, Morocco; k.azzaoui@yahoo.com (K.A.); hammoutib@gmail.com (B.H.)

4 Engineering Laboratory of Organometallic, Molecular Materials and Environment, Faculty of Sciences, Sidi Mohammed Ben Abdellah University, Fez 30000, Morocco

5 Laboratory of Bioresources, Biotechnology, Ethnopharmacology and Health, Faculty of Sciences, Mohammed First University, Oujda 60000, Morocco; iy.meryem@ump.ac.ma (M.I.Y.); asehraou@yahoo.fr (A.A.)

6 Laboratory of Polymeric & Composite Materials, Materia Nova Research Center, 3 Avenue Nicolas Copernic, B-7000 Mons, Belgium; fouad.laoutid@materianova.be

7 Department of Pharmaceutical Chemistry, College of Pharmacy, King Saud University, Riyadh 11451, Saudi Arabia; mmalanazi@ksu.edu.sa

* Correspondence: r.sabbahi@uiz.ac.ma

Abstract: This article presents a new method for preparing multifunctional composite biomaterials with applications in advanced biomedical fields. The biomaterials consist of dicalcium phosphate (DCPD) and bioactive silicate glasses (SiO_2/Na_2O and SiO_2/K_2O), containing the antibiotic streptomycin sulfate. Materials were deeply characterized by X-ray diffraction and attenuated total reflectance Fourier transform infrared spectroscopy, and zeta potential analysis, UV–visible spectrophotometry, and ion-exchange measurement were applied in a simulating body fluid (SBF) solution. The main results include an in situ chemical transformation of dicalcium phosphate into an apatitic phase under the influence of silicate solutions and the incorporation of the antibiotic. The zeta potential showed a decrease in surface charge from $\zeta = -24.6$ mV to $\zeta = -16.5$ mV. In addition, a controlled and prolonged release of antibiotics was observed over a period of 37 days, with a released concentration of up to 755 ppm. Toxicity tests in mice demonstrated good tolerance of the biomaterials, with no significant adverse effects. Moreover, these biomaterials have shown potent antibacterial activity against various bacterial strains, including *Listeria monocytogenes*, *Staphylococcus aureus*, *Escherichia coli*, and *Pseudomonas aeruginosa*, suggesting their potential use in tissue engineering, drug delivery, and orthopedic and dental implants. By integrating the antibiotic into the biomaterial composites, we achieved controlled release and prolonged antibacterial efficacy. This research contributes to advancing biomaterials by exploring innovative synthetic routes and showcasing their promise in regenerative medicine and controlled drug delivery.

Keywords: antimicrobial; biomaterials; co-precipitation; drugs; hydroxyapatite; multifunctional

1. Introduction

The restoration of bone defects has been a central concern in regenerative medicine, captivating the attention of many researchers for years. Various studies have been carried out to develop biomaterials for clinical applications [1,2]. These biomaterials must be bioactive and composed of polymers, whether synthetic or natural, ceramics, or metals [3,4].

Among them, hydroxyapatite (HAp), a calcium phosphate, is widely recognized for its excellent compatibility with bone tissue due to its similarity to natural bone minerals [5,6].

HAp is valued for its ability to adjust its crystallinity and microstructure to meet specific needs, thanks to its biodegradable properties and biocompatibility, ensuring that it is non-toxic, non-inflammatory, and enhances the immune response [5,7]. However, HAp can present certain limitations, particularly in terms of mechanical and chemical properties. Traditional synthesis methods require extremely high purity [8,9], which can result in the loss of crucial elements such as sodium, silicon, and potassium, essential for bone growth and biological functions [10–12]. In contrast, brushite (dicalcium phosphate dihydrate, DCPD) is metastable under physiological conditions and resorbs faster than apatitic cements, while having the ability to transform into hydroxyapatite in vivo [13,14].

This study proposes a new approach by developing "HAp/bio-glass" biocomposites by precipitating HAp in silicate solutions based on the hydrolysis of dicalcium phosphate dihydrate. This process aims to strengthen interactions between the final phases of composite biomaterials, create a favorable chemical environment for the deposition of apatitic particles, and promote synergy between biocomposite components. This method also enables the material to be consolidated at low temperatures, facilitating the integration of active ingredients, unlike conventional bioceramics which require sintering at very high temperatures [15–17].

Research on sustained-release delivery systems plays a key role in the mitigation of antibiotic resistance. In the context of anti-infective treatments, which often require prolonged treatment durations, adequate exposure to antibiotics is essential for the eradication of microorganisms [18]. However, patient compliance remains a challenge. Patients often discontinue treatment once they feel better, contributing inadvertently to incomplete antibiotic treatment [19]. This incomplete treatment can exacerbate the development of antibiotic resistance. In addition, many antibiotics have a short half-life, requiring frequent administration. To solve these problems, adaptable drug delivery systems have emerged [18,19]. These innovative systems not only overcome biological barriers, but also ensure precise, prolonged and controlled drug release at the target site. Furthermore, they have the ability to incorporate multiple drugs in the same delivery vehicle.

One of the greatest challenges facing contemporary medicine in the treatment of chronic diseases such as osteomyelitis and osteoporosis is antibiotic resistance and the control of drug release [20,21]. A major effort has been made by specialists to develop materials capable of releasing drugs precisely and with reproducible and predictable kinetics. Although most of these drug carriers are polymers, certain inorganic materials can also play an important role.

The aim of this integrated approach is to deepen our understanding of the properties and performance of multifunctional biocomposites, with a view to exploring their potential applications in medicine. Various strategies have been investigated for combining antibiotics with phosphocalcic materials to extend the release period, with the aim of optimizing integration methods to regulate the release rate. This study will address several key steps, from the synthesis of the composite biomaterial to the analysis of its drug release, as well as structural and surface characterization, and will conclude with the exploration of its antibacterial efficacy, thus fostering a deeper understanding of the multifunctional biocomposite and its potential biomedical applications.

2. Results and Discussion

2.1. Characterization of Multifunctional Composite Biomaterials

2.1.1. Characterization by X-ray Diffraction

X-ray diffraction characterization of the engineered biomaterials was carried out on DCPD samples synthesized using the double decomposition method, which had previously been chosen at the start of this study, in the presence of bio-glasses (SiO_2/Na_2O

and SiO_2/K_2O), followed by consolidation. The X-ray diffraction pattern is shown in Figures 1 and 2, where it can be seen that in both the SiO_2/Na_2O and SiO_2/K_2O bio-glass cases, dicalcium phosphate evolves in situ towards a poorly crystallized apatitic phase.

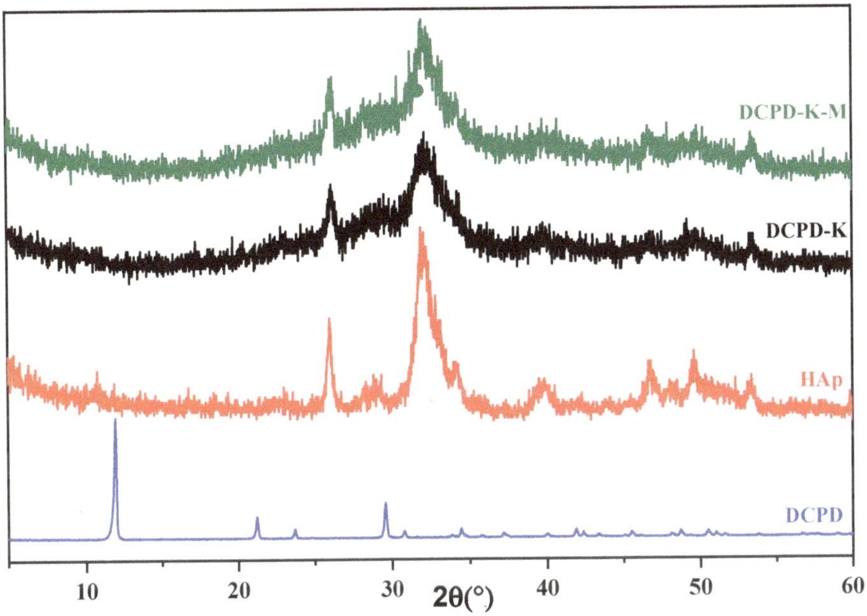

Figure 1. Diffractograms of DCPD-K and DCPD-K-M composite biomaterials, HAp, and DCPD.

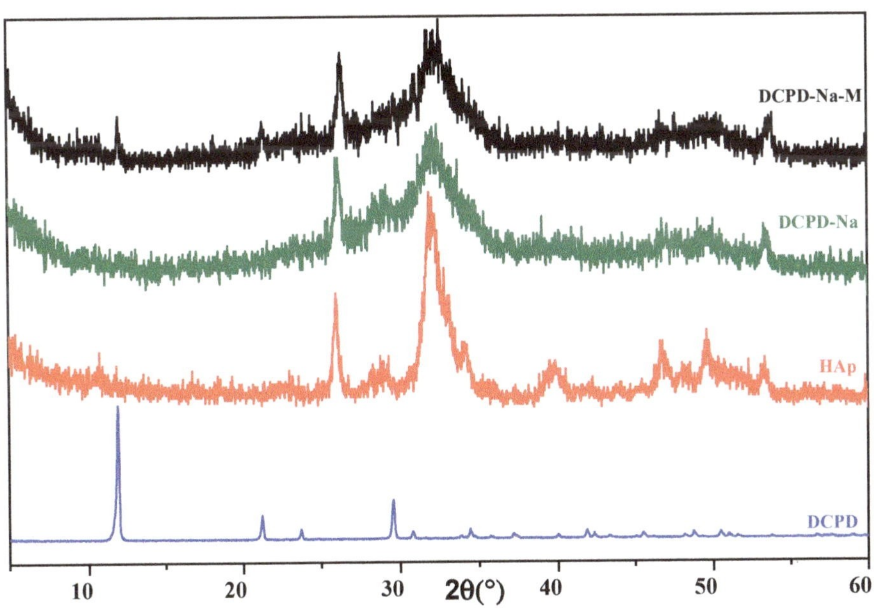

Figure 2. Diffractograms of DCPD-Na and DCPD-Na-M composite biomaterials, HAp, and DCPD.

Combining the XRD diagrams of the composite biomaterials after the drug has been introduced into the different silicate solutions, for the DCPD/SiO_2-Na_2O and DCPD/SiO_2-Na_2O/cured antibiotic composite biomaterials (Figure 1), we see an in situ chemical transformation towards the apatitic phase. The diffractograms reveal broad peaks at $2\theta = 26.42°$ and $2\theta = 32°$, characteristic of the apatitic phase, in both cases, whether in the absence of antibiotic (DCPD-K) or in its presence (DCPD-K-M). For the cured DCPD-Na and DCPD-Na-M biocomposites (Figure 2), their XRD spectra clearly demonstrate in situ chemical transformation towards a poorly crystallized apatitic phase.

The results of X-ray diffraction analysis highlight the importance of the chemical conditions imposed by silicate media, in particular pH conditions, on the nature of composite biomaterials. Similarly, the nature of the cations (Na+ and K+) plays a significant role in the in situ chemical evolution of dicalcium phosphate towards the apatitic phase in the presence or absence of the antibiotic.

2.1.2. Characterization by Infrared Spectroscopy

In this study, we explored the characteristics of HAp/bio-glass composite biomaterials, incorporating the antibiotic streptomycin sulfate, using infrared spectroscopy analysis (Figures 3 and 4). Our main objective was to understand how the various dicalcium phosphate groups evolve in situ in the presence of various silicate solutions, and the impact of the presence or absence of antibiotics.

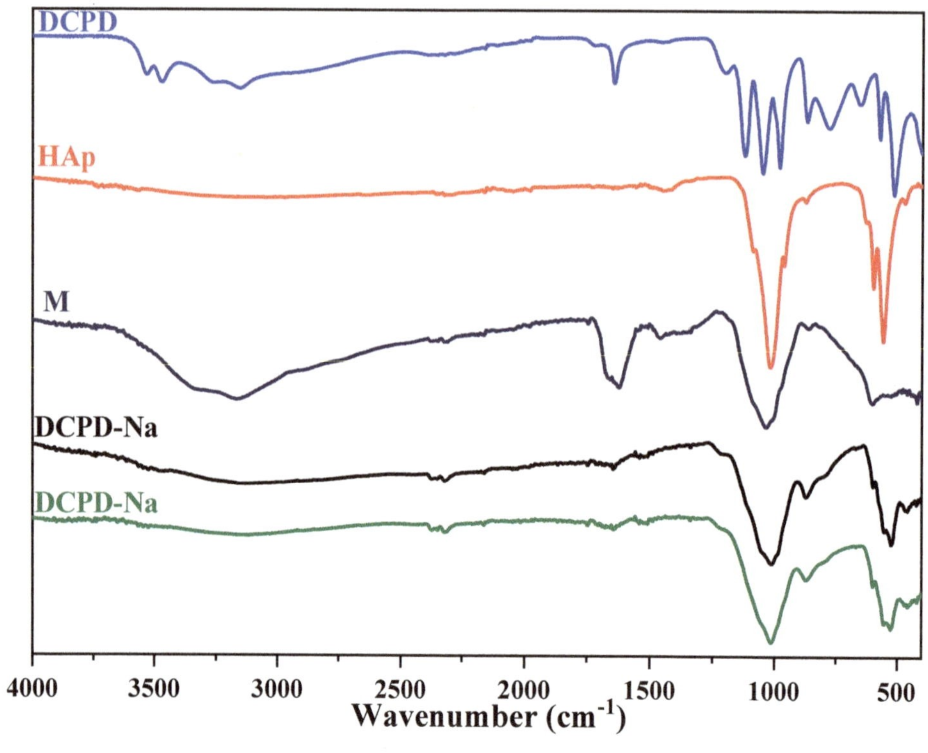

Figure 3. IR spectra of DCPD-Na and DCPD-Na-M composites, antibiotic M, HAp, and DCPD.

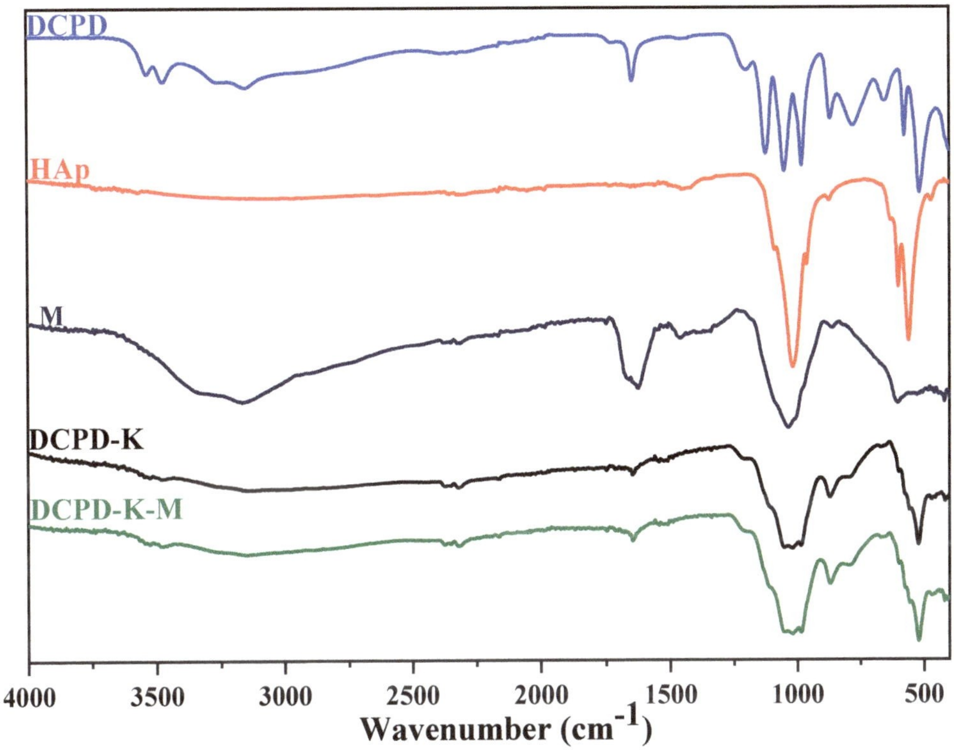

Figure 4. IR spectra of DCPD-K and DCPD-K-M composites, antibiotic M, HAp, and DCPD.

The infrared absorption spectra depicted in Figures 3 and 4 illustrate the in situ evolution of brushite towards an apatitic phase. This transformation occurs in the absence of antibiotics but in the presence of various silicate solutions. Analyzing these FTIR spectra reveals several key features: First, the characteristic DCPD bands between ν = 550 cm^{-1} and ν = 1500 cm^{-1} vanish. Second, the band width increases between ν = 1200 cm^{-1} and ν = 700 cm^{-1}. Third, HAp bands emerge [22]. These results clearly indicate an in situ chemical conversion of DCPD to an apatitic phase in the presence of SiO_2/Na_2O and SiO_2/K_2O bio-glasses. These findings align with previous observations from X-ray diffraction, confirming the formation of HAp/SiO_2/Na_2O and HAp/SiO_2/K2O composite biomaterials.

With regard to the specific DCPD-Na composite biomaterial, whether or not associated with streptomycin sulfate (Figures 3 and 4), several important observations were made: (i) the shift of the band at 3151 to 3143 cm^{-1}, associated with elongations of the O-H bond in hydroxyapatite, suggests changes in the chemical environment of the hydroxyl groups [23], (ii) the presence of C-H group vibrations at 3100 cm^{-1} confirms the incorporation of these groups into the HAp/SiO_2/Na_2O structure, and (iii) the appearance of the band at 1679 cm^{-1}, corresponding to the stretching vibrations of the amide group (−C=O−NH−) present in streptomycin sulfate, confirms the presence of this antibiotic in the composite biomaterial.

Other band shifts, notably at 1648, 1340, 1213, and 871 cm^{-1}, as well as bands at 525, 553, and 597 cm^{-1}, correspond to vibrations characteristic of the carbonate ions (CO_3^{2-}) [24,25] introduced into the apatite structure and the phosphate ions (PO_4^{3-}) of apatite [26].

These observations clearly demonstrate the complex interactions between bio-glass, apatite, and streptomycin sulfate, confirming changes in the chemical environment of these compounds and validating the formation of the HAp/SiO_2/Na_2O-M composite biomaterial.

The infrared spectra of the DCPD-K and DCPD-K-M composite biomaterials (Figures 3 and 4) also reveal a chemical transformation of the DCPD phase in situ towards an apatitic phase in both cases. Furthermore, the observation of absorption bands between 1250 and 750 cm^{-1}, as well as the appearance of bands associated with antibiotic and apatite in the interval between 3700 and 2500 cm^{-1}, confirms the formation of the HAp/SiO_2/K_2O-M composite biomaterial, implying the combined presence of apatite, silicate, and antibiotic.

2.2. Study of Biomaterial Surface Charges

Zeta potential, an important measurement in materials science and surface chemistry, is used to assess the surface charge of composite biomaterials. In our study, the surfaces of the biomaterials are negatively charged (Table 1). We observed a significant difference between the zeta potential of the phosphate/bio-glass composite biomaterial and that of the two/bio-glass-M composite biomaterials.

Table 1. Zeta potentials of engineered composite biomaterials.

	Charged Particle		
Composite Biomaterial	**Average Zeta Potential ζ [mV]**	**Distribution Peak [mV]**	**Electron Mobility [μm × cm/Vs]**
DCPD	−26.6	−24.0	−2.076
DCPD-Na	−23.9	−0.0202	−1.8658
DCPD-Na-M	−19.7	−0.0158	−1.5318
DCPD-K	−24.6	−19.5	−1.9183
DCPD-K-M	−16.5	−0.0125	−1.2847

In contrast, other analytical techniques, such as IR spectroscopy and X-ray diffraction (XRD) of DCPD-Na and DCPD-K composites, show an in situ evolution towards an apatite phase. This transition to an apatite phase leads to the formation of agglomerates, highlighted by zeta potential values. This conclusion is reinforced by our preceding results.

After insertion of the antibiotic, values of zeta potentials decreased in the case of DCPD-Na composite biomaterials ($\zeta = -23.9$ mV) compared to the presence of the antibiotic (DCPD-Na-M, $\zeta = -19.7$ mV). Similarly, for DCPD-K composite biomaterials, the values of zeta potentials decreased from $\zeta = -24.6$ mV to $\zeta = -16.5$ mV (DCPD-K-M). This could be attributed to interactions between the biomaterials and the antibiotic, as well as to the formation of particles with a greater tendency to agglomerate due to the presence of the antibiotic [27,28].

2.3. Antibiotic Release Into SBF Solution

To monitor the kinetics of antibiotic release from the composite (Figure 5), we used a UV–visible spectrophotometer. This method enabled us to assess the concentration of the antibiotic in the SBF solution. These measurements were obtained using a calibration curve correlating the absorbance at 203 nm, derived from the UV–visible spectrum, with the concentration of the antibiotic "streptomycin sulfate" in ppm.

It is noticeable that after three days of incubation at 37 °C, the DCPD-Na-M composite biomaterial (326 ppm) rapidly releases more antibiotic than the DCPD-K-M composite biomaterial (244 ppm). Both DCPD-Na-M and DCPD-K-M biocomposites have the advantage of trapping the antibiotic within the apatite formed in situ, which is characterized by the presence of tunnels. In addition, electrostatic interactions between the antibiotic and the apatite are formed, reinforced by the presence of silicate in the form of bio-glass surrounding the apatite.

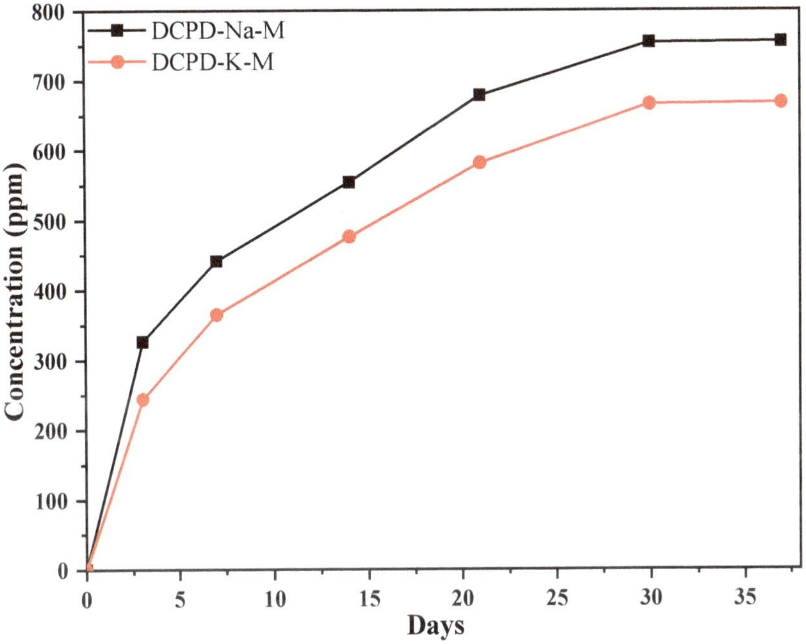

Figure 5. Kinetics of streptomycin sulfate release from the DCPD-Na-M and DCPD-K-M composite biomaterials.

The DCPD-K-M composite releases less antibiotic due to the presence of potassium silicate, compared to the DCPD-Na-M composite. This difference could be explained by the difference in ionic radii between potassium and sodium. On the other hand, the controlled long-term release may be attributed to in situ precipitation of hydroxyapatite in the presence of silicate solutions, which could further promote phosphate/bio-glass interactions and synergy between the constituents of the phosphate/bio-glass/antibiotic composite.

2.4. Ion Exchange with SBF Medium

The use of ICP-AES enables highly sensitive measurements to be carried out, and precise data to be obtained (sensitivity of approximately 1 ppm, depending on the matrix analyzed). This technique can be used to determine the ion exchange between composite biomaterials and the SBF solution. The measurements were carried out on the SBF solution used during the immersions. The results show variations in the concentration of the following elements: silicon, calcium, potassium, and sodium (Figure 6). Silicon content is an indicator of bio-glass dissolution, while calcium content is an indicator of phosphocalcic exchange, leading to the formation of an apatitic layer favored by favorable pH conditions.

In addition, the rapid release of sodium ions (Figure 7) and potassium ions can be observed over the course of 15 days, caused by the dissolution of the silicate phase present in the composite biomaterial. The increase in silicon concentration is attributed to the loss of SiO_4^{4-} tetrahedral units from the material surface and the formation of silanol (Si-OH) groups. Overall, the rapid dissolution rate observed can be directly attributed to the high amount of sodium strongly disrupting Si-O-Si connectivity in the bio-glass network, thus reducing its integrity and leading to a higher and more constant dissolution rate [4].

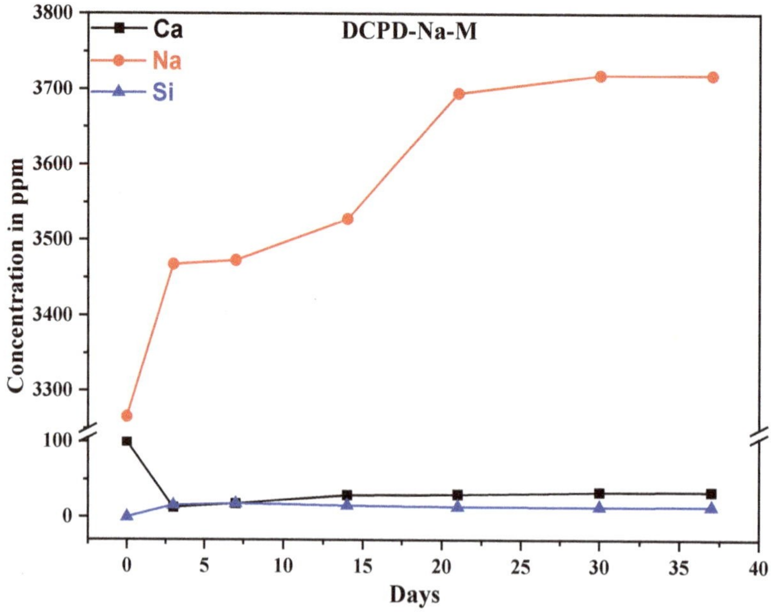

Figure 6. Concentrations of the elements Ca, Na, and Si released by the DCPD-Na-M composite biomaterial.

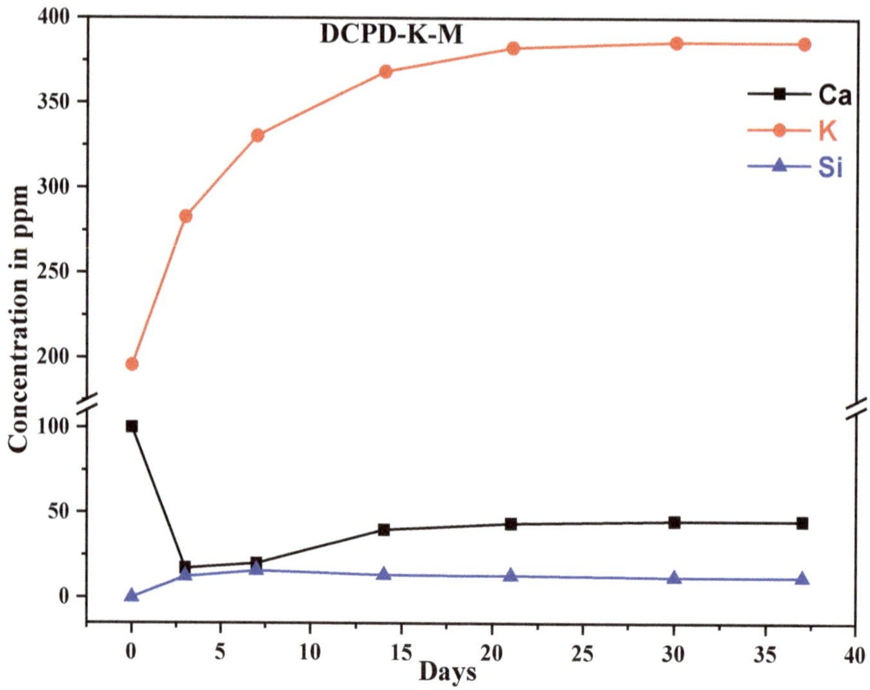

Figure 7. Concentrations of the elements Ca, K and Si released by the DCPD-K-M composite biomaterial.

The results show the following concentration variations: calcium concentration decreases over time, while silicon concentration increases due to dissolution of the glass surface over the first 21 days, followed by significant stabilization.

These results are due to the dissolution of the glass in contact with the SBF solution, the formation of a silica gel layer, and finally the formation of a calcium phosphate crystal. This mechanism can be summarized in three successive phases: dissolution of the glass matrix, formation of silica gel, and precipitation of calcium phosphate with an apatitic structure. Based on the results obtained, we can emphasize that this new composite support could be a promising bone substitute due to its bioactivity and dissolution capacity.

2.5. Element Distribution on the Surface of Composite Biomaterials

Scanning electron microscopy reveals significant changes in the biomaterials after 37 days immersion in the SBF solution. Typical needle-shaped apatite crystals and large blocky sodium silicate gel formations surrounding small crystals are observed in all composite biomaterials, confirming the formation of interpenetrating matrices where the polymerized gel fills the pores of the composite biomaterial.

In the case of the DCPD-Na-M composite biomaterial (Figure 8A), an increased porosity is observed compared to the biomaterial before immersion in the SBF solution (Figure 8B). This observation can be attributed to the dissolution of the biocomposite constituents in the SBF solution, including the antibiotic. Similarly, for the DCPD-K-M composite biomaterial (Figure 8C), porosity became greater compared to the biomaterial before immersion in the SBF solution (Figure 8D). This increase in porosity can also be attributed to ionic and molecular exchange with the SBF solution [29].

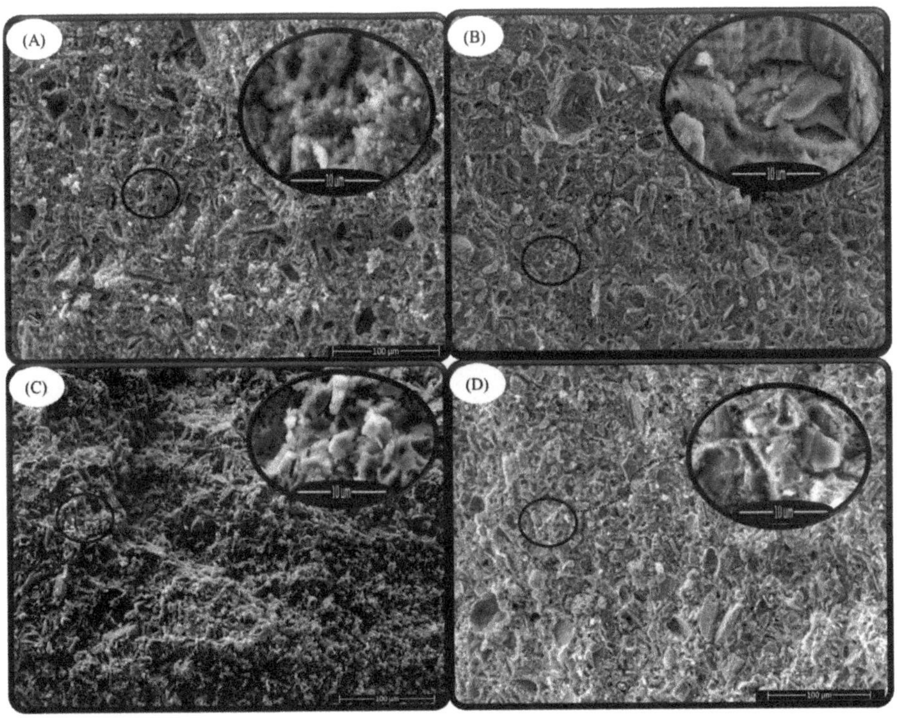

Figure 8. SEM images of composite biomaterials before immersion in SBF (DCPD-Na-M (**A**), DCPD-K-M (**C**)) and after immersion in SBF (37 days) (DCPD-Na-M (**B**), DCPD-K-M (**D**)).

Scanning electron microscopy thus highlights the structural changes in biomaterials after immersion in the SBF solution. Mapping clearly reveals the distribution of elements on the surface of composite biomaterials after 37 days of immersion in the SBF solution. The signal intensity of each ion is reflected in the intensity of each image. As illustrated in Figures 9 and 10, the elements calcium (Ca), phosphorus (P), sodium (Na), oxygen (O), silicon (Si), potassium (K), chlorine (Cl), carbon (C) and magnesium (Mg) are represented by different colors on the distribution maps. The distribution of the composite biomaterial particles was found to be homogeneous.

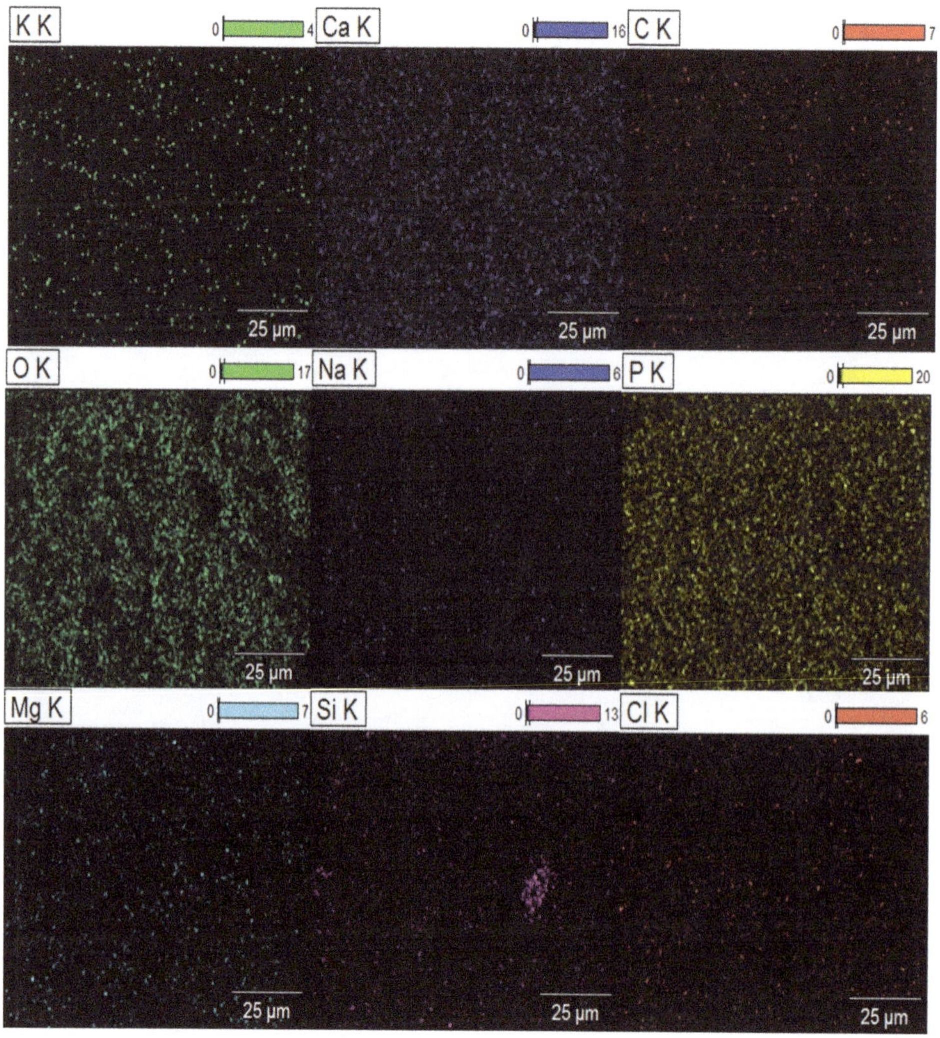

Figure 9. Mapping of DCPD-K-M composite biomaterial after 37 days immersion in SBF solution.

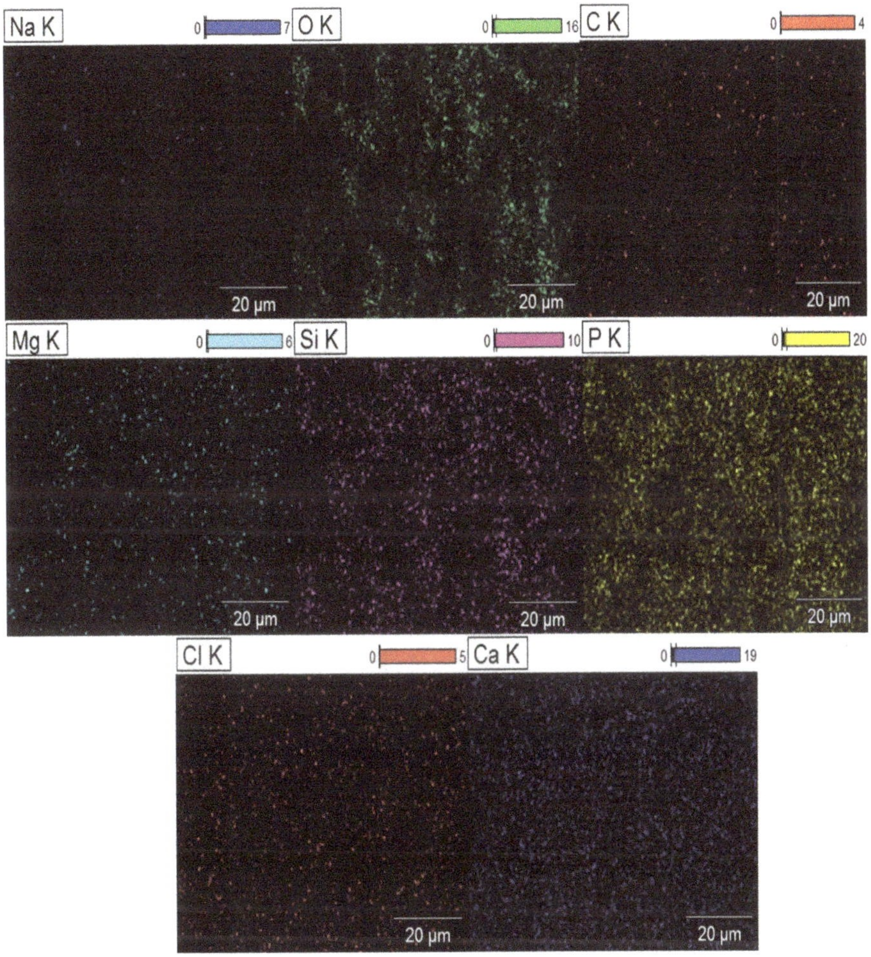

Figure 10. Mapping of DCPD-Na-M composite biomaterial after 37 days immersion in SBF solution.

The results highlight ionic exchange between the SBF solution and the composites, characterized by the appearance of the elements chlorine (Cl), magnesium (Mg), and sodium (Na) in the DCPD-K-M biocomposite and potassium (K) in the DCPD-Na-M biocomposites.

2.6. *Toxicity Study*

To ensure the suitability of developed biomaterials for applications involving human contact, it is essential to verify that they exhibit no signs of toxicity or adverse health effects. Conducting toxicity tests on these biomaterials is crucial in this regard, as it helps assess any potential harmful or toxic effects they may have on living organisms. These toxicity assays help determine whether the biomaterials can induce adverse reactions such as skin irritation, allergic responses, hormonal disruptions, or other health complications.

In order to assess the toxicity of our composite biomaterial, a series of rigorous experiments were conducted involving three groups (G1, G2, and G3) of albino mice to which different doses of the biomaterial were administered. The doses were meticulously selected within a range of 5 mg/kg (G1), 10 mg/kg (G2), and 15 mg/kg (G3) to allow for precise observation of potential effects over a 15-day period. This duration was deemed adequate to detect any signs of short-term toxicity. The results obtained are promising, as no mortality or significant weight changes were observed in the treated mice during the course of the experiment. This finding is particularly significant as it suggests a favorable tolerance of the composite biomaterial by the mice, thereby reinforcing its potential viability for future applications. Furthermore, the absence of any notable adverse effects, as well as the stability of the mice's behavior throughout the experiment, also indicate the acceptability of the composite biomaterial by the animals. These observations are crucial for evaluating the safety and suitability of the biomaterial, not only from a toxicological standpoint but also in terms of practical applicability.

2.7. Antibacterial Activity

A comparative study of the activity of the DCPD-Na and DCPD-K composite biomaterials in the presence and absence of medication after a 37-day release was conducted on four different bacterial strains: *Listeria monocytogenes*, *Staphylococcus aureus*, *Escherichia coli*, and *Pseudomonas aeruginosa*. Table 2 revealed that both medication-free biomaterials showed no antibacterial activity. However, in the case of the DCPD-Na-M biocomposite, inhibition zones of 10.1, 10.1, 10.5, and 9.5 mm were measured, respectively, against *L. monocytogenes*, *S. aureus*, *E. coli*, and *P. aeruginosa*, indicating medication release. Similarly, antibacterial tests of DCPD-K-M showed inhibition zones of 8.5, 8.5, 12.1, and 8.1 mm, respectively, against *L. monocytogenes*, *S. aureus*, *E. coli*, and *P. aeruginosa*. These results suggest that the prolonged release of medication from the composite biomaterials leads to effective antibacterial activity.

Table 2. Inhibition diameter (mm) of composite biomaterial tested four bacterial strains.

	DCPD-Na	DCPD-K	DCPD-Na-M	DCPD-K-M	Cycloheximide	DMSO
Escherichia coli	ND *	ND	10.5 ± 0.1	12.1 ± 0.3	31 ± 0.1	ND
Pseudomonas aeruginosa	ND	ND	9.5 ± 0.1	8.1 ± 0.1	21 ± 0.2	ND
Staphylococcus aureus	ND	ND	10.1 ± 0.2	8.5 ± 0.1	30.7 ± 0.3	ND
Listeria monocytogenes	ND	ND	10.1 ± 0.3	8.5 ± 0.2	30.3 ± 0.2	ND

* Not determined.

This sustained antibiotic release from the composite biomaterials offers potential benefits in medical applications, particularly in the field of bone surgery. Indeed, it may help prevent post-operative infections by providing continuous antibacterial protection over an extended period, thereby reducing the risk of complications and improving clinical outcomes for patients. Unlike antibiotics administered alone, which are rapidly eliminated by the body.

3. Materials and Methods

3.1. Materials

The reagents used in this study are calcium nitrate tetrahydrate $Ca(NO_3)_2$, $4H_2O$ (99%), ammonium hydrogen phosphate $(NH_4)_2HPO_4$ (99%), high-purity SiO_2 grade, Davisil Grade 633, NaOH pellets, and KOH pellets. They were all purchased from Sigma-Aldrich, Saint-Quentin-Fallavier, France, and were used without further purification.

3.2. Attenuated Total Reflectance Fourier Transform Infrared Spectroscopy (ATR-FTIR)

ATR-FTIR was used to evaluate the formation of composite biomaterials. The spectra were obtained using a FT/IR-4700 spectrometer (JASCO International Ltd., Tokyo, Japan). The spectral range was 400–4000 cm^{-1}, and each spectrum was an average of 32 scans at a resolution of 4 cm^{-1}. A background check was performed before each analysis.

3.3. UV–Visible Spectrophotometry

The analysis of antibiotic concentration in the museum study was carried out by UV–visible spectrophotometry, using a high-performance dual-beam spectrophotometer, the Shimadzu UV-1900 I PC spectrometer manufactured by Shimadzu Duisburg, Germany. This spectrometer covers a spectral range from 190 to 1100 nm.

3.4. X-ray Diffraction Analysis (XRD)

To study the crystal structure of the scaffolds and confirm the formation of HAp particles in situ, XRD was performed using the Panalytical X'Pert Pro instrument (Malvern Panalytical GmbH, Kassel, Germany) with a Cu Kα X-ray source at 40 kV and 30 mA, and a scan speed of 2°/min.

3.5. Scanning Electron Microscopy (SEM) with Energy-Dispersive X-ray Spectroscopy (EDX)

SEM images were obtained using a Thermo ScientificTM Quattro ESEM (ThermoFisher Scientific, Paisley, UK) at an accelerating voltage of 15 kV. The films were sputter coated with gold before imaging to improve the electron beam conductivity. EDX spectra were acquired using an attached detector on the same instrument.

3.6. Inductively Coupled Plasma Atomic Emission Spectrometer (ICP-AES)

ICP analyses were performed using a Horiba Jobin Yvon Ultima 2 ICP-AES spectrometer equipped with a temperature-controlled optical system comprising two back-to-back 4343 tr/mm and 2400 tr/mm gratings covering the spectral range from 120 to 800 nm, with nitrogen scanning. The detection system consists of two photomultipliers.

3.7. Zeta Potential

The zeta potential of biomaterial particles was measured using the Anton Paar Litesizer 500 instrument at 25°. Zeta potential values were obtained automatically using the instrument's software, Kalliope version 2.22.2, which converts the measured electrophoretic mobility into zeta potential in order to evaluate variations in the latter for particles of the materials processed.

3.8. Preparation of Antibiotic-Loaded Composite Biomaterials

3.8.1. Synthesis of Dicalcium Phosphate by the Double Decomposition Method

The double decomposition method is often used to obtain a solid precipitate from two clear reactive solutions. It is based on the reaction of two salts dissolved in separate solutions, which exchange ions to form an insoluble precipitate.

In this case, a two-stage synthesis process is used. In the first stage, two solutions, (A) and (B), are prepared and used as reagents. A certain mass of diammonium phosphate is dissolved in distilled water to obtain phosphate solution (A). At the same time, one mass of calcium nitrate is dissolved in one volume of distilled water to obtain calcium solution (B). Both solutions are stirred until they are completely clear. Once the two solutions have been prepared, they are mixed, and the reaction medium is left to stir for 15 min. Then, stop stirring and leave the solution to mature for 2 h. The reaction is as follows:

$$(NH_4)_2HPO_4 + Ca(NO_3)_2.4H_2O \xrightarrow{H_2O} CaHPO_4.2H_2O + 2NH_4NO_3 \quad (1)$$

After ripening, the resulting dicalcium phosphate is filtered and dried overnight at 40 °C.

3.8.2. Synthesis of Sodium Silicate and Potassium Silicate Solutions

Silicate solutions are generally presented as a dispersion of colloidal silica species in an alkaline aqueous solution. In this study, we focused on a concentrated sodium silicate or potassium silicate solution with a low molar ratio (SiO_2/Na_2O = 1 or SiO_2/K_2O = 1) due to the high reactivity of their non-condensed silica species.

For this purpose, a solution of sodium silicate or potassium silicate (Na_2SiO_3, H_2O or K_2SiO_3, H_2O) with a molar ratio of 1 was prepared at 90 °C. Pure NaOH (or pure KOH) pellets were dissolved in deionized water, and then an appropriate amount of commercial silica gel was added. This yielded a liquid glass containing 25% SiO_2 by weight, 25% Na_2O (or 25% K_2O) and 50% water, with a pH of approximately 12. The resulting solution was aged for a short period to ensure the stability of the final state.

3.8.3. Synthesis of Antibiotic-Loaded Composite Biomaterials

The active ingredients are introduced into the initial composition of the dicalcium phosphate/bio-glass solution, undergoing in situ evolution towards the apatite phase, according to the following process:

A solution (A) is prepared by dissolving a precise quantity of drug powder in the corresponding silicate solution. The dicalcium phosphate powder is then gradually added to the solution, paying particular attention to homogenizing the mixture. Solution (A) contains a 1% concentration of the bioactive molecule. The paste is then placed in an airtight container in a humid atmosphere and cured in an oven at 37 °C. The biomaterials synthesized are listed in Table 3.

Table 3. Prepared composite biomaterials.

Composite	SiO_2/M_2O	Antibiotic 1%
DCPD-Na	SiO_2/Na_2O	0%
DCPD-K	SiO_2/K_2O	0%
DCPD-Na-M *	SiO_2/Na_2O	1%
DCPD-K-M *	SiO_2/K_2O	1%

* M refers to streptomycin sulfate.

3.8.4. Study of the Release of Active Ingredients from Engineered Composite Biomaterials

The ability to exchange ions with the immersion medium is crucial in assessing a biomaterial's ability to promote bonding with living tissue. In vitro tests are therefore carried out to assess this ability. These tests involve immersing samples in a synthetic physiological liquid, SBF (simulated body fluid), whose ionic composition is designed to be similar to that of human blood plasma [30]. SBF is adjusted to a pH of 7.4. Table 4 compares the ionic concentrations of SBF with those of human blood plasma.

Table 4. Ionic concentrations of SBF and human blood plasma in mM [30].

Ions (mM)	Na^+	K^+	Mg^{2+}	Ca^{2+}	Cl^-	HCO^{3-}	HPO_4^{2-}	SO_4^{2-}
SBF	142.0	5.0	1.5	2.5	147.8	4.2	1.0	0.5
Plasma	142.0	5.0	1.5	2.5	103.0	27.0	1.0	0.5

The multifunctional composite biomaterials studied are mainly in the form of cylindrical blocks measuring 16.5 mm in diameter by 5 mm in height (Figure 11). This specific configuration was chosen to enable a precise evaluation of the bioactivity kinetics of the various composite biomaterials produced at different points in time.

For in vitro testing, the blocks were placed in hermetically sealed vials and then immersed in 60 mL of SBF. The temperature was maintained at 37 °C under controlled stirring in incubators. The immersion times chosen for the cylinder studies were 5, 7, 14, 21, and 37 days.

After immersion, the cylinders were immersed in SBF solution. These solutions were then analyzed by UV–visible spectroscopy to monitor the variation in drug concentration over time in the SBF solution. We also monitored ion exchange by ICP-AES and observed possible surface modifications by scanning electron microscopy and possible surface mapping of chemical element distribution in blocks after antibiotic release into the SBF solution.

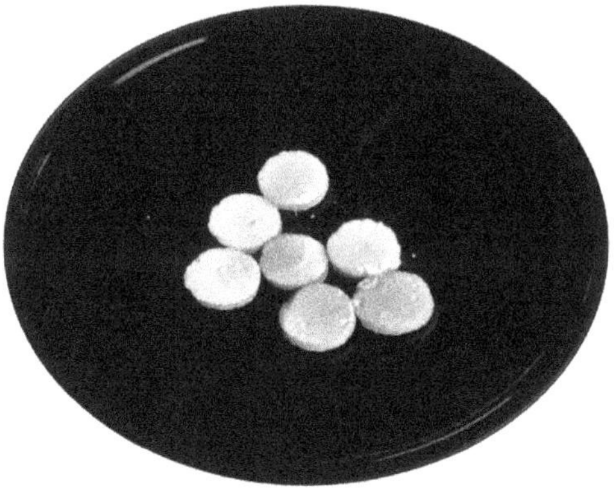

Figure 11. Shaping the sample before immersion in SBF.

3.9. Test In Vitro

3.9.1. Antibacterial Activity

The in vitro evaluation of antibacterial activity was conducted with two strains of Gram-negative bacteria (*Escherichia coli* ATCC 10536 and *Pseudomonas aeruginosa* ATCC 49189) and two strains of Gram-positive bacteria (*Listeria monocytogenes* ATCC 12117 and *Staphylococcus aureus* ATCC 6538), obtained from the Laboratory of Bioresources, Biotechnologies, Ethnopharmacology, and Health (LBBEH), Faculty of Sciences, Oujda. The bacteria were cultured in Muller-Hinton broth (MHB; BIOKAR, Beauvais, France) [31].

For each bacterial strain, 1 mL of liquid bacterial suspension was added to 9 mL of MHB and incubated at 37 °C for 24 h until the microbial suspension reached the exponential growth phase. Bacterial cultures were adjusted to 0.5 McFarland's standard to achieve a concentration of 1.5×108 CFU/mL.

The antibacterial activity was evaluated using the well method. This involved punching Muller–Hinton agar (MHA) inoculated with the test bacteria (100 µL) to create wells, which were then filled with 60 µL of extract. Negative controls were performed using dimethyl sulfoxide (DMSO), and positive controls were performed using gentamicin.

Cultures were incubated for 18 h at 37 °C after a 30 min pre-diffusion at room temperature [32]. The zone of inhibition around the well was measured in mm using a sliding caliper after incubation.

3.9.2. Toxicity Tests

Swiss albinos were maintained at a temperature of 25 °C with a relative humidity of 45–50% on a 12 h light/dark cycle, with free access to food and water. Prior to the experiments, mice were compared in terms of body weight (between 35 and 30 g). All animals were treated in full compliance with internationally recognized standards for the care and use of laboratory animals, as published by the US National Institutes of Health (NIH Publication No. 85-23, revised 1985).

An initial group of 16 mice was divided into 4 groups of 4 (comprising 2 males and 2 females). The first group served as a control, receiving distilled water. The other three groups were treated with increasing doses of the product. The doses administered were selected on the basis of the maximum volume that could be administered orally. For chemical toxicity studies, doses should be between 5 and 5000 mg/kg.

4. Conclusions

In our study, we explored a novel approach to the synthesis of multifunctional composite biomaterials. This consolidation method, based on controlled in situ dissolution and precipitation, enabled the creation of complex biocomposites with remarkable properties. We characterized these biomaterials using a variety of techniques, including infrared spectroscopy, X-ray diffraction, scanning electron microscopy, and zeta potential analysis. These analyses revealed chemical transformations, surface changes, and complex interactions between the composites' constituent elements. Toxicity tests showed good acceptability. In vitro tests revealed the ability of these biomaterials to exchange ions and active ingredients with a medium simulating body fluid, demonstrating their potential bioactivity. In addition, antibiotic release kinetics were studied, revealing significant differences between composites in terms of antibiotic release and retention. Finally, our experiments demonstrated the antibacterial efficacy of these composites, paving the way for promising applications in the biomedical field. By incorporating the antibiotic into the biomaterial composites, we were able to control its release and prolong its antibacterial activity over time, enabling the development of biocomposites capable of simultaneously playing an osteogenerative role and releasing active ingredients in a continuous and prolonged manner for medical purposes. This research contributes to the advancement of biomaterials by exploring new synthetic routes and demonstrating their potential in the fields of regenerative medicine and controlled drug release. Future studies will further develop these results and explore the practical applications of these innovative biomaterials.

Author Contributions: Conceptualization, E.M. and M.A.; methodology, M.A., R.E.Y. and M.I.Y.; software, R.E.Y.; validation, B.H., R.S. and K.A.; formal analysis, R.S. and F.L.; investigation, A.A.; resources, E.M.; data curation, M.A.; writing—preparation of original version, M.A.; writing—revision and editing, R.S., K.A. and M.A.; visualization, F.L.; supervision, E.M. and B.H.; project administration, E.M. and M.M.A.; fund acquisition, M.M.A. All authors have read and agreed to the published version of the manuscript.

Funding: This research was supported by the Researchers Supporting Project number (RSPD2024R628), King Saud University, Riyadh, Saudi Arabia.

Institutional Review Board Statement: Not applicable.

Informed Consent Statement: Not applicable.

Data Availability Statement: The data presented in this study are available upon request from the corresponding author.

Acknowledgments: The authors extend their appreciation to the Researchers Supporting Project number (RSPD2024R628), King Saud University, Riyadh, Saudi Arabia for supporting this research. The authors would also like to thank Abdelmonaem El Talhaoui, for making the analytical platform of the Chemistry Department available to them.

Conflicts of Interest: The authors declare no conflict of interest.

References

1. Dornelas, J.; Dornelas, G.; Rossi, A.; Piattelli, A.; Di Pietro, N.; Romasco, T.; Mourão, C.F.; Alves, G.G. The Incorporation of Zinc into Hydroxyapatite and Its Influence on the Cellular Response to Biomaterials: A Systematic Review. *J. Funct. Biomater.* **2024**, *15*, 178. [CrossRef]
2. Abdelhamid, M.A.; Khalifa, H.O.; Ki, M.-R.; Pack, S.P. Nanoengineered Silica-Based Biomaterials for Regenerative Medicine. *Int. J. Mol. Sci.* **2024**, *25*, 6125. [CrossRef] [PubMed]
3. Alizadeh-Osgouei, M.; Li, Y.; Wen, C. A comprehensive review of biodegradable synthetic polymer-ceramic composites and their manufacture for biomedical applications. *Bioact. Mater.* **2019**, *4*, 22–36. [CrossRef] [PubMed]
4. Kargozar, S.; Ramakrishna, S.; Mozafari, M. Chemistry of biomaterials: Future prospects. *Curr. Opin. Biomed. Eng.* **2019**, *10*, 181–190. [CrossRef]
5. Swetha, M.; Sahithi, K.; Moorthi, A.; Srinivasan, N.; Ramasamy, K.; Selvamurugan, N. Biocomposites containing natural polymers and hydroxyapatite for bone tissue engineering. *Int. J. Biol. Macromol.* **2010**, *47*, 1–4. [CrossRef] [PubMed]
6. Azzaoui, K.; Jodeh, S.; Mejdoubi, E.; Hammouti, B.; Taleb, M.; Ennabety, G.; Berisha, A.; Aaddouz, M.; Youssouf, M.; Shityakov, S. Synthesis of hydroxyapatite/polyethylene glycol 6000 composites by novel dissolution/precipitation method: Optimization of the adsorption process using a factorial design: DFT and molecular dynamic. *BMC Chem.* **2023**, *17*, 150. [CrossRef]
7. Magnaterra, G. Additive Manufacturing of Hydroxyapatite Scaffolds for Bone Repair. Ph.D. Thesis, Politecnico di Torino, Turin, Italy, 2020.
8. Pu'ad, N.M.; Haq, R.A.; Noh, H.M.; Abdullah, H.; Idris, M.; Lee, T. Synthesis method of hydroxyapatite: A review. *Mater. Today Proc.* **2020**, *29*, 233–239.

9. DileepKumar, V.; Sridhar, M.S.; Aramwit, P.; Krut'ko, V.K.; Musskaya, O.N.; Glazov, I.E.; Reddy, N. A review on the synthesis and properties of hydroxyapatite for biomedical applications. *J. Biomater. Sci. Polym. Ed.* **2022**, *33*, 229–261. [CrossRef] [PubMed]
10. El-Ghannam, A. Bone reconstruction: From bioceramics to tissue engineering. *Expert Rev. Med. Devices* **2005**, *2*, 87–101. [CrossRef]
11. Pantulap, U.; Arango-Ospina, M.; Boccaccini, A.R. Bioactive glasses incorporating less-common ions to improve biological and physical properties. *J. Mater. Sci. Mater. Med.* **2022**, *33*, 3. [CrossRef]
12. El Hammari, L.; Latifi, S.; Saoiabi, S.; Azzaoui, A.; Hammouti, B.; Chetouani, A.; Sabbahi, R. Toxic heavy metals removal from river water using a porous phospho-calcic hydroxyapatite. *Moroc. J. Chem.* **2022**, *10*, 62–72.
13. Apelt, D.; Theiss, F.; El-Warrak, A.; Zlinszky, K.; Bettschart-Wolfisberger, R.; Bohner, M.; Matter, S.; Auer, J.A.; von Rechenberg, B. In vivo behavior of three different injectable hydraulic calcium phosphate cements. *Biomaterials* **2004**, *25*, 1439–1451. [CrossRef] [PubMed]
14. Şahin, E. *Synthesis and Characterization of Calcium Phosphate Cement Based Macroporous Scaffolds*; Izmir Institute of Technology: Urla, Turkey, 2012.
15. Dorozhkin, S.V. Calcium orthophosphate-based bioceramics and its clinical applications. In *Clinical Applications of Biomaterials*; Kaur, G., Ed.; Springer: Cham, Switzerland, 2017; pp. 123–226. [CrossRef]
16. Nabiyouni, M.; Brückner, T.; Zhou, H.; Gbureck, U.; Bhaduri, S.B. Magnesium-based bioceramics in orthopedic applications. *Acta Biomater.* **2018**, *66*, 23–43. [CrossRef] [PubMed]
17. Atila, D.; Dalgic, A.D.; Krzemińska, A.; Pietrasik, J.; Gendaszewska-Darmach, E.; Bociaga, D.; Lipinska, M.; Laoutid, F.; Passion, J.; Kumaravel, V. Injectable Liposome-Loaded Hydrogel Formulations with Controlled Release of Curcumin and α-Tocopherol for Dental Tissue Engineering. *Adv. Healthc. Mater.* **2024**, 2400966. [CrossRef]
18. Mansour, A.; Romani, M.; Acharya, A.B.; Rahman, B.; Verron, E.; Badran, Z. Drug delivery systems in regenerative medicine: An updated review. *Pharmaceutics* **2023**, *15*, 695. [CrossRef] [PubMed]
19. Gao, P.; Nie, X.; Zou, M.; Shi, Y.; Cheng, G. Recent advances in materials for extended-release antibiotic delivery system. *J. Antibiot.* **2011**, *64*, 625–634. [CrossRef] [PubMed]
20. Chindamo, G.; Sapino, S.; Peira, E.; Chirio, D.; Gonzalez, M.C.; Gallarate, M. Bone diseases: Current approach and future perspectives in drug delivery systems for bone targeted therapeutics. *Nanomaterials* **2020**, *10*, 875. [CrossRef]
21. Liang, W.; Zhou, C.; Jin, S.; Fu, L.; Zhang, H.; Huang, X.; Long, H.; Ming, W.; Zhao, J. An update on the advances in the field of nanostructured drug delivery systems for a variety of orthopedic applications. *Drug Deliv.* **2023**, *30*, 2241667. [CrossRef]
22. Aaddouz, M.; Azzaoui, K.; Akartasse, N.; Mejdoubi, E.; Hammouti, B.; Taleb, M.; Sabbahi, R.; Alshahateet, S. Removal of methylene blue from aqueous solution by adsorption onto hydroxyapatite nanoparticles. *J. Mol. Struct.* **2023**, *1288*, 135807. [CrossRef]
23. Azzaoui, K.; Aaddouz, M.; Akartasse, N.; Mejdoubi, E.; Jodeh, S.; Hammouti, B.; Taleb, M.; ES-Sehli, S.; Berisha, A.; Rhazi, L. Synthesis of β-Tricalcium Phosphate/PEG 6000 Composite by Novel Dissolution/Precipitation Method: Optimization of the Adsorption Process Using a Factorial Design—DFT and Molecular Dynamic. *Arab. J. Sci. Eng.* **2023**, *49*, 711–732. [CrossRef]
24. Degli Esposti, L.; Adamiano, A.; Siliqi, D.; Giannini, C.; Iafisco, M. The effect of chemical structure of carboxylate molecules on hydroxyapatite nanoparticles. A structural and morphological study. *Bioact. Mater.* **2021**, *6*, 2360–2371. [CrossRef] [PubMed]
25. Walsh, D.; Kingston, J.L.; Heywood, B.R.; Mann, S. Influence of monosaccharides and related molecules on the morphology of hydroxyapatite. *J. Cryst. Growth* **1993**, *133*, 1–12. [CrossRef]
26. Aaddouz, M.; Azzaoui, K.; Sabbahi, R.; Youssoufi, M.H.; Yahyaoui, M.I.; Asehraou, A.; El Miz, M.; Hammouti, B.; Shityakov, S.; Siaj, M. Cheminformatics-based design and synthesis of hydroxyapatite/collagen nanocomposites for biomedical applications. *Polymers* **2023**, *16*, 85. [CrossRef] [PubMed]
27. Khin, S.Y.; Soe, H.M.S.H.; Chansriniyom, C.; Pornputtapong, N.; Asasutjarit, R.; Loftsson, T.; Jansook, P. Development of fenofibrate/randomly methylated β-cyclodextrin-loaded Eudragit® RL 100 nanoparticles for ocular delivery. *Molecules* **2022**, *27*, 4755. [CrossRef] [PubMed]
28. Cerchiara, T.; Abruzzo, A.; Di Cagno, M.; Bigucci, F.; Bauer-Brandl, A.; Parolin, C.; Vitali, B.; Gallucci, M.; Luppi, B. Chitosan based micro-and nanoparticles for colon-targeted delivery of vancomycin prepared by alternative processing methods. *Eur. J. Pharm. Biopharm.* **2015**, *92*, 112–119. [CrossRef] [PubMed]
29. Đošić, M.S.; Mitrić, M.; Mišković-Stanković, V.B. The porosity and roughness of electrodeposited calcium phosphate coatings in simulated body fluid. *J. Serbian Chem. Soc.* **2015**, *80*, 237–251. [CrossRef]
30. Kokubo, T.; Kushitani, H.; Sakka, S.; Kitsugi, T.; Yamamuro, T. Solutions able to reproduce in vivo surface-structure changes in bioactive glass-ceramic A-W3. *J. Biomed. Mater. Res.* **1990**, *24*, 721–734. [CrossRef] [PubMed]
31. Celiktas, O.Y.; Kocabas, E.H.; Bedir, E.; Sukan, F.V.; Ozek, T.; Baser, K. Antimicrobial activities of methanol extracts and essential oils of Rosmarinus officinalis, depending on location and seasonal variations. *Food Chem.* **2007**, *100*, 553–559. [CrossRef]
32. Pundir, C.S.; Rawal, R. Determination of sulfite with emphasis on biosensing methods: A review. *Anal. Bioanal. Chem.* **2013**, *405*, 3049–3062. [CrossRef]

molecules

MDPI

Article

Sol–Gel Synthesis of Silica–Poly (Vinylpyrrolidone) Hybrids with Prooxidant Activity and Antibacterial Properties

Albena Bachvarova-Nedelcheva [1,*], Yoanna Kostova [2], Lilia Yordanova [3], Elena Nenova [3], Pavletta Shestakova [4], Iliana Ivanova [3] and Elitsa Pavlova [5]

1 Institute of General and Inorganic Chemistry, Bulgarian Academy of Sciences, Acad. G. Bonchev Str., Bl. 11, 1113 Sofia, Bulgaria

2 Institute of Metal Science, Equipment and Technologies with Hydro- and Aerodynamics Centre "Acad. A. Balevski", Bulgarian Academy of Sciences, Shipchenski Prohod Str., 67, 1574 Sofia, Bulgaria; y_kostova@ims.bas.bg

3 Faculty of Biology, Sofia University "St. Kliment Ohridski", 8 Dragan Tsankov Blvd., 1164 Sofia, Bulgaria; lilijapj@uni-sofia.bg (L.Y.); nenova@uni-sofia.bg (E.N.); iaivanova@biofac.uni-sofia.bg (I.I.)

4 Institute of Organic Chemistry with Centre of Phytochemistry, Bulgarian Academy of Sciences, Acad. G. Bonchev Str., Bl. 9, 1113 Sofia, Bulgaria; pavletta.shestakova@orgchm.bas.bg

5 Faculty of Physics, Sofia University "St. Kliment Ohridski", 5 James Boucher Blvd., 1164 Sofia, Bulgaria; elli_pavlova@abv.bg

* Correspondence: albenadb@svr.igic.bas.bg

Abstract: The present work deals with the sol–gel synthesis of silica–poly (vinylpyrrolidone) hybrid materials. The nanohybrids (Si-PVP) have been prepared using an acidic catalyst at ambient temperature. Tetramethyl ortosilane (TMOS) was used as a silica precursor. Poly (vinylpyrrolidone) (PVP) was introduced into the reaction mixture as a solution in ethanol with a concentration of 20%. The XRD established that the as-prepared material is amorphous. The IR and ^{29}Si MAS NMR spectra proved the formation of a polymerized silica network as well as the hydrogen bonding interactions between the silica matrix and OH hydrogens of the silanol groups. The TEM showed spherical particle formation along with increased agglomeration tendency. The efficacy of SiO_2/PVP nanoparticles as a potential antimicrobial agent against a wide range of bacteria was evaluated as bacteriostatic, using agar diffusion and spot tests. Combined effects of hybrid nanomaterial and antibiotics could significantly reduce the bactericidal concentrations of both the antibiotic and the particles, and they could also eliminate the antibiotic resistance of the pathogen. The registered prooxidant activity of the newly synthesized material was confirmative and explicatory for the antibacterial properties of the tested substance and its synergetic combination with antibiotics. The effect of new hybrid material on Crustacea *Daphnia magna* was also estimated as harmless under concentration of 0.1 mg/mL.

Keywords: sol–gel; silica hybrids; antibacterial properties; ROS; prooxidant activity; *Daphnia magna*

1. Introduction

A wide range of materials, such as thin films, particles, or aerogels with numerous possible uses, can be produced using sol–gel chemistry [1]. Nowadays, this process is still being developed and it is used in many different industries to produce sophisticated materials, biomaterials, sensors, smart coatings, and optical devices [2]. The synthesis of organic–inorganic hybrids has been facilitated by the sol–gel method over the past three decades. Its key advantages over alternative methods include low processing temperature and pressure, adaptability, and flexibility [3]. It has been shown that the properties of the hybrid materials include a synergy at the nanometer level with the properties of the starting materials, making these materials appropriate for future technological applications [4]. For this reason, they are usually considered to be innovative advanced materials, with promising applications in many fields, such as optics, biology, mechanics, sensors, electronics, and coatings [5]. Hybrid properties strongly depend on the nature and strength of the interactions between the organic and inorganic components [6]. The bioactivity of sol–gel hybrids was found to be higher than that of materials obtained by other methods [7]. The presence of –OH groups on their surface is responsible for their bioactivities.

A large group of sol–gel materials is based on silicon alkoxides, e.g., tetramethoxysilane ($Si(OCH_3)_4$) or tetraethoxysilane ($Si(OC_2H_5)_4$). Applying appropriate conditions such as precursor/solvent ratio, precursor/water ratio, and catalyst (pH) leads to the formation of a gel composed of a silica network [8–10]. These gels are highly desirable for a variety of applications due to their low density, low thermal conductivity, low dielectric constant, and high specific area [11–13]. It has to be noted that native silica aerogels are very brittle, which limits their applications. However, several methods used to strengthen their structure have already been developed, and others are still in the works [14]. These include the gels' aging process, the use of silica precursors to increase the network's flexibility, and the addition of polymers to silica aerogel networks [1]. Applying the sol–gel processes, silicon alkoxides are also used for the synthesis of hybrid materials which are organic–inorganic ones. The creation of hybrids, which combine the advantageous aspects of inorganic and organic materials, was aided by developments in materials science. The inorganic phase in the hybrids can change the mechanical and thermal properties of pure organic materials and vice versa. Additionally, hybrid materials exhibit new functionalities such as magnetic and electric properties, increased adsorption, or better structural properties [15,16]. In the past, researchers proposed that the characteristics of the resulting hybrid material are significantly influenced by the ratio of the applied polymer, metal alcoholate, water, and catalysts [17]. The silica-based sol–gel functional products are generally based on polymers. Polyvinylpyrrolidone (PVP) is a macromolecular compound which is often used for the sol–gel production of silica hybrids and the first primary results have been reported by several authors [18,19]. Among polymers, PVP is a preferable compound due to its solubility in water and organic solutions, low toxicity, and high physiological compatibility. Its excellent qualities make it widespread, especially in the fields of medicine, foods, cosmetics, and other areas relevant to human health [20].

The synthesis of alternative materials is a highly favored strategy due to the outbreak of infectious diseases and antibiotic resistance [21,22]. Since the discovery of penicillin, β-lactam antibiotics have been widely used as antibacterial agents because of their broad spectrum of activity and low toxicity. However, the overuse of antibiotics has led to bacteria adapting by developing resistance. Due to this fact, pharmaceutical companies and researchers have devoted efforts to find compounds that do not cause such resistance in bacteria. The strategies adopted so far are not particularly effective and new alternatives are being explored to prevent bacterial resistance [23,24]. And this is where nanomaterials come in. They are used as antimicrobial agents due to their unique physical and chemical properties [25]. Considering the growing problem of bacterial resistance to antibiotics, nanoparticle-based antimicrobial agents are expected to provide alternatives to conventional antibiotics and biocidal chemicals. Due to their toxic properties, metal-containing nanocomposites are good candidates for new antimicrobial products for consumers and patient care [26]. A great potential in nanomedicine has been discovered in the past decade due to the effectiveness of various nanoconjugates against pathogenic microbes. One approach to counter bacterial drug resistance is the application of metal composites, especially at the nanoscale, to control bacterial infections [27]. Several enzymes and mutations in genetic sequences can impede multidrug resistance mechanisms by altering drug efflux from cells, thereby reducing bacterial vulnerability to antibacterial agents [28,29]. Therefore, scientists are developing new ways to control resistant pathogens. Advances in nanotechnology have prompted microbiologists to apply metal nanoparticles as an effective way to control certain pathogenic microbes involved in infectious diseases [30,31]. The combination of antibiotics and metal nanoparticles can enhance the efficacy of antibiotics against resistant pathogens. Furthermore, nanoparticle–antibiotic conjugates reduce the amount of both agents in the dose, which reduces toxicity and increases antimicrobial properties [32,33].

These conjugates can be very effective against resistant bacteria. Furthermore, due to this conjugation, antibiotic concentrations are decreased at the site of antibiotic–bacteria contact, and thus the association between microorganisms and antibiotics is accelerated [22,33,34].

The generation of reactive oxygen species (ROS) is an important biomarker about the redox properties of substances. By following the kinetics of the generation of free radicals and ROS, the properties of newly synthesized materials and their effects on the cascade of reactions causing the formation and accumulation of antibacterial free radicals and ROS can be evaluated [35,36]. Chemiluminescence analysis is a rapid and sensitive method for such studies. It is applied to follow the dynamics of free radical and ROS generation and to determine the prooxidant/antioxidant activity of various materials. The responses are recorded in the range of 480–580 nm and can be used to estimate the quantum yield [37,38].

Daphnia are a fundamental ecological species utilized for various biological applications including acute and chronic (eco)toxicology assessment and in fundamental research on ecology, genetics, and evolution. Due to their position in the food chain, and their filter-feeding capabilities, they are exposed to everything in their environment. Scientific data on *D. magna* related to immobilization, lethality, reproductive, behavioral, physiological and biochemical parameters used in the toxicity assessment of pharmaceuticals were presented by Tkaczyk et al. [39]. They demonstrated the role of these invertebrate model organisms for evaluating the toxicity of different therapeutic classes of pharmaceuticals. The growing need for environmental protection has led to the development of alternative biofuels. Hubai et al. [40] conducted studies related to their ecotoxicity by conducting an acute immobilization test on *Daphnia magna*. The toxic effect of CeO_2 and ZnO nanoparticles of the same size that were stabilized by a capping agent polyvinylpyrrolidone (10 k PVP) was investigated by Briffa et al. [41]. The authors found that ZnO nanoparticles were more toxic than CeO_2 nanoparticles and demonstrated that PVP encapsulation had no effect on toxicity. Other authors proposed a refractive index gel permeation chromatography (GPC) method for the quantification of PVP [35]. The method was applied to *Daphnia magna* exposed to PVP for 48 h. It was suggested that PVP is ingested by *Daphnia magna*, which warrants that the bioaccumulation of PVP could cause the sublethal effects observed in other studies [42,43].

The present work deals with the sol–gel synthesis and characterization of silica–poly (vinylpyrrolidone) hybrid material (SiO_2/20PVP). Our goal was to evaluate the efficacy and toxicity of the prepared material as a potential antimicrobial agent against a broad spectrum of bacteria, including those with novel resistance mechanisms. This hybrid was tested for antibacterial efficacy alone and in combination with different conventional antibiotics against four different bacterial isolates. In addition, we started to study their redox properties and ROS-generating activity, explaining their antibacterial properties. Moreover, a toxicity test with *Daphnia magna* predicted possible maximum permissible concentration in the environment without harm for water inhabitants.

2. Results and Discussion

2.1. Phase Transformations, SEM and TEM Observations

X-ray diffraction patterns of pure TMOS and PVP samples along with that containing 20% PVP amount are shown in Figure 1. As is seen from the figure, all gels are amorphous, which proves the hybrid material formation.

SEM images of the prepared gels are shown in Figure 2a,b. It is observed that the sample's surface is homogeneous and smooth for the pure TMOS and other sample too (Figure 2a,b). This is a proof for the successful progress of the co-condensation reactions. The SEM micrographs of the hybrids containing PVP looks similar and their surface are small-grained (Figure 2b). Moreover, the surface texture of SiO_2/20PVP (Figure 2b) shows bigger SiO_2 grains. Obviously, the higher PVP amount leads to the increase in particle size which is about 5 μm. This was also observed by other authors [20]. Generally, it is considered that PVP belongs to the group of selective capping agents and, in a reaction, it controls the growth rates of various faces of metal oxide nanoparticles throughout the adsorption on the surfaces. In other studies, it was shown that PVP enhanced the growth rate along [100] directions [44].

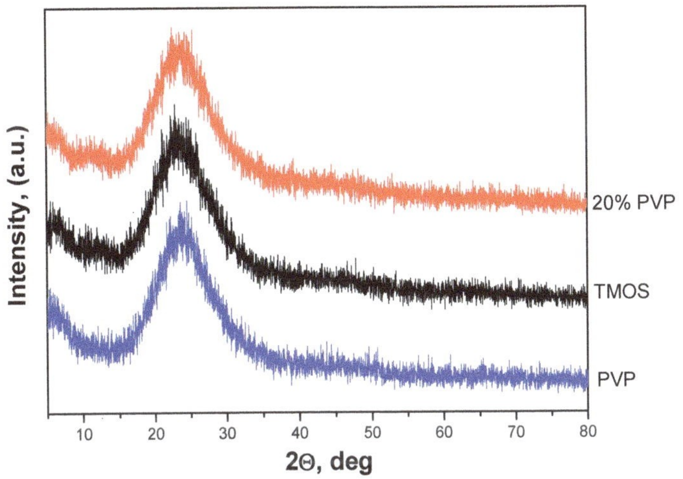

Figure 1. XRD patterns of SiO_2/20PVP, TMOS, and PVP.

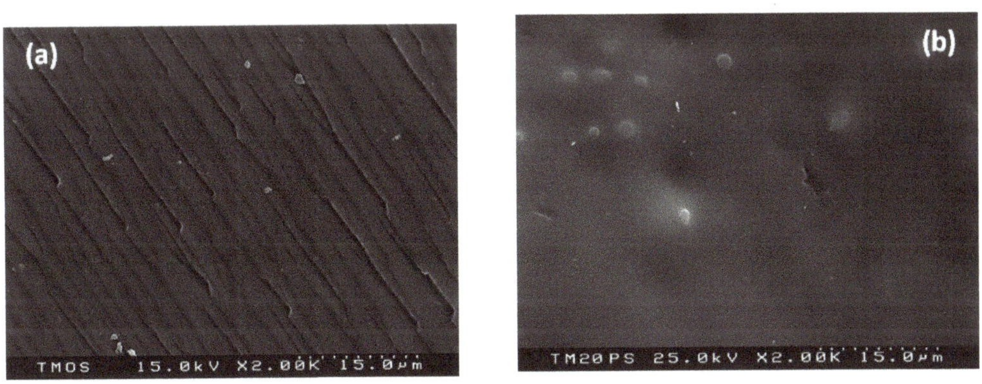

Figure 2. SEM micrographs of pure TMOS/SiO_2 (**a**) and sample with 20PVP (**b**).

The morphology of the hybrids was also characterized by TEM. Figure 3a,b shows the TEM micrographs of the investigated samples. The images exhibit the presence of agglomeration in the material, but only in some sections, not the entire volume. As is seen from the figures, all samples—pure TMOS along with that containing 20% PVP—showed spherical particles. The particle size distribution histogram determined from TEM micrographs is shown in Figure 3c,d. It was found that the average particle size for pure TMOS was 60–65 nm while the SiO_2/20PVP sample exhibited large amount of nanoparticles with a size of 115–125 nm. It is obvious that the increase in the PVP amount leads to an increase in the agglomeration of the samples. The obtained data through electron microscopy studies are in accordance with those obtained by other authors [45–49].

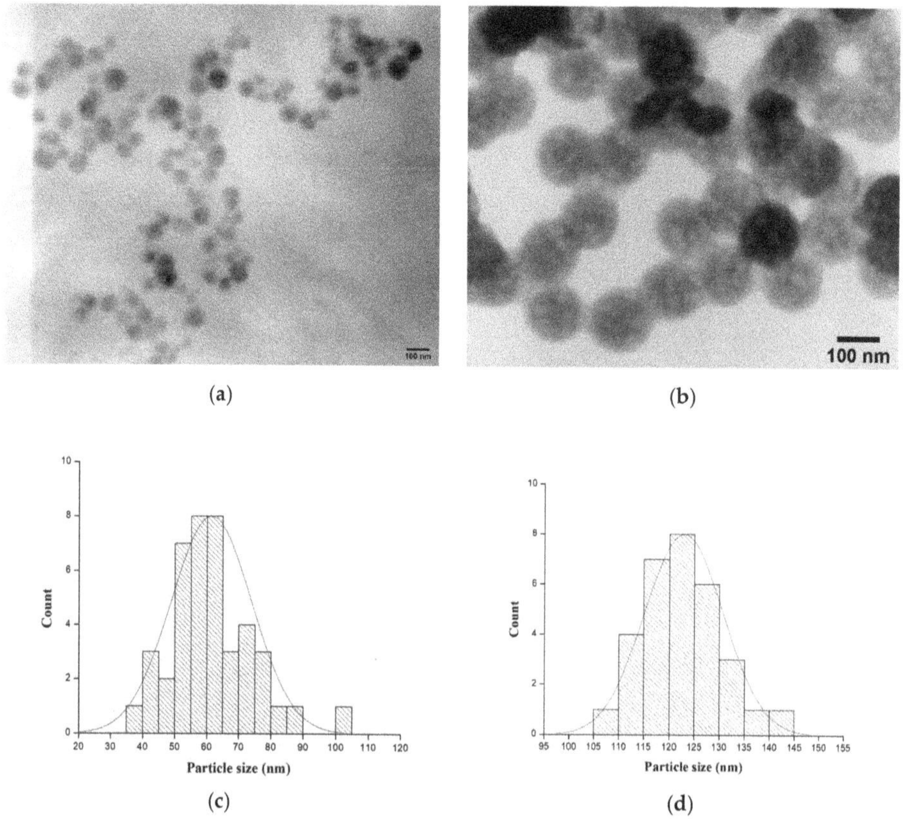

Figure 3. TEM images with corresponding histograms of TMOS (**a**,**c**) and SiO_2/20PVP (**b**,**d**).

2.2. IR Structural Investigations

The IR spectroscopy is commonly used in the analysis of hybrids of organic and inorganic materials [2]. By this approach, the existence of a novel organic–inorganic network could be verified. The analysis of the absorption bands provided useful information for the molecular structure of the as-prepared materials.

The IR spectra of pure PVP and the sample containing 20% PVP are shown in Figure 4. In these spectra, there are several main absorption regions: 3460–2150 cm^{-1}, 1700–960 cm^{-1}, and 800–440 cm^{-1}. It is obvious that the structures of pure TMOS, PVP, and the hybrid material are different. Typical silica bands are present in the spectra of SiO_2/20PVP. Generally, the bands at 430, 1075, and 1180 cm^{-1} could be assigned to the bending vibrations of siloxane (Si-O-Si) bonds [50]. The characteristic band of the Si-OH is seen at about 960 cm^{-1}. The absorption band at 650–640 cm^{-1} can be assigned to the Si-CH_2 stretching [51]. Generally, the band about 1080 cm^{-1} is typical of the polymerized silica network. As is seen from the figure, this band is present and well defined in the IR spectra of the hybrid, which is an indication that the polymerized silica network was formed in the amorphous state.

In the spectra of pure PVP, a band at 1440 cm^{-1}, associated with the deformations of CH_2 groups, could be noticed. This band is shifted and transformed into a broad one centered at about 1470 cm^{-1} in the IR spectrum of the SiO_2/20PVP hybrid. That shifting indicates a change in interchain forces in the PVP molecule. The band at 1660 cm^{-1} is present in all IR spectra, but its strongest absorption is observed in the pure PVP spectrum. This could be related to the vibrations of the C=O group which was also observed and reported by other authors [52,53]. The strong decrease in the band at 1660 cm^{-1} in the

IR spectrum of the SiO_2/20PVP sample is a proof for the presence of hydrogen bonding between PVP and SiO_2 [54]. On the other hand, the band around 1660–1650 cm^{-1} could be also associated with the angular vibration of water molecules bonded to the inorganic framework. The wide band centered at 3500 cm^{-1} is attributed to the OH stretching frequency of the silanol groups in the inorganic framework. These findings are in good correlation with those obtained by other authors [55,56]. Overall, the spectral features show strong interactions between PVP and TMOS provoked by the contact during the sol–gel reaction.

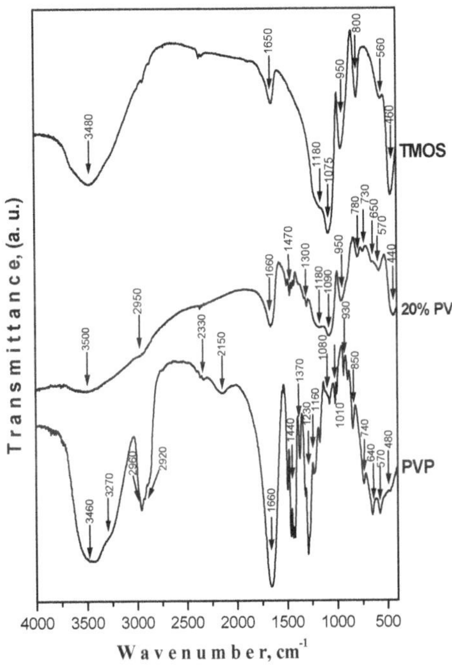

Figure 4. IR spectra of SiO_2/20PVP, TMOS, and PVP.

2.3. ^{29}*Si MAS NMR Spectra*

In the present study, solid-state ^{29}Si NMR spectroscopy was used to investigate the structural characteristics of the silica matrix in the parent silicate and in the hybrid SiO_2/20PVP material, while ^{1}H→^{13}C cross-polarization magic-angle-spinning NMR spectroscopy (^{1}H→^{13}C CP-MAS) was applied to get an insight into possible interactions between the PVP and the silicate framework in the hybrid SiO_2/20PVP material [57–60].

Chemical shifts and relative intensities of the signals in the direct-excitation (single-pulse) ^{29}Si NMR spectra provide qualitative and quantitative information about the type and the distribution of the different $(SiO)_n$ $Si(OH)_{4-n}$ species (n = 1, 2, 3; e.g Q^n species) of the silica matrix. The single-pulse ^{29}Si NMR spectrum of the parent silicate (Figure 5a) displays three partially overlapping resonances. The signal at −110.6 ppm is characteristic of the Q^4 species [Si(0OH) structural units] that represent the main building blocks of the bulk silicate framework. The resonance at around—101 ppm is assigned to Q^3 centers [Si(1OH) units], while the third lower intensity signal at around—91.7 ppm indicates the presence of a small amount of Q^2 structures [Si(2OH) units]. The Q^3 and Q^2 units represent defect sites located on the silica surface and/or at pore edges. The relative fractions of the three types of structures were calculated by means of the deconvolution of the spectral pattern and are as follows: Q^4:Q^3:Q^2 = 65:32:3. The single-pulse ^{29}Si spectrum of the hybrid SiO_2/20PVP material demonstrates a similar spectral pattern (Figure 5b); however, higher structural heterogeneity was registered in this case. The enhanced structural diversity of the hybrid material is reflected by (i) a redistribution of the intensities of the resonances for the different Si structural units, and (ii) the appearance of additional low-intensity resonances, denoted as Q^{4b} (−116 ppm) and Q^{2b} (−88 ppm), with different chemical shifts as compared to the main resonances for these type of species, denoted as Q^{4a} (−110.4 ppm) and Q^{2a} (−101 ppm). These additional resonances could be assigned to Q^4 and Q^2 species with distorted bond lengths and valence angles due to the incorporation of the polymer in the silica matrix. The relative fractions of the different types of Si structures in the hybrid SiO_2/PVP material calculated by means of the deconvolution of the spectral pattern are as follows: Q^{4b}:Q^{4a}:Q^3:Q^{2a}:Q^{2b} = 10:40:45:4:1.

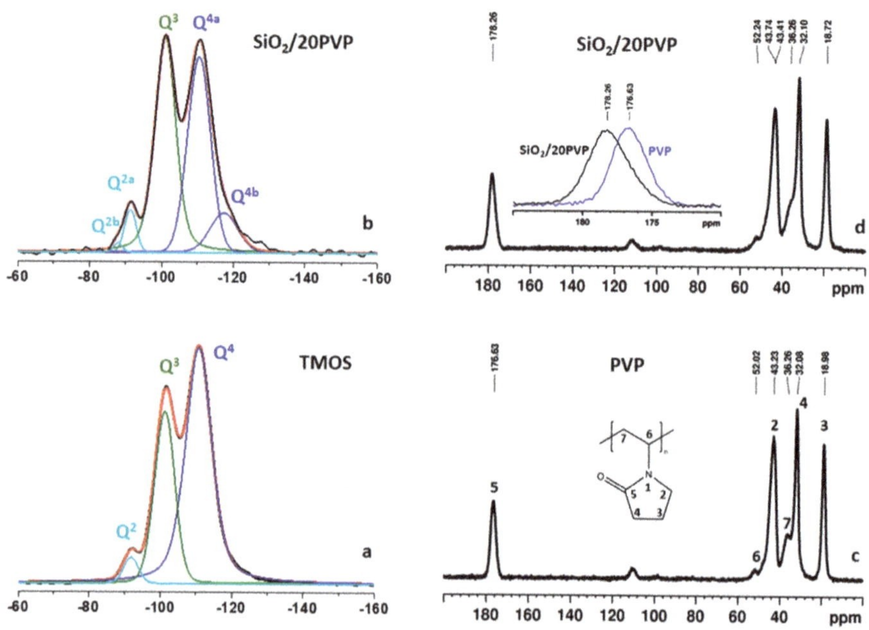

Figure 5. Experimental (black) and simulated (red) direct-excitation ^{29}Si NMR spectra of (**a**) TMOS and (**b**) SiO_2/20PVP. The individual contributions of the different Si environments obtained after the deconvolution are given with colored lines (Q^4 blue, Q^3 green, and Q^2 light blue). (**c**) $^1H{\rightarrow}^{13}C$ CP MAS spectrum of PVP. (**d**) $^1H{\rightarrow}^{13}C$ CP MAS spectrum of SiO_2/20PVP. The insert in (**d**) shows an overlay of the expanded regions of the C=O signal in the pure (blue) and hybrid (black) materials for comparison.

In a next step, we applied $^1H{\rightarrow}^{13}C$ cross-polarization magic-angle-spinning NMR spectroscopy ($^1H{\rightarrow}^{13}C$ CP-MAS) to investigate the nature of the possible interactions between the PVP and the silicate in the hybrid SiO_2/20PVP material. Figure 5c shows the $^1H{\rightarrow}^{13}C$ CP-MAS spectrum of the pure PVP along with the PVP structure and the chemical shift assignment of the characteristic resonances of the respective PVP structural fragments. The spectrum of the PVP in the hybrid SiO_2/20PVP material is given in Figure 5d. The comparison of the ^{13}C chemical shifts of the two samples shows that in the spectrum of the hybrid material, the resonance of the C=O groups is shifted by 1.63 ppm toward a lower field (see the insert in Figure 5d). The signals of the other structural fragments are also shifted to a lower field; however, the chemical shift changes are either minor (up to 0.22 ppm) or remain unchanged. These observations imply that the C=O groups of the pyrrolidone polymer fragment are localized in the vicinity of the Q^3 and Q^2 Si centers of the silica matrix via hydrogen bonding interactions with the OH hydrogens of the silanol groups.

2.4. Antibacterial Properties

As shown in Figure 6, the testing of the silica–poly (vinylpyrrolidone) hybrid material started at concentrations of 15 mg/mL, 20 mg/mL, and 50 mg/mL. No obvious bactericidal effect was found at these concentrations. A slight bacteriostatic effect is observed in the highest concentration (50 mg/mL) of the SiO_2/20PVP sample. This suggested the consecutive testing of SiO_2/20PVP in a synergistic effect with an antibiotic acting specific to Gram-negative bacteria (Ciprofloxacin) and Gram-positive bacteria (Vancomycin).

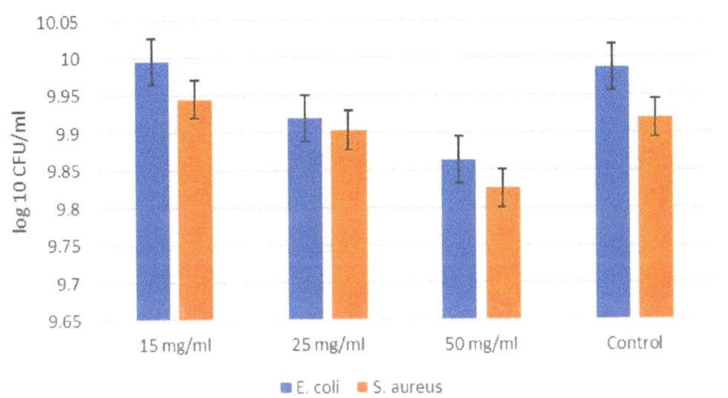

Figure 6. Concentration-dependent antibacterial effect of SiO_2/20PVP on Gram-positive bacterium *Staphylococcus aureus* and Gram-negative bacterium *Escherichia coli* at 24 h.

A spot-test scheme was utilized to assess the antibacterial potential of the antibiotics, the newly synthesized SiO_2/20PVP hybrid, and their combined inhibition. The minimum bactericidal concentration (MBC) of the sample alone and in combination with antibiotics against pathogenic bacteria was examined using the broth microdilution method as described above.

The MBC of the single action of the antibiotic against *S. aureus* was clearly determined—50 μg/mL, while in the combination of Vancomycin with the highest concentration of SiO_2/20PVP, the MBC already decreased to only 12.5 μg/mL for the antibiotic concentration. The results in Figure 7 show that the minimum bactericidal concentration (MBC) in combination with Vancomycin (12.5 μg/mL) of the SiO_2/20 PVP was at a concentration of 100 mg/mL.

The results for the Bacillus cereus are similarly presented in Figure 8. As is well known, spores of bacilli are extremely resistant to all physical and chemical agents. However, when combining 100 mg/mL of the hybrid material with the antibiotic Vancomycin at a concentration of 125 μg/mL, a bactericidal effect of two orders of magnitude was observed. It is interesting to mention that the single action of SiO_2/20PVP at a concentration of 25 mg/mL and an antibiotic at a concentration between 30 and 60 μg/mL has a stimulating effect on this bacterium known as hormesis.

The experiments with the Gram-negative bacteria *Escherichia coli* and *Pseudomonas aeruginosa* and the antibiotic Ciprofloxacin showed similar results in the resistance of the bacteria against the antibiotic alone, and in the combination of Ciprofloxacin with the highest concentration of the hybrid. But these microorganisms are significantly more sensitive to the combination of both the antibiotic and the SiO_2/20PVP sample. This can be explained by the difference in cell walls between Gram-positive and Gram-negative bacteria.

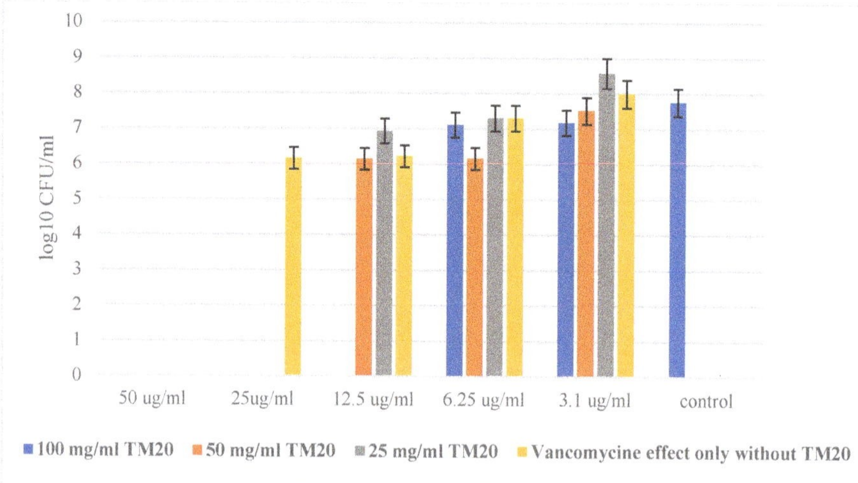

Figure 7. SiO_2/20PVP in combination with Vancomycin against *Staphylococcus aureus* at 24 h.

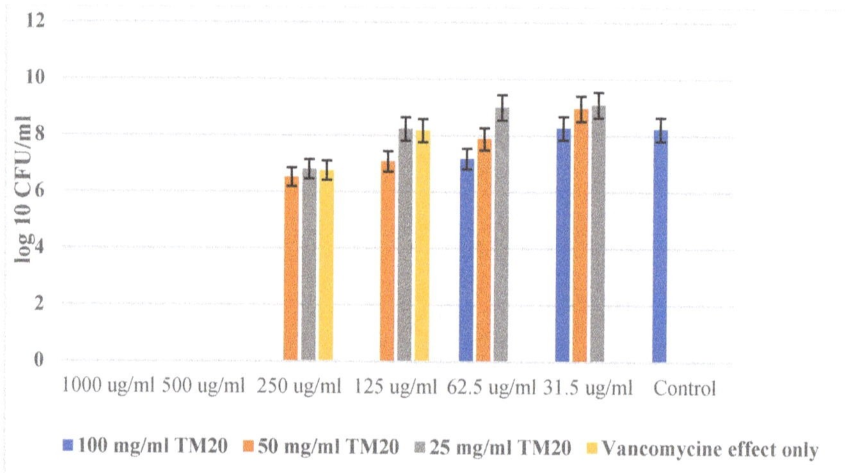

Figure 8. New SiO_2/20PVP in combination with Vancomycin against *Bacillus cereus*.

Figure 9 shows a significantly higher MBC of Ciprofloxacin alone than in combination with 100 mg/mL of the hybrid material. The MBC of the antibiotic against *Escherichia coli* was found to be 3.5 μg/mL, while that for the combination of Ciprofloxacin and the highest concentration (100 mg/mL) of SiO_2/20PVP was 0.7 μg/mL.

Pseudomonas aeruginosa showed higher resistance to the concentration of antibiotics. Here, the MBC of Ciprofloxacin alone was 6.25 μg/mL, while in a synergistic effect with the new hybrid material at a concentration of 100 mg/mL, the MBC decreased to 1.5 μg/mL, as is shown in Figure 10.

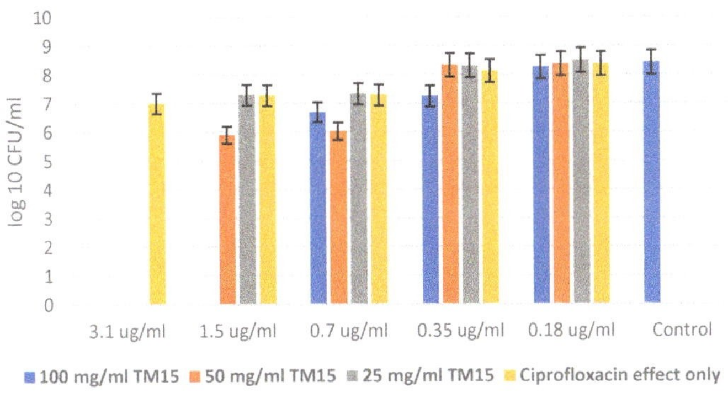

Figure 9. SiO_2/20PVP in combination with Ciprofloxacin against *E. coli*.

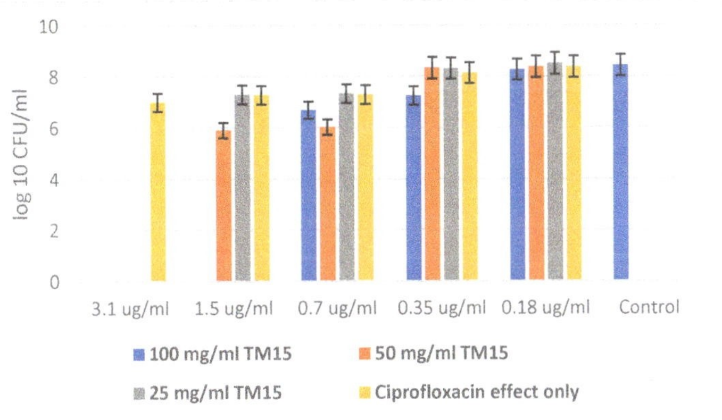

Figure 10. SiO_2/20PVP in combination with Ciprofloxacin against *Pseudomonas aeruginosa*.

2.5. Chemiluminescence Assay

Figure 11 presents the results about the chemiluminescence assay and the capability of the tested hybrid to generate ROS and present antibacterial properties. As a suitable, highly sensitive, and relatively inexpensive method, it allows to monitor the dynamics of free radical reactions. Thus, the prooxidant/antioxidant activity of the investigated material can be estimated [36,37].

As is seen at pH 7.4 (physiological), the kinetic curves keep a plateau shape. The Ciprofloxacin antibiotic does not affect the generation or neutralization of ROS in this model reaction. This result confirms the safe administration of the tested antibiotic in vivo and other than a free-radical generation activity mechanism. In all other cases, the recorded signal is higher than the control (more than 32,000 RLU), which is indicative of the stimulation of the generation of ·OH and ·OOH radicals. The registered effects are as follows: TMOS—340%; PVP—more than 220%; SiO_2/20PVP—almost 33%; and SiO_2/20PVP+ciprofloxacin—almost 78%. The as-prepared hybrid SiO_2/20PVP shows a significant prooxidant effect, which is preserved with time, and an almost twice higher chemiluminescent signal than the control reaction. This is indicative of definite antibacterial activity. The obtained results are in agreement with the antibacterial tests conducted with all Gram-positive and Gram-negative bacteria. On the other hand, it is necessary to confirm the observed effects in additional redox model systems using the method of activated luminescence (ex vivo), at physiological pH and pH 8.5, in order to completely define the action mechanism of the tested hybrid. This will be performed in our future investigations as the obtained information will predict its effect in vivo.

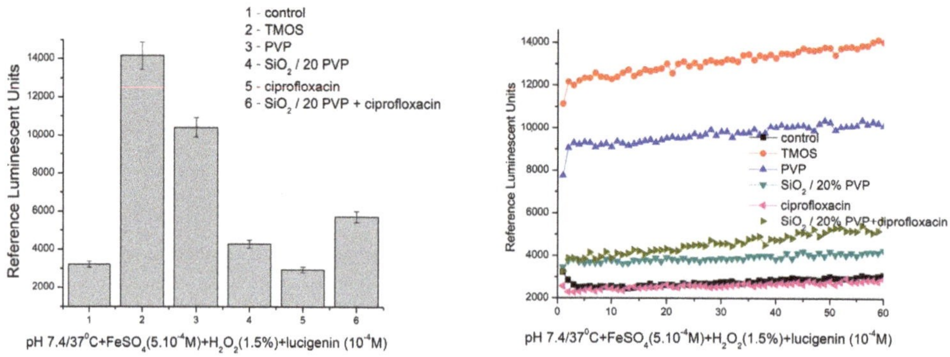

(a) (b)

Figure 11. Chemiluminescence induced by ·OH and ·OOH radicals at pH 7.4 and the effect of materials: (**a**) maximum effects and (**b**) Fenton's reaction in time ($p \leq 0.05$).

2.6. Daphnia Magna Toxicity

Aiming to estimate the toxicity of the as-prepared SiO_2/PVP hybrid, an acute toxicity test with *Daphnia magna* was performed that allows predicting the possible maximum permissible concentration in the environment without harm for water inhabitants. The experiments were performed using four concentrations of the substance—0.1 mg/mL; 0.05 mg/mL; 0.01 mg/mL and 0.001 mg/mL with three replicates of each concentration and two controls as shown in Figure 12. Generally, *D. magna* are extremely sensitive organisms in the aquatic environment, which also allows conclusions to be drawn from the obtained results about the influence of the as-prepared hybrid on other aquatic organisms. The results of the survival of *Daphnia* were 97% at a concentration of 0.01 and 0.001 mg/mL and 93% at a concentration of 0.1 and 0.05 mg/mL of the substance. Since 95% *D. magna* survival was observed in the controls, it can be speculated that low concentrations below 0.01 mg/mL have a slight stimulatory effect, while the higher concentration of 0.05 mg/mL has a weak inhibitory effect. Therefore, at these concentrations, the substance used can be discharged into surface waters without harm to organisms.

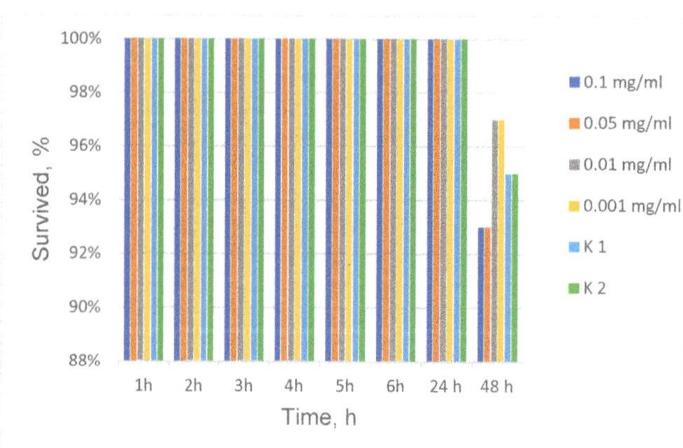

Figure 12. Survival of *Daphnia magna* treated with SiO_2/20%PVP.

2.7. Analysis of the Results

Bearing in mind the obtained results, it has to be noted that one experimental fact still provokes scientific interest. Irrespective of the absence of antibacterial activity of the sol–gel-prepared pure SiO_2/20PVP hybrid, in a synergistic effect with antibiotics, it acts specific to both Gram-negative and Gram-positive bacteria. It is evident that the functionalization of the silica hybrid with small molecules such as vancomycin and ciprofloxacin provokes the antibacterial activity of the hybrid. Despite the differences in the cell wall of the tested Gram-positive (*Staphylococcus aureus* and *Bacillus cereus*) and Gram-negative (*Escherichia coli* and *Pseudomonas aeruginosa*) bacteria, it was established that the combination of both the antibiotic and the SiO_2/20PVP sample led to a significant increase in the antibacterial properties. According to Bernardos et al. [61], this experimental result could be ascribed to the fact that the antibiotic reacts with the outer surface of the hybrid, forming a hydrogen bonding interaction with the terminal functional groups on the cell membrane. Supporting this suggestion are the performed IR and NMR analyses which prove the presence of hydrogen bonding interactions between the silica matrix and the OH hydrogens of the silanol groups (Figures 4 and 5). Moreover, the registered prooxidant activity coincides well with the suggested antibacterial properties of the tested substance and its combination with antibiotics. On the other hand, it has already been stated that the size, shape, pore diameter, surface properties, composition, and concentration features can all contribute to these properties of the synthesized material [62–64]. For example, some authors established that sol–gel-derived PVP powders composed of spherical particles exhibited higher antibacterial properties as compared to ellipsoid ones [65]. This experimental fact corresponds well to the results obtained by us. Moreover, the investigated hybrid exhibited good killing efficiency at the 24th hour.

One complementary investigation concerning the *D. magna* toxicity test highlights this paper's originality. It was observed that the effect of the hybrid material on Crustacea *D. magna* is estimated to be harmless at a concentration of 0.1 mg/mL. This could be related with the fact that the silica-based compounds are hydrolytically unstable and they progressively transform into harmless silicic acid or polysilicic acid that the body can safely absorb or excrete [61]. It is evident that, at these concentrations, the sol–gel-derived substance can be discharged into surface waters without harm to aquatic organisms.

Thus, it could be generalized that the present study, which is devoted to obtaining a SiO_2-containing hybrid material and evaluating its antibacterial properties, represents an attempt to elucidate the composition–structure–property relationship. Based on the above discussed results, it could be suggested that the as-prepared material can be used in further research related to other possible applications of SiO_2/20PVP for environmental protection.

3. Experimental Procedure

3.1. Materials

The gels were prepared using a combination of the alkoxid—tetramethyl orthosilane (TMOS)—Sigma Aldrich Chemical (Burlington, MA, USA) and poly(vynyl pyrrolidon) K25-(PVP), Fluka Chemie AG (Buchs, Switzerland). The preparation procedure is described in details below.

3.2. Preparation of Silica–Polyvinylpyrrolidone (SiO_2-PVP) Hybrids

The precursor tetramethyl orthosilicate {TMOS, $Si(OCH_3)_4$}, distilled H_2O, and 0.1 M HCl in the molar ratio 4:1:1 were mixed and stirred together. Aiming to obtain a hybrid material with improved properties, the added amount of PVP was 20wt %. It was dissolved in ethanol and added dropwise to the stirred solution. Stirring continued until the mixture became clear. The gelation occurred at room temperature and it took about 20 h. All steps of the hybrid preparation are shown in Figure 13. The investigated samples were denoted as TMOS, PVP, and SiO_2/20PVP.

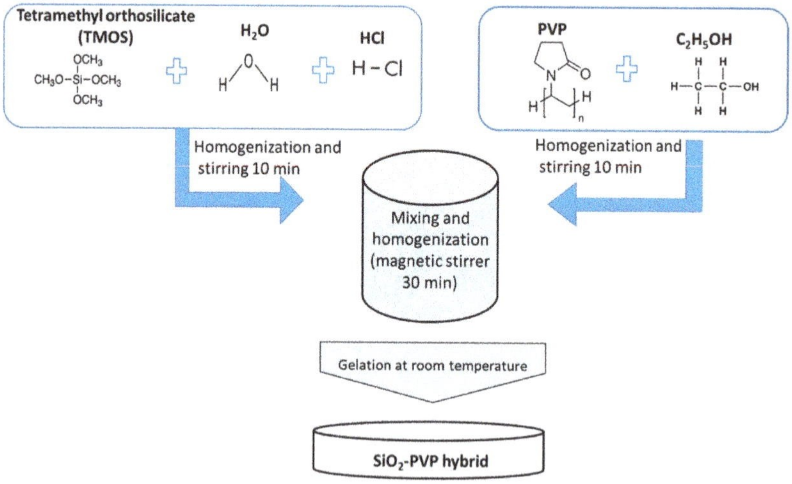

Figure 13. Scheme for the synthesis of SiO_2/PVP hybrids.

3.3. Methods of Characterization

Powder X-ray diffraction data were obtained on a Philips PW1730/10 diffractometer using Ni-filtered CuKα radiation (Philips Corporation, Almelo, the Netherlands). The scanning rate for crystallinity was 1.2° 2θ/min. SEM images were obtained on a Hitachi S-4100 (Hitachi Ltd., Tokyo, Japan) microscope at an accelerating voltage of 25.0 kV. TEM images were taken on a Hitachi H-600A (Tokyo, Japan). A powdered hybrid sample was suspended in a mixture of ethanol and polysorbate 80 (1:1 *v/v*) using an ultrasonic generator (with an intensity of 250 W) for 3 min. One or two drops of the resulting dispersion were dropped on a 300-mesh copper grid (Tedpella, Inc., Redding, CA, USA) coated with carbon film and left to evaporate. FTIR spectra were registered using the KBr pellet technique on an FTIR spectrophotometer—Nicolet 6700 FT (Matson, UK). ^{29}Si MAS NMR spectra were recorded on a Bruker Avance HD III 600 NMR spectrometer (Billerica, MA, USA) operating at 599.98 MHz proton frequency (150.84 MHz for ^{13}C, 119.18 MHz for ^{29}Si), using 4 mm solid state i-CP/MAS dual ^{1}H/^{31}P-^{15}N probehead (Billerica, MA, USA). The samples were loaded in 4 mm zirconia rotors and spun at a magic-angle-spinning (MAS) rate of 10 kHz for both the ^{13}C and ^{29}Si measurements. ^{1}H$\rightarrow$^{13}C cross-polarization MAS (CP MAS) spectra were acquired with the following experimental parameters: 8 K time domain data points, a spectrum width of 50 kHz, an ^{1}H excitation pulse of 3.6 μs, a contact time of 2 ms, 2048 scans, and a recycle delay of 5 s. The ^{1}H SPINAL-64 decoupling scheme was used during the acquisition of the CP experiments. The spectra were processed with an exponential window function (line broadening factor 10) and zero-filled to 32 K data points. The quantitative direct-excitation ^{29}Si NMR spectra were recorded with one-pulse sequence, a 90° pulse length of 4.5 μs, 3 K time domain data points, a spectrum width of 70 kHz, 1024 scans, and a relaxation delay of 60 s. Exponential window function was applied (line broadening factor 10) prior to Fourier transformation.

3.4. Antimicrobial Activity Testing

The tested microbial strains, Gram-negative bacteria *Escherichia coli* ATCC 25922 and *Pseudomonas aeruginosa* ATCC 27853, and Gram-positive bacteria *Staphylococcus aureus* ATCC 25923 and *Bacillus cereus* NBIMCC 1090, were provided by the National Bank of Microorganisms and Cell Cultures (NBIMCC), Bulgaria, and cultured in the nutrient medium (Conda, Spain). The pure culture of every strain was prepared as a bacterial suspension in exponential phase with OD 0.5 McFarland.

The $SiO_2/20PVP$ sample was tested for antibacterial efficacy alone and in combination with conventional antibiotics in liquid medium too. Antibiotics were selected from five groups with a different mode of action, including vancomycin (Glycopeptide) and ciprofloxacin (Quinolone). Vancomycin is a tricyclic glycopeptide antibiotic used for the treatment of Gram-positive bacterial infections. It belongs to the cell-wall-synthesis inhibitor class of antimicrobial drugs. Almost all quinolone antibiotics used are fluoroquinolones, which contain a fluorine atom in their chemical structure and are effective against both Gram-negative and Gram-positive bacteria [66].

3.5. Methodology for the Evaluation of the Minimum Inhibitory and Minimum Bactericidal Concentration (MBC) and Antibacterial Mode of Inhibition of SiO_2/20PVP

The MBC of the $SiO_2/20PVP$ hybrid combined with antibiotics was determined using the broth microdilution method and spot-test on agar. A standard suspension of bacterial pathogens (100 µL/0.5 MFU) was added to micro dilution wells containing 50 µL of the corresponding concentration of the investigated sample (25 mg/mL, 50 mg/mL, and 100 mg/mL) and 50 µL of different concentrations of the antibiotic for each well to obtain a final volume of 200 µL in 11 variants. The final (12th) column was left for control (100 µL bacterial suspension and 100 µL autoclaved physiological saline solutions). After 24 h incubation at 36 ± 1 °C, the wells were examined for growth. The lowest concentration that showed no growth was assessed as a minimum bactericidal concentration (MBC). It can be determined from broth tests by sub-culturing to agar plates that do not contain the tested agent [30]. Experiments were performed with three independent runs of three replicates per run.

3.6. Chemiluminescence Assay

3.6.1. Materials

Purchased with high purity: iron sulphate (p. a.) (Merck, Darmstadt, Germany), hydrogen peroxide (30%) (Merck, Darmstadt, Germany), lucigenin (bis-N-methylacridinium nitrate) (p. a.) (Sigma-Aldrich, St. Louis, MI, USA and Burlington, MA, USA), dimethyl sulfoxide (p. a.) (DMSO, Sigma-Aldrich, St. Louis, MI, USA), and buffer pH 7.4 (Sigma-Aldrich, St. Louis, MI, USA and Burlington, MA, USA). All chemicals were used as purchased.

3.6.2. Method

The redox activity of the newly synthesized material was tested in Fenton's model chemical reaction system, generating free radicals and ROS, at pH 7.4 (physiological), by means of the activated chemiluminescence method [67]. The chemical probe that we applied for signal amplification was lucigenin. Thus, reliable, comparable differences were achieved.

Fenton's system generates $^{\cdot}OOH$ and $^{\cdot}OH$ radicals. The control samples do not contain the tested material (active concentration 100 mg/mL). The reactions are monitored for 3 min, every 3 s, at 37 °C, and measured in triplicate. All materials are sonicated for 20 min prior to testing to ensure good dispersion.

Fenton's system:

$$Fe^{2+} + H_2O_2 \rightarrow Fe^{3+} + {}^{\cdot}OH + {}^{-}OH \quad (1)$$

$$Fe^{3+} + H_2O_2 \rightarrow Fe^{2+} + {}^{\cdot}OOH + H^+ \quad (2)$$

In general, the higher the signal, the more ROS are formed and a prooxidant effect is described. On the contrary, if the signal is below the control level, antioxidant activity can be described.

3.6.3. Statistics

All experiments were performed using LUMIstar Omega (BMG Labtech GmbH, Ortenberg, Germany, 2020) in triple reproducible measurements; statistical analysis was performed using OriginPro 8 and Microsoft Office Excel 2010.

3.7. *Daphnia Magna*

A toxicity test was conducted according to the acute lethality toxicity protocol OECD (2004) and the guidelines for the testing of chemicals' acute immobilization test (2012), Test No: 211 [68]. The experiments used 4 concentrations of the hybrid SiO_2/20PVP nanoparticles (0.1 mg/mL; 0.05 mg/mL; 0.01 mg/mL; and 0.001 mg/mL) with 3 replicates of each concentration and 2 controls.

4. Conclusions

Hybrid nanocomposites containing TMOS and PVP were synthesized via the sol–gel method at room temperature. The obtained products were characterized using several methods. They established homogeneous and amorphous samples which showed useful structural properties. The IR and ^{29}Si MAS NMR spectra proved the formation of a polymerized silica network as well as the hydrogen bonding interactions between the silica matrix and the OH hydrogens of the silanol groups. The TEM showed spherical particle formation along with increased agglomeration tendency.

The minimum bactericidal concentration (MBC) in the synergistic effect of the hybrid material (SiO_2/20PVP) with the corresponding antibiotic was three to five times lower than in the case of the antibiotic action alone. These findings suggest that the synthesized SiO_2/20PVP hybrid may be a new, effective, and broad-spectrum antibacterial agent, even at lower doses than those currently used in clinical trials to treat bacterial infections. The observed prooxidant activity confirmed and explained the registered antibacterial properties of the tested substance and its combination with antibiotics, especially ciprofloxacin. The low concentrations below 0.01 mg/mL had a slight stimulatory effect on *Daphnia magna*, while the higher concentration of 0.05 mg/mL had a weak inhibitory effect. Therefore, at these concentrations, the substance can be discharged into surface waters without harm to water organisms.

Author Contributions: Conceptualization, Y.K. and A.B.-N.; methodology, Y.K. and A.B.-N.; sample characterization, Y.K. and A.B.-N.; antibacterial properties, I.I. and L.Y.; NMR investigation, P.S.; chemiluminescence assay, E.P.; toxicity test with Daphnia magna, E.N.; writing, Y.K., A.B.-N., P.S., I.I. and E.P. All authors have read and agreed to the published version of the manuscript.

Funding: The team from the Faculty of Biology, Sofia University, is grateful for the financial support of project 80-10-176/18.4.2024. The author E.P. is thankful for the financial support to the project "Clean technologies for sustainable environment—waters, waste, energy for circular economy", Ministry of Education and Science, Bulgaria, Contract Number: BG05M2OP001-1.002-0019.

Institutional Review Board Statement: Not applicable.

Informed Consent Statement: Not applicable.

Data Availability Statement: Data are contained within the article.

Acknowledgments: The author A.B.-N. is thankful to the Project CoE "National Center of Mechatronics and Clean Technologies" (BG05M2OP001-1.001-0008). Research equipment of distributed research infrastructure INFRAMAT, supported by the Bulgarian Ministry of Education and Science, was used. The team from the Faculty of Biology, Sofia University, is grateful to the funds allocated specifically from the state budget of SU "Kliment Ohridski" for scientific research on a project 80-10-176/18.4.2024. The author E.P. is thankful to the project "Clean technologies for sustainable environment—waters, waste, energy for circular economy", Ministry of Education and Science, Bulgaria, Contract Number: BG05M2OP001-1.002-0019.

Conflicts of Interest: The authors declare no conflicts of interest.

References

1. Babiarczuk, B.; Lewandowski, D.; Szczurek, A.; Kierzek, K.; Meffert, M.; Gerthsen, D.; Jerzy, K.; Krzak, J. Novel approach of silica-PVA hybrid aerogel synthesis by simultaneous sol-gel process and phase separation. *J. Supercrit. Fluids* **2020**, *166*, 104997. [CrossRef]
2. Barrino, F. Hybrid Organic–Inorganic Materials Prepared by Sol–Gel and Sol–Gel-Coating Method for Biomedical Use: Study and Synthetic Review of Synthesis and Properties. *Coatings* **2024**, *14*, 425. [CrossRef]
3. Catauro, M.; Ciprioti, S.V. Characterization of Hybrid Materials Prepared by Sol-Gel Method for Biomedical Implementations. A Critical Review. *Materials* **2021**, *14*, 1788. [CrossRef]
4. Castrillo, P.; Olmos, D.; Amador, D.; González-Benito, J. Real dispersion of isolated fumed silica nanoparticles in highly filled PMMA prepared by high energy ball milling. *J. Colloid Interface Sci.* **2007**, *308*, 318–324. [CrossRef] [PubMed]
5. Ogoshi, T.; Chujo, Y. Organic–inorganic polymer hybrids prepared by the sol-gel method. *Compos. Interfaces* **2005**, *11*, 539–566. [CrossRef]
6. Sanchez, C.; Julián, B.; Belleville, P.; Popall, M. Applications of hybrid organic–inorganic nanocomposites. *J. Mater. Chem.* **2005**, *15*, 3559–3592. [CrossRef]
7. Rejab, M.R.; Hamdan, M.H.; Quanjin, M.; Siregar, J.P.; Bachtiar, D.; Muchlis, Y. Historical Development of Hybrid Materials. *Mat. Sci. Mat. Eng.* **2020**, *4*, 445–455.
8. Vichery, C.; Nedelec, J.-M. Bioactive glass nanoparticles: From synthesis to materials design for biomedical applications. *Materials* **2016**, *9*, 288. [CrossRef]
9. Brinker, C.J. Hydrolysis and condensation of silicates: Effects on structure. *J. Non Cryst. Solids* **1988**, *100*, 31–50. [CrossRef]
10. Innocenzi, P. *The Sol to Gel Transition*; Springer International Publishing: Cham, Switzerland, 2016.
11. Schmidt, M.; Schwertfeger, F. Applications for silica aerogel products. *J. Non Cryst. Solids* **1998**, *225*, 364–368. [CrossRef]
12. Kuttor, A.; Szalóki, M.; Rente, T.; Kerényi, F.; Bakó, J.; Fábián, I.; Lázár, I.; Jenei, A.; Hegedü, C. Preparation and Application of Highly Porous Aerogel-based Bioactive Materials in Dentistry. *Front. Mater. Sci.* **2014**, *8*, 46–52. [CrossRef]
13. Pajonk, G.M. Some applications of silica aerogels. *Colloid Polym. Sci.* **2003**, *281*, 637–651. [CrossRef]
14. Maleki, H.; Durães, L.; Portugal, A. An overview on silica aerogels synthesis and different mechanical reinforcing strategies. *J. Non Cryst. Solids* **2014**, *385*, 55–74. [CrossRef]
15. Babooram, K.; Francis, B.; Bissessur, R.; Narain, R. Synthesis and characterization of novel (amide–imide)-silica composites by the sol–gel process. *Compos. Sci. Technol.* **2008**, *68*, 617–624. [CrossRef]
16. Seo, S.-J.; Kim, J.-J.; Kim, J.-H.; Lee, J.-Y.; Shin, U.S.; Lee, E.-J.; Kim, H.-W. Enhanced mechanical properties and bone bioactivity of chitosan/silica membrane by functionalized-carbon nanotube incorporation. *Compos. Sci. Technol.* **2014**, *96*, 31–37. [CrossRef]
17. Gadalla, A.M.; Yun, S.J. Characterization of gels prepared from silicon ethoxide in presence of HCl and HF. *J. Non-Cryst. Solids* **1992**, *143*, 121–132. [CrossRef]
18. Haraguchi, K.; Usami, Y.; Ono, Y. The preparation and characterization of hybrid materials composed of phenolic resin and silica. *J. Mater. Sci.* **1998**, *33*, 3337–3344. [CrossRef]
19. Morikawa, A.; Lyoku, Y.; Kakimoto, M.; Mai, Y. Preparation of Silica-Containing Polyvinylpyrrolidone Films by Sol-Gel Process Polymer. *J. Mater. Sci.* **1992**, *24*, 689–692.
20. Hsiao, C.N.; Huang, K.S. Synthesis, Characterization, and Applications of Polyvinylpyrrolidone/SiO_2. Hybrid Materials. *J. Appl. Polym. Sci.* **2005**, *96*, 1936–1942. [CrossRef]
21. Bhattacharyya, D.; Singh, S.; Satnalika, N.; Khandelwal, A.; Jeon, S.H. Nanotechnology, big things from a tiny world: A review. *Int. J. U E Serv. Sci. Technol.* **2009**, *2*, 29–38.
22. Gupta, A.; Mumtaz, S.; Li, C.H.; Hussain, I.; Rotello, V.M. Combatting antibiotic-resistant bacteria using nanomaterials. *Chem. Soc. Rev.* **2019**, *48*, 415–427. [CrossRef]
23. Makabenta, J.M.V.; Nabawy, A.; Li, C.H.; Schmidt-Malan, S.; Patel, R.; Rotello, V.M. Nanomaterial-based therapeutics for antibiotic-resistant bacterial infections. *Nat. Rev. Microbiol.* **2021**, *19*, 23–36. [CrossRef]
24. Chakraborty, N.; Jha, D.; Roy, I.; Kumar, P.; Gaurav, S.S.; Marimuthu, K.; Ng, O.-T.; Lakshminarayanan, R.; Verma, N.K.; Gautam, H.K. Nanobiotics against antimicrobial resistance: Harnessing the power of nanoscale materials and technologies. *J. Nanobiotechnology* **2022**, *375*, 1477–3155. [CrossRef]
25. Hetta, H.F.; Ramadan, Y.N.; Al-Harbi, A.I.; Ahmed, E.; Battah, B.; Abd Ellah, N.H.; Zanetti, S.; Donadu, M.G. Nanotechnology as a Promising Approach to Combat Multidrug Resistant Bacteria: A Comprehensive Review and Future Perspectives. *Biomedicines* **2023**, *11*, 413. [CrossRef]
26. Skłodowski, K.; Chmielewska-Deptuła, S.J.; Piktel, E.; Wolak, P.; Wollny, T.; Bucki, R. Metallic Nanosystems in the Development of Antimicrobial Strategies with High Antimicrobial Activity and High Biocompatibility. *Int. J. Mol. Sci.* **2023**, *24*, 2104. [CrossRef] [PubMed]
27. Wahab, S.; Salman, A.; Khan, Z.; Khan, S.; Krishnaraj, C.; Yun, S.-I. Metallic Nanoparticles: A Promising Arsenal against Antimicrobial Resistance-Unraveling Mechanisms and Enhancing Medication Efficacy. *Int. J. Mol. Sci.* **2023**, *24*, 14897. [CrossRef] [PubMed]
28. Bondarenko, O.M.; Sihtmäe, M.; Kuzmičiova, J.; Ragelienė, L.; Kahru, A.; Daugelavičius, R. Plasma membrane is the target of rapid antibacterial action of silver nanoparticles in Escherichia coli and Pseudomonas aeruginosa. *Int. J. Nanomed.* **2018**, *13*, 6779–6790. [CrossRef] [PubMed]

29. Kamat, S.; Kumari, M. Emergence of microbial resistance against nanoparticles: Mechanisms and strategies. *Front. Microbiol.* **2023**, *14*, 1102615. [CrossRef] [PubMed]
30. Breijyeh, Z.; Jubeh, B.; Karaman, R. Resistance of gram-negative bacteria to current antibacterial agents and approaches to resolve it. *Molecules* **2020**, *25*, 1340. [CrossRef]
31. Moradi, F.; Ghaedi, A.; Fooladfar, Z.; Bazrgar, A. Recent advance on nanoparticles or nanomaterials with anti-multidrug resistant bacteria and anti-bacterial biofilm properties: A systematic review. *Heliyon* **2023**, *9*, e22105. [CrossRef]
32. Karnwal, A.; Kumar, G.; Pant, G.; Hossain, K.; Ahmad, A.; Alshammari, M.B. Perspectives on Usage of Functional Nanomaterials in Antimicrobial Therapy for Antibiotic-Resistant Bacterial Infections. *ACS Omega* **2023**, *8*, 13492–13508. [CrossRef] [PubMed]
33. Naqvi, S.Z.H.; Kiran, U.; Ali, M.I.; Jamal, A.; Hameed, A.; Ahmed, S.; Ali, N. Combined efficacy of biologically synthesized silver nanoparticles and different antibiotics against multidrug-resistant bacteria. *Int. J. Nanomed.* **2013**, *8*, 3187–3195. [CrossRef] [PubMed]
34. Adeniji, O.O.; Nontongana, N.; Okoh, J.C.; Okoh, A.I. The Potential of Antibiotics and Nanomaterial Combinations as Therapeutic Strategies in the Management of Multidrug-Resistant Infections: A Review. *Int. J. Mol. Sci.* **2022**, *23*, 15038. [CrossRef] [PubMed]
35. Abebe, B.; Zereffa, E.A.; Tadesse, A.; Murthy, H.C. A Review on Enhancing the Antibacterial Activity of ZnO: Mechanisms and Microscopic Investigation. *Nanoscale* **2020**, *15*, 190. [CrossRef]
36. Pavlova, E.L.; Toshkovska, R.D.; Doncheva, T.E.; Ivanova, I.A. Prooxidant and antimicrobic effects of iron and titanium oxide nanoparticles and thalicarpine. *Arch. Microbiol.* **2020**, *202*, 1873–1880. [CrossRef] [PubMed]
37. Pavlova, E.L.; Savov, V.M. Chemiluminescent in vitro estimation of the inhibitory constants of antioxidants ascorbic and uric acids in Fenton's reaction in urine. *Biochemistry* **2006**, *71*, 861–863. [CrossRef] [PubMed]
38. Faulkner, K.; Fridovich, I. Luminol and lucigenin as detectors for O2ṡ−. *Free. Radic. Biol. Med.* **1993**, *15*, 447–451. [CrossRef] [PubMed]
39. Tkaczyk, A.; Bownik, A.; Dudka, J.; Kowal, K.; Ślaska, B. Daphnia magna model in the toxicity assessment of pharmaceuticals: A review. *Sci. Total Environ.* **2021**, *763*, 143038. [CrossRef] [PubMed]
40. Hubai, K. Daphnia magna Acute Immobilization Test: An Opportunity to Test the Ecotoxicity of Alternative Fuels. *Hung. J. Ind. Chem.* **2021**, *49*, 77–82. [CrossRef]
41. Briffa, S.M.; Nasser, F.; Valsami, E.; Jones, I.L. Uptake and impacts of polyvinylpyrrolidone (PVP) capped metal oxide nanoparticles on Daphnia magna: Role of core composition and acquired corona. *Environ. Sci. Nano* **2018**, *7*, 1745–1756. [CrossRef]
42. Tarring, E.C.; Robison-Smith, C.; Cable, J.; Durance, I.; Harbottle, M.; Ward, B.D. Detection of Polyvinylpyrrolidone in Daphnia Magna: Development of a Refractive Index Quantification Method for Water-Soluble Polymers in Aquatic Organisms. *Sci. Total Environ.* **2024**, *935*, 173428. [CrossRef] [PubMed]
43. Mondellini, S.; Schott, M.; Löder, M.G.J.; Agarwal, S.; Greiner, A.; Laforsch, C. Beyond microplastics: Water soluble synthetic polymers exert sublethal adverse effects in the fresh water cladoceran Daphnia magna. *Sci. Total Environ.* **2022**, *847*, 157608. [CrossRef] [PubMed]
44. Shahmiri, M.; Bayat, S.; Kharrazi, S. Catalytic performance of PVP-coated CuO nanosheets under environmentally friendly conditions. *RSC Adv.* **2023**, *13*, 13213–13223. [CrossRef] [PubMed]
45. Wang, L.; Shen, C.; Cao, Y. PVP modified Fe_3O_4@SiO_2 nanoparticles as a new adsorbent for hydrophobic substances. *J. Phys. Chem. Solids* **2019**, *133*, 28–34. [CrossRef]
46. Ghobashy, M.M.; Elbarbary, A.M.; Hegazy, D.E. Synthesis of poly (vinylpyrrolidone)/Fe_3O_4@SiO_2 nanoporous catalyst by γ-rays and evaluation their sono-photo-Fenton degradation of toluidine blue under magnetic field. *Appl. Organomet. Chem.* **2021**, *35*, e6388. [CrossRef]
47. Ding, D.; Yu, J.; Guo, Q.; Guo, X.; Xiao, X.; Mao, D.; Lu, G. The effects of PVP-modified SiO_2 on the catalytic performance of CO hydrogenation over Rh–Mn–Li/SiO_2 catalyst. *RSC Adv.* **2017**, *7*, 48420. [CrossRef]
48. Velikova, N.; Vueva, Y.; Ivanova, Y.; Georgieva, R.; Detcheva, A. Synthesis and characterization of sol-gel mesoporous organosilicas functionalized with amine groups. *J. Non-Cryst. Solids* **2013**, *378*, 89–95. [CrossRef]
49. Aengjun, N.; Vibulyaseak, K.; Ogawa, M. Heterostructural transformation of mesoporous silica–titania hybrids. *Sci. Rep.* **2021**, *11*, 3210. [CrossRef]
50. Yang, S.M.; Coombs, N.; Ozin, G.A. Micromolding in inverted polymer opals (MIPO): Synthesis of hexagonal mesoporous silica opals. *Adv. Mater.* **2000**, *12*, 1940–1944. [CrossRef]
51. Diaz, J.F.; Balkus, J.K.; Bedioui, F.; Kurshev, V.; Kevan, L. Synthesis and Characterization of Cobalt-Complex Functionalized MCM-41. *Chem. Mater.* **1997**, *9*, 61–67. [CrossRef]
52. Linsenbuhler, M.; Werth, J.H.; Dammer, S.M.; Knudsen, H.A.; Hinrichsen, H.; Wirth, K.-E.; Wolf, D.E. Cluster size distribution of charged nanopowders in suspensions. *Powder Technol.* **2006**, *167*, 124–133. [CrossRef]
53. Al-Harbi, L.M.; Kosa, S.A.; Baloch, M.K.; Bhatti, Q.A.; El-Mossalamy, E.S. Adsorption of Polyvinylpyrrolidone over the Silica Surface: As Affected by Pretreatment of Adsorbent and Molar Mass of Polymer Adsorbate. *Int. J. Polym. Sci.* **2016**, *2016*, 2417292. [CrossRef]
54. Wahab, M.A.; Kim, I.I.; Ha, C.S. Hybrid periodic mesoporous organosilica materials prepared from 1,2-bis(triethoxysilyl)ethane and (3-cyanopropyl)triethoxysilane. *Microporous Mesoporous Mater.* **2004**, *69*, 19–27. [CrossRef]
55. Kuo, S.W.; Chang, F.C. POSS related polymer nanocomposites. *Progress. Polym. Sci.* **2011**, *36*, 1649–1696. [CrossRef]

56. Shalaby, A.; Angelova, T.; Bachvarova-Nedelcheva, A.; Georgieva, N.; Iordanova, R.; Staneva, A.; Dimitriev, Y. Sol-gel synthesis of materials in the system $SiO_2/ZnO/TiO_2/RGO$ and their antimicrobial efficiency against *E. coli* K12. *Comptes Rendus L'academie Bulg. Des. Sci.* **2016**, *69*, 25–30.
57. Marchetti, A.; Yin, J.; Su, Y.; Kong, X. Solid-state NMR in the field of drug delivery: State of the art and new perspectives. *Magn. Reson. Lett.* **2021**, *1*, 28–70. [CrossRef]
58. Popova, M.; Mihaylova, R.; Momekov, G.; Momekova, D.; Lazarova, H.; Trendafilova, I.; Mitova, V.; Koseva, N.; Mihályi, J.; Shestakova, P.; et al. Verapamil delivery systems on the basis of mesoporous ZSM-5/KIT-6 and ZSM-5/SBA-15 polymer nanocomposites as a potential tool to overcome MDR in cancer cells. *Eur. J. Pharm. Biopharm.* **2019**, *142*, 460–472. [CrossRef]
59. Szegedi, Á.; Shestakova, P.; Trendafilova, I.; Mihályi, J.; Tsacheva, I.; Mitova, V.; Kyulavska, M.; Koseva, N.; Momekova, D.; Konstantinov, S.; et al. Modified mesoporous silica nanoparticles coated by polymer complex as novel curcumin delivery carriers. *J. Drug Deliv. Sci. Technol.* **2019**, *49*, 700–712. [CrossRef]
60. Trendafilova, I.; Szegedi, Á.; Yoncheva, K.; Shestakova, P.; Mihály, J.; Ristic, A.; Konstantinov, S.; Popova, M. A pH dependent delivery of mesalazine from polymer coated and drug-loaded SBA-16 systems. *Eur. J. Pharm. Sci.* **2016**, *81*, 75–81. [CrossRef] [PubMed]
61. Bernardos, A.; Piacenza, E.; Sancenón, F.; Hamidi, M.; Maleki, A.; Turner, R.J.; Martínez-Máñez, R. Mesoporous Silica-Based Materials with Bactericidal Properties. *Small* **2019**, *15*, e1900669. [CrossRef]
62. Llopis-Lorente, A.; Lozano-Torres, B.; Bernardos, A.; Martínez-Máñez, R.; Sancenón, F.J. Mesoporous silica materials for controlled delivery based on enzymes. *Mater. Chem. B* **2017**, *5*, 3069–3083. [CrossRef] [PubMed]
63. Wu, S.-H.; Mou, C.-Y.; Lin, H.-P. Synthesis of mesoporous silica nanoparticles. *Chem. Soc. Rev.* **2013**, *42*, 3862. [CrossRef] [PubMed]
64. Hao, N.; Li, L.; Tang, F. Roles of particle size, shape and surface chemistry of mesoporous silica nanomaterials on biological systems. *Int. Mater. Rev.* **2017**, *62*, 57–77. [CrossRef]
65. Stanković, A.; Dimitrijević, S.; Uskoković, D. Influence of size scale and morphology on antibacterial properties of ZnO powders hydrothemally synthesized using different surface stabilizing agents. *Colloids Surf. B Biointerfaces* **2013**, *102*, 21–28. [CrossRef] [PubMed]
66. Dove, A.S.; Dzurny, D.I.; Dees, W.R.; Qin, N.; Nunez, R.C.C.; Alt, L.A.; Ellward, G.L.; Best, J.A.; Rudawski, N.G.; Fujii, K.; et al. Silver nanoparticles enhance the efficacy of aminoglycosides against antibiotic-resistant bacteria. *Front. Microbiol.* **2023**, *13*, 1064095. [CrossRef] [PubMed]
67. Pavlova, E.L.; Ivanova, I.A.; Staneva, A.D.; Kostadinova, A.S.; Kichukova, D.G.; Yocheva, L.D. Prooxidant, antioxidant and biological activity of nanocomposites of reduced graphene oxide, silver, copper and their combinations. *Chem. Pap.* **2022**, *76*, 6789–6800. [CrossRef]
68. Poirier, D.G.; Westlake, G.F.; Abernethy, S.G. *Daphnia Magna Acute Lethality Toxicity Protocol*; Ontario Ministry of the Environment: Toronto, ON, Canada, 1988.

molecules

MDPI

Article

Luminescent Alendronic Acid-Conjugated Micellar Nanostructures for Potential Application in the Bone-Targeted Delivery of Cholecalciferol

Federica Rizzi [1,2], Annamaria Panniello [1], Roberto Comparelli [1,2], Ilaria Arduino [3], Elisabetta Fanizza [1,2,4], Rosa Maria Iacobazzi [3], Maria Grazia Perrone [5], Marinella Striccoli [1], Maria Lucia Curri [1,2,4], Antonio Scilimati [5], Nunzio Denora [3,*] and Nicoletta Depalo [1,2,*]

1 CNR-Institute for Chemical and Physical Process, 70125 Bari, Italy; f.rizzi@ba.ipcf.cnr.it (F.R.); a.panniello@ba.ipcf.cnr.it (A.P.); r.comparelli@ba.ipcf.cnr.it (R.C.); elisabetta.fanizza@uniba.it (E.F.); m.striccoli@ba.ipcf.cnr.it (M.S.); marialucia.curri@uniba.it (M.L.C.)
2 Consorzio Interuniversitario Nazionale per la Scienza e Tecnologia dei Materiali (INSTM), 50121 Firenze, Italy
3 Department of Pharmacy—Pharmaceutical Sciences, University of Bari, 70125 Bari, Italy; ilaria.arduino@uniba.it (I.A.); rosa.iacobazzi@uniba.it (R.M.I.)
4 Department of Chemistry, University of Bari, 70125 Bari, Italy
5 Research Laboratory for Woman and Child Health, Department of Pharmacy—Pharmaceutical Sciences, University of Bari, 70125 Bari, Italy; mariagrazia.perrone@uniba.it (M.G.P.); antonio.scilimati@uniba.it (A.S.)
* Correspondence: nunzio.denora@uniba.it (N.D.); n.depalo@ba.ipcf.cnr.it (N.D.)

Abstract: Vitamin D, an essential micronutrient crucial for skeletal integrity and various non-skeletal physiological functions, exhibits limited bioavailability and stability in vivo. This study is focused on the development of polyethylene glycol (PEG)-grafted phospholipid micellar nanostructures co-encapsulating vitamin D3 and conjugated with alendronic acid, aimed at active bone targeting. Furthermore, these nanostructures are rendered optically traceable in the UV–visible region of the electromagnetic spectrum via the simultaneous encapsulation of vitamin D3 with carbon dots, a newly emerging class of fluorescents, biocompatible nanoparticles characterized by their resistance to photobleaching and environmental friendliness, which hold promise for future in vitro bioimaging studies. A systematic investigation is conducted to optimize experimental parameters for the preparation of micellar nanostructures with an average hydrodynamic diameter below 200 nm, ensuring colloidal stability in physiological media while preserving the optical luminescent properties of the encapsulated carbon dots. Comprehensive chemical-physical characterization of these micellar nanostructures is performed employing optical and morphological techniques. Furthermore, their binding affinity for the principal inorganic constituent of bone tissue is assessed through a binding assay with hydroxyapatite nanoparticles, indicating significant potential for active bone-targeting. These formulated nanostructures hold promise for novel therapeutic interventions to address skeletal-related complications in cancer affected patients in the future.

Keywords: micellar nanostructures; luminescent carbon dots; cholecalciferol; alendronate; hydroxyapatite nanoparticles; active bone targeting

1. Introduction

In the advanced stages of various types of cancers, such as breast, prostate, lung, and multiple melanoma, the occurrence of bone metastases is quite common. These bone metastases give rise to several significant skeletal-related events (SREs), which include issues such as fractures, severe pain, limited mobility, spinal compression, and hypercalcemia. These complications not only significantly affect the quality of life for oncology patients but also reduce their overall survival rate. Additionally, patients experiencing SREs require extended hospital stays, resulting in substantial healthcare costs [1].

In the context of standard clinical practice, while a multidisciplinary approach is often employed to provide the best therapeutic outcomes for bone metastasis treatments, the primary treatment option for patients with SREs is the use of anti-resorptive agents, such as bisphosphonates (BPs) [1,2]. BPs are synthetic analogues of naturally pyrophosphate compounds that inhibit bone resorption and bone formation [3]. In vitro studies have reported that BPs may have a direct action on tumour cells by inducing apoptosis, inhibiting the adhesion of tumour cells within the bone [4]. Although prolonged BP administration is generally well-tolerated by oncology patients, it can lead to the development of hypocalcaemia due to the BPs' sustained anti-resorptive effects. Another risk factor for hypocalcaemia is vitamin D deficiency. Therefore, it is recommended to supplement with calcium and vitamin D during the BP treatment to mitigate the risk of hypocalcaemia [1,5]. Vitamin D plays crucial roles in skeletal health, including bone strength and calcium absorption, as well as in various non-skeletal functions. Proper levels of vitamin D have been associated with a reduced risk of conditions such as diabetes, cardiovascular diseases, and certain cancers [6–9]. Between the two primary forms of vitamin D, namely ergocalciferol (vitamin D2) and cholecalciferol (vitamin D3, VitD3), in humans, VitD3 is more effective than vitamin D2, primarily because it is more efficient in elevating blood serum levels of biologically active vitamin D metabolites, thanks to its higher affinity for the vitamin-D-binding protein [10]. The physiological benefits and functionality of VitD3 are constrained due to its classification as a fat-soluble micronutrient, characterized by its limited water solubility, heightened vulnerability to environmental factors, and susceptibility to oxidation. In accordance with a multitude of research studies, it was observed that a significant proportion exceeding 75% of ingested VitD3 undergoes processes of catabolism and excretion prior to its conversion into its biologically active form [11]. The clinical utilization of VitD3 is further marked by its notably brief half-life in the circulatory system and its susceptibility to the first-pass effect. Furthermore, excessive consumption of VitD3 may induce toxic effects associated with the development of hypervitaminosis syndrome [12]. To address these inherent constraints, novel drug delivery nanosystems have been designed for the formulation of VitD3, encompassing polymeric- or lipid-based nanovectors, as recently reported [11–16]. The primary objective of these nanosystems is to encapsulate VitD3, thereby not only augmenting its bioavailability and in vivo stability but also facilitating the administration of the optimal dosages, thereby mitigating the potential risks associated with toxicity.

While several studies have been conducted to explore the encapsulation of VitD3, there is a paucity of research focusing on the utilization of nanocarriers for the targeted delivery of VitD3 to the skeletal system [17]. It is important to recognize that bones are encased by lining cells that serve as a protective blood–marrow barrier, consequently limiting direct contact between bone surfaces and exogenous compounds. Furthermore, in mineralized tissues, the expression of biomolecules with specific targeting capabilities, such as enzymes or antigens, remains relatively low, thereby limiting the opportunities for active targeting. In the realm of drug delivery nanosystems tailored for bone targeting, only certain agents have emerged as the most commonly utilized. These include the arginine–glycine–aspartic acid peptide, as well as two notable members of the BP family, namely alendronic (ALE) and zoledronic acids [18–20]. Extensive research has revealed the substantial potential of these agents in the development of pharmaceuticals with a bone-targeted focus [21–28]. The distinctive composition of bone, characterized by high concentrations of calcium and phosphorus, contributes to its supramolecular structure, rendering it a unique and specific target for binding by BPs. The presence of hydroxyapatite (HA) during bone remodelling further enhances the affinity of mineral-binding drugs for sites exhibiting high turnover rates, often associated with pathological conditions [29]. Compounds such as BPs exploit these inherent characteristics to facilitate robust and precise in vivo binding to bone tissue [30,31]. Indeed, BPs, among which ALE is notable, possess a unique capability to chelate with calcium ions present in HA crystals, which constitute a fundamental mineral component within the bone microenvironment [32]. This distinctive property renders HA crystals ideal and specific binding sites for drugs designed for bone targeting [33].

This study aims to elucidate the use of polyethylene glycol (PEG)-grafted phospholipids in combination with luminescent carbon dots (C-dots) to fabricate optically traceable micellar nanostructures for encapsulating VitD3, which are further conjugated with ALE (VitD3/C-dot/ALE–micelles). C-dots are renowned for their intense photoluminescence (PL) characteristics in the visible range, marked by exceptional biocompatibility and robust photostability. Consequently, C-dots have extensive applications in diverse fields such as live cell imaging, biosensing, targeted drug delivery, and various biomedical applications [34]. The incorporation of functional nanoparticles (NPs) such as C-dots into the hydrophobic core of polymer-grafted lipid micelles represents an effective approach for the co-encapsulation of a wide spectrum of poorly water-soluble therapeutic agents. This approach yields multifunctional nanoformulations characterized by noteworthy colloidal stability, a high degree of biocompatibility, and stealth properties, thereby enhancing their suitability for various biomedical applications [35–40].

Here, a comprehensive characterization of the micellar nanostructures specifically designed for the bone-targeted delivery of VitD3 was conducted at each stage of the preparation process using a combination of optical and morphological techniques. The optical properties of the C-dots were investigated both before and after their integration into the micellar cores, as well as following their conjugation with ALE. This investigation aimed to evaluate the preservation of their PL, which is crucial for achieving optical traceability. This information will be valuable for future in vitro studies. Here, the PL properties of the ALE-conjugated micellar nanostructures were investigated in this study to assess their binding affinity for HA NPs, with the aim of demonstrating the robust affinity of the novel formulation for the primary inorganic component of bone. This validation underscores its potential for actively targeting bone tissue.

2. Results and Discussion

2.1. Preparation of PEGylated Phospholipid-Based Micellar Nanostructures

Oil-soluble C-dots were obtained using a one-step synthetic method as the preliminary step in the preparation of luminescent micellar nanostructures. In the synthetic process, citric acid served as the carbon precursor, while 1-octadecene (ODE) and 1-hexadecylamine (HDA) were employed as a high-boiling point solvent and surface-passivating agent, respectively [41].

The TEM analysis (Figure 1B) exhibited the formation of spherical-shaped C-dots with an average diameter of approximately 3.5 nm ($\sigma = 23\%$). The UV-Vis absorption spectrum of a chloroform dispersion of 'as synthesized' C-dots (Figure 1A inset) displayed a distinctive peak in the range of 300 to 400 nm. This peak was attributed to the n-π^* transition, which was associated with both the C=O bonds and surface chemical functional groups. Furthermore, the spectrum revealed a broadened absorption band centred around 450 nm, ascribed to the formation of molecular fluorophore aggregates during the carbonization process [41].

The PL spectroscopic measurements of the chloroform dispersion of C-dots (Figure 1A) indicated a consistent dependence of the emission band from the excitation wavelength in the visible range up to 540 nm, where the signal appeared sensibly quenched. Notably, the highest PL quantum yield (QY) of $(25.3 \pm 0.1)\%$ was achieved for excitation at $\lambda = 360$ nm (Figure S1B, see Supplementary Materials (SM)).

To encapsulate oil-soluble C-dots within the hydrophobic micellar cores, an experimental procedure previously established for the preparation of PEG-stabilized micellar nanostructures that incorporate luminescent quantum dots or superparamagnetic NPs [35,36,38–40] was followed. Specifically, PEG-stabilized micellar nanostructures were obtained using mainly PEG-2-PE (1,2-Dipalmitoyl-sn-glycero-3-phosphoethanolamine-N-[methoxy (poly (ethylene glycol))-2000; 16:0), with only a very low percentage (molar ratio of 4:1) of the lipid mixture composed of DSPE-PEG-COOH (1,2-distearoyl-sn-glycero-3-

phosphoethanolamine-N-[carboxy(polyethylene glycol)-2000), ensuring the presence of carboxylic groups on the micellar surface for conjugation with ALE. Here, PEG-2-PE-based micelles were selected as suitable nanovectors for drug delivery based on the findings of Wang et al., who demonstrated the safety of PEG-2-PE in normal cells and its toxicity in cancer cells. The same report also clarified the molecular mechanism of the cytotoxicity in cancer cells, demonstrating that PEG-2-PE micelles insert into cell membranes without compromising the membrane integrity. The micelles disassemble at the membrane level and the resulting disassembled PEG-PE molecules can be internalized into cells through non-specific endocytosis and accumulate in the endoplasmic reticulum (ER), leading to ER stress. Notably, cancer cells initiate proapoptotic signaling under PEG-2-PE-induced ER stress, while normal cells activate pro-survival signaling pathways. This suggests that PEG-2-PE micelles can safely serve as suitable nanocarriers for delivering anticancer drugs [42].

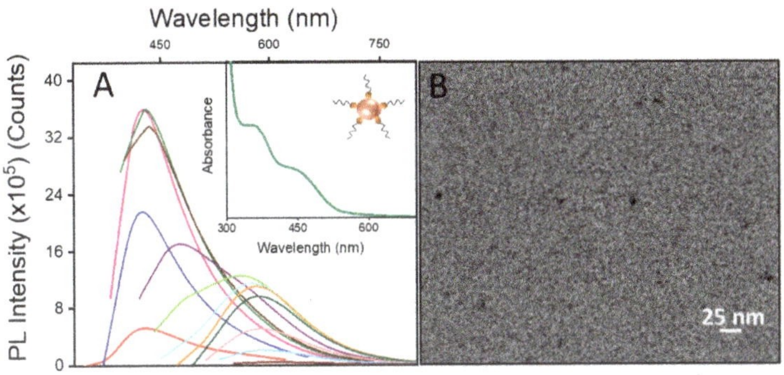

Figure 1. (**A**) PL spectra of the 'as synthesized' C-dots dispersed in organic solvent and recorded at increasing excitation wavelengths (λ) of 300 nm (black line), 320 nm (red line), 340 nm (blue line), 360 nm (magenta line), 375 nm (olive line), 380 nm (brown line), 400 nm (violet line), 420 nm (lime green line), 440 nm (light blue line), 460 nm (orange line), 480 nm (dark blue line), 500 nm (pink line), 520 nm (heavenly blue line), and 540 nm (purple line). Inset: UV-Vis absorption spectrum. (**B**) TEM micrograph of oil-soluble C-dots cast from chloroform.

Different starting percentages of the C-dot/PEG–phospholipid weight ratio, ranging from 7% to 42% (samples A, B, C, D, E, and F), as indicated in Figure 2A, were systematically explored in the preparation of the luminescent PEG-stabilized micellar nanostructures. This investigation aimed to pinpoint the optimal experimental conditions to both preserve the distinctive optical characteristics of the C-dots and yield micellar aggregates with an average hydrodynamic diameter below 200 nm (Figure 2A–D) [43,44].

Prior to their characterization in terms of the dimensional, morphological, and optical properties, the 'as-prepared' luminescent micellar nanostructures underwent purification steps. These included centrifugation to recover the non-encapsulated oil-soluble C-dots as a pellet, followed by filtration to remove the excess lipids not assembled in the micellar structures, as described in the Section 3.

The dynamic light scattering (DLS) analysis revealed that the different samples exhibited a bimodal size distribution. Specifically, the size distribution profile exhibited a peak range centred at 15–20 nm, attributed to the formation of empty micelles, in addition to a peak due to micellar structures of a larger size (Figure 2A), encapsulating the C-dots.

The recorded average hydrodynamic diameters ranged from 110 to 150 nm for samples B–E and increased as the C-dot/phospholipid weight ratio percentage increased from 21 to 42%. Conversely, sample A, obtained at the lowest investigated C-dot/phospholipid weight ratio percentage, exhibited a larger average hydrodynamic diameter. However, the presence of a peak at sizes larger than empty micelles suggests the formation of micellar nanostructures with multiple C-dots embedded within the micellar core.

A

Sample	C-dot/PEG-Lipid weight ratio (%)	Size Peak 1 (nm)	Size Peak 2 (nm)	PDI	ζ-potential (mV)
A	7	245±7	20±1	0.37±0.03	−2.4±0.1
B	14	128±6	21±2	0.35±0.01	−12.4±1.4
C	21	110±6	15±3	0.20±0.02	−29.8±0.6
D	25	118±2	20±1	0.27±0.04	−27.2±2.2
E	28	125±5	16±5	0.29±0.03	−28.3±0.2
F	42	148±4	18±8	0.33±0.04	−27.4±0.4

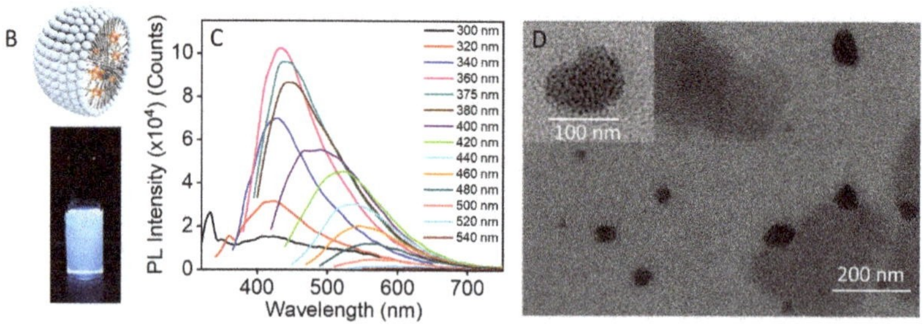

Figure 2. (**A**) DLS analysis and ζ-potential values for micellar nanostructures prepared at different starting C-dot/PEG–phospholipid weight ratio percentages. (**B**) Picture of the vial containing micellar nanostructures encapsulating C-Dots, acquired under 400 nm light exposure along with a representative scheme. (**C**) PL emission spectra recorded at excitation wavelengths ranging from 300 to 540 nm (1:3 dilution of sample C in PBS) and (**D**) representative TEM micrograph and corresponding close-up view in the inset cast from the water from sample C.

The ζ-potential analysis revealed, for all investigated samples, the presence of a negative surface charge on the PEG–micelle surface, which was decorated with carboxylic groups. It also demonstrated significant colloidal stability in a physiological medium (phosphate-buffered solution (PBS), 10 mM, pH 7.4), for samples C and D, while lower ζ-potential values were recorded for samples A and B, indicating poorer colloidal stability in aqueous environments compared to samples C and D (Figure 2A). Based on the DLS and ζ-potential measurements, samples A and B were not further considered. The PL characterization spectroscopy was performed on samples C–E. In Figure 2B,C, the UV-Vis and PL spectra of sample C are reported, while in Figure S1 of the Supplementary Materials the spectra resulting from the PL characterization of samples D and E can be observed. The findings demonstrated that despite the manipulation undergone by the C-dots in the encapsulation process into the micellar nanosystems and the considerable variation of the chemical surroundings they experienced, the peculiar optical properties of the C-dots were retained. No significant difference in the emission properties of samples C, D, and E was observed (Figure S1, Supplementary Materials), indicating that further increasing the C-dot/phospholipid weight ratio percentage is not necessary to improve the emission properties of the micellar nanostructures.

Therefore, the sample labelled as 'C', prepared using a C-dot/phospholipid weight ratio percentage of 21%, was demonstrated to retain the optical emission properties and have the smallest average hydrodynamic diameter and highest degree of size uniformity (polydispersity index (PDI) = 0.20 ± 0.02). Considering such findings, this sample was selected for further characterization and experimentation. The rationale behind this choice was that since the typical gaps between mineralized bone fibers (lamellae) are of the order of a few hundred nanometers, only NPs with dimensions falling within the range of 100 to 200 nm can effectively accomplish bone tissue targeting and penetration [40].

The PL QY was assessed for sample C. Due to the processing steps involved and the change in dispersion medium (PBS, 10 mM, pH 7.4), a slight decrease in PL quantum yield (QY = 12.2 ± 0.1%) was observed compared to the PL QY of the 'as-synthesized'

C-dots (Figure S2B, see Supplementary Materials). A detailed examination of sample C, performed via a transmission electron microscopy (TEM) investigation (inset of Figure 2D), revealed the presence of numerous black spots, each measuring only a few nanometers in size. These dimensions are consistent with the anticipated size of the C-dots and were visibly contained within the round-shaped nanostructures. In the broader view in Figure 2D, the round-shaped nanostructures, attributed to micellar aggregates, exhibit sizes ranging approximately from 40 to 100 nm. Concurrently, the empty micelles appear as smaller nanospheres of approximately 10 nm in diameter. This observation is in good agreement with the findings of the DLS analysis, accounting for the shrinkage of the micellar nanostructures that occurred during the drying process on the grid before the TEM measurements.

In the formulation of micellar nanostructures loaded with both VitD3 and C-dots, using a starting C-dot/phospholipid weight ratio percentage of 21%, various nanoformulations were developed by varying the starting amount of VitD3. Specifically, different weight ratio percentages of VitD3 to phospholipids were examined, with values of 2.6%, 3.3%, 4.0%, 5.3%, and 6.6%, corresponding to 0.4 mg, 0.5 mg, 0.6 mg, 0.8 mg, and 1 mg of VitD3, respectively. The actual amount of VitD3 effectively incorporated within the micellar nanostructures was determined via UV-Vis absorption spectroscopy (Figure 3A). This analysis was performed after freeze-drying and subsequent re-dispersing the samples in methanol. The results were expressed as EE% and DL% for each sample, as illustrated in Figure 3A and Figure S3C (see Supplementary Materials). These findings indicate that the maximum values of DL% and EE% were attained when the initial feed of the drug was 0.5 mg. As a result, this specific formulation, selected among those prepared with various initial amounts of VitD3, was chosen for subsequent conjugation with ALE.

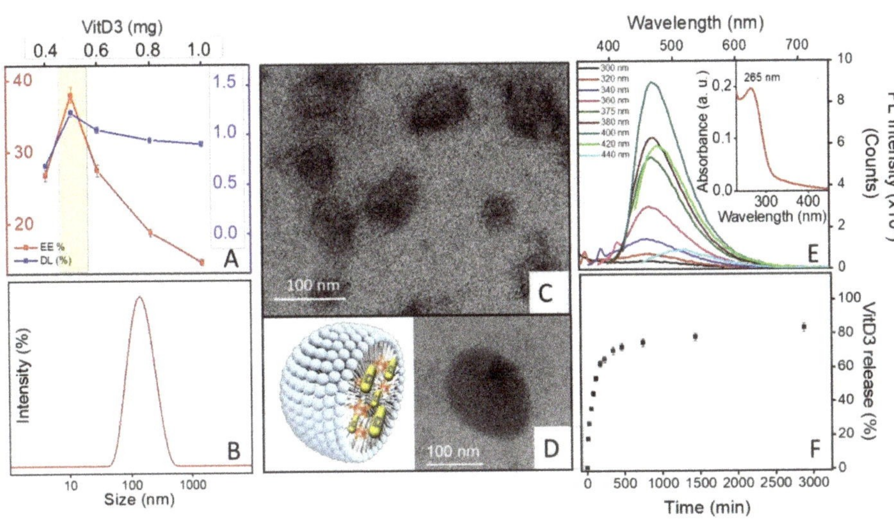

Figure 3. (**A**) Encapsulation efficiency (EE%) and loading (DL%) percentages of the VitD3 for samples of micellar nanostructures co-encapsulating VitD3 and C-Dots, prepared at different starting VitD3/phospholipid weight ratio percentages. (**B**) Size distribution by intensity of the micellar nanostructures co-encapsulating VitD3 and C-Dots obtained by using a VitD3/phospholipid weight ratio percentage of 3.3% and dispersed in PBS (10 mM, pH 7.4). (**C**) representative TEM micrograph along with (**D**) corresponding close-up and schematic sketch. (**E**) PL emission spectra recorded at excitation wavelengths ranging from 300 to 440 nm. Inset: UV-Vis absorbance spectrum. (**F**) In vitro release profile of the VitD3 recorded for the VitD3/C-dot micellar nanostructures (VitD3/phospholipid weight ratio percentage of 3.3%, C-dot/phospholipid weight ratio percentage of 21%).

The concentration of C-dots incorporated into the formulation, which was prepared at a VitD3/phospholipid weight ratio percentage of 3.3%, was determined to be 37.5 μg/mL. Such an evaluation was carried out by creating a calibration curve based on PL emission spectra under excitation at 375 nm of chloroform dispersion of previously freeze-dried formulations. The PL spectra of the formulations showed the same peculiar emission profiles for the pristine C-dots (Figure 3E), thereby suggesting that C-dots, after their co-encapsulation into the micellar nanostructures with VitD3 (Figure 3B), retain their emission properties, although in this case an additional decrease in their PL QY was detected (7.2 ± 0.2%; Figure S2B, see Supplementary Materials), due to both the further processing and environmental changes that C-dots undergo by passing from the original organic solvent to the hydrophobic micellar cores where they are also co-loaded with VitD3. The absorption spectrum (inset, Figure 3E) of the formulations was dominated by a band at 265 nm attributed to the VitD3 (Figure S3A, see Supplementary Materials) within the micellar system. The absorption features, characteristic of the C-dots, covering the range between 300 and 400 nm (see the spectrum of the 'as-synthesized' C-dots inset in Figure 1A as a comparison) were poorly visible, since they fell in the same spectral region of VitD3 absorption or due to the altered chemical environment experienced by the C-dots' surfaces.

The TEM analysis performed on the VitD3/C-dot micellar nanostructures (Figure 3C,D) revealed the formation of spherical NPs with sizes ranging from 60 nm to 100 nm. The DLS investigations unveiled that the VitD3/C-dot micellar nanostructures exhibited an average hydrodynamic diameter of approximately 130 nm, with a polydispersity index (PDI) of (0.262 ± 0.133). The monomodal size distribution in Figure 3B indicates the complete elimination of empty micelles as a result of the ultracentrifugation process (see experimental section for more details). The ζ-potential value measured for this formulation was (−24.1 ± 3.0) mV, underscoring the good colloidal stability in aqueous solutions and highlighting a negative surface charge, attributed to outer exposed phosphate and carboxylate groups on the surfaces of the micellar structures.

The in vitro release of VitD3 from the micellar nanostructures (sampled at a VitD3/phospholipid weight ratio percentage of 3.3% and C-dot/phospholipid weight ratio percentage of 21%) was monitored using UV-Vis spectroscopy under physiological conditions (PBS 10 mM, pH = 7.4). The release profile in Figure 3F indicates that a payload fraction of about 50% is released into the medium within the first 4 h, followed by more sustained release of vitamin D3, reaching up to (81 ± 3)% at 50 h.

2.2. Conjugation with ALE of the Luminescent Micellar VitD3 Containing Nanostructures

The ALE was synthesized by reacting the 4-aminobutyric acid (**1**) with phthalic anhydride to afford the *N*-phthaloyl butyric acid (**2**). The *N*-phthaloyl butyric acid (**2**) was converted into (**3**) using a modified Arbuzov's reaction. Specifically, **2** was first converted into the corresponding acyl chlorides by thionyl chloride and then used as a reagent in the modified Arbuzov's reaction, in which the phosphorylating agent was the tris(trimethylsilyl)phosphite. The silyl esters of the geminal bisphosphonic acid intermediate were hydrolyzed into compound **3**. The deprotection of the amino group hydrolyzing the phthalimide moiety, achieved with 12 N HCl at reflux, afforded the alendronic acid **4** (Scheme 1) [41,43–47].

ALE was then used for conjugation onto the surfaces of the micellar nanostructures. The conjugation process promoted the formation of covalent bonds between the carboxylic groups on the micellar surface and the amine groups present in the ALE structure. This strategic approach was adopted with the aim of creating nanosystems that have the potential to target bone tissue [38,48].

The effective conjugation of the ALE with the micellar nanoformulations was assessed using an FTIR-ATR (Fourier transform infrared spectroscopy–attenuated total reflection) analysis (Figure 4A). For comparison, the pure VitD3 encapsulated in the nanoformulations and ALE and the bare micellar nanostructures were analyzed. The FTIR spectrum of the luminescent micellar nanostructures loaded with VitD3 revealed two distinct peaks at 3480 and 3350 cm^{-1}, corresponding to stretching vibrations of N-H attributable to the primary amine groups within the molecular structure of ALE. In the spectrum of the luminescent micellar nanostructures loaded with VitD3 and conjugated with ALE, a singular N-H peak stretching vibration at 3480 cm^{-1} was evident, indicative of amide bond formation. Additionally, the signal of VitD3 at 3330 cm^{-1}, associated with the stretching of the hydrogen bond O-H, and peaks within the 2990 to 2880 cm^{-1} range, attributed to symmetric stretching of aliphatic C-H, were discernible in conjunction with a peak centered at 1110 cm^{-1} arising from C-O-C stretching of the PEG–phospholipid chains within the spectrum of the micellar nanoformulations loaded with VitD3 and conjugated with ALE. A broad band spanning the 1200 to 800 cm^{-1} range, corresponding to phosphate functional groups, was observed in the ALE-conjugated sample due to the overlapping of phosphate esters (1100 cm^{-1}) and phosphonate vibrations from lipids and ALE, respectively [49,50]. Consequently, the FTIR-ATR analysis indicated the successful conjugation of ALE onto the micellar surfaces. The spectroscopic investigation of the conjugated sample demonstrated that similarly to previous findings, while the emission properties were retained, a slight decrease in the PL QY (5.2 ± 0.2)% was observed (see Figure S2B, see Supplementary Materials).

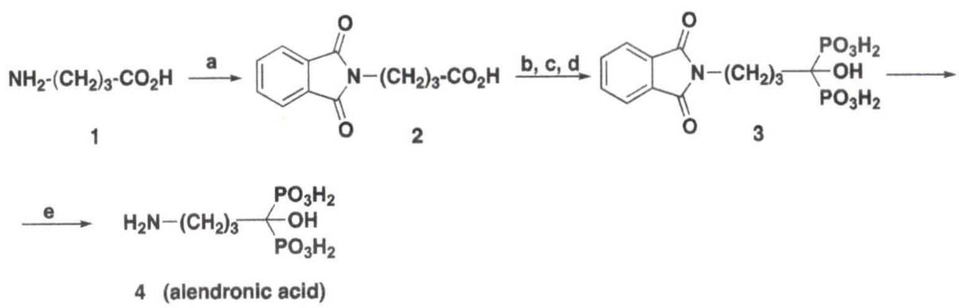

Scheme 1. Reaction scheme: (a) phthalic anhydride, triethylamine ($Et_3N_{(cat \cdot)}$), toluene, reflux, 5 h; (b) thionyl chloride, reflux, 2 h; (c) tris(trimethylsilyl)phosphite, tetrahydrofuran (THF), 0 °C to r. t., 15 min–15 h; (d) methanol (MeOH), r. t., 1 h; (e) 12 N HCl, reflux, 5.5–20 h.

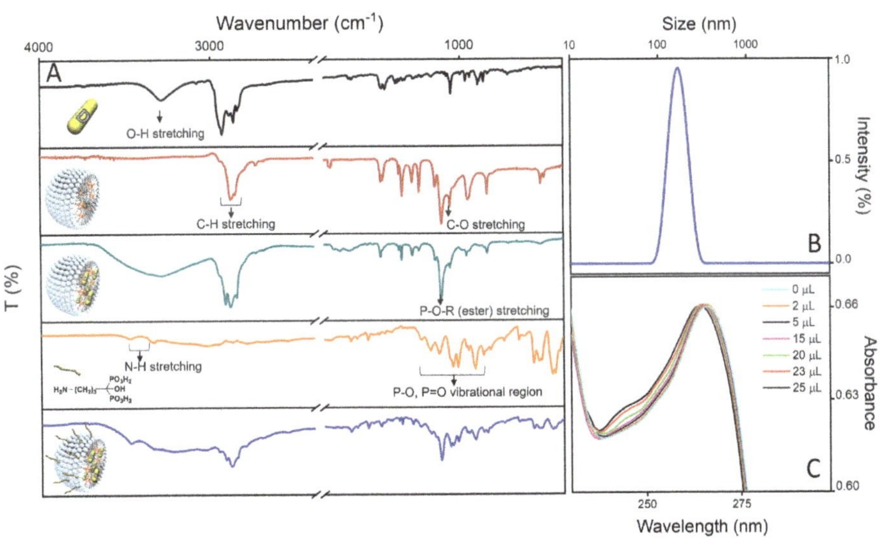

Figure 4. (**A**) FT-IR spectra of free VitD3, luminescent micellar structures and loaded with VitD3, synthesized ALE and ALE conjugated to the surface of the luminescent micellar formulation loaded with VitD3. (**B**) Representative size distribution based on intensity. (**C**) Determination of the ALE concentrations in the micellar formulations based on complexation with Fe(III) ions in acidic conditions.

DLS analysis performed on the conjugated samples reveals a monomodal size distribution and an increase in the average hydrodynamic diameter that shifts from 130 to about 150 nm (PDI 0.298 ± 0.065) passing from nude micellar to conjugated structures (Figure 4B), while ζ-potential measurements results (−28 ± 4) mV, highlighting relevant colloidal stability in the aqueous solution of the resulting nanoformulations and suggesting that residual negatively charged phosphate and carboxylate groups are still present on the micellar surface.

According to the procedure reported by Kuljanin et al. [46], the ALE conjugated on the surface of the micellar formulations was colorimetrically determined through a complexation reaction with Fe(III) ions, as ALE does not absorb in the UV-Vis spectral region. It is well known that bisphosphonates, including ALE, exhibit strong chelating properties towards metals, including iron, owing to the excellent complexing ability of the O=P-C-P=O moiety, which facilitates the formation of stable metal complexes [46]. The pH condition is a critical parameter for this complex formation, as it heavily depends on the deprotonation degree of the phosphonic acid groups. Since the pKa1 of ALE is approximately 2.43 [51], the complex formation was promoted under highly acidic conditions (pH < 2). The progress of the complex formation was monitored using UV-Vis spectroscopy in the wavelength range of 200 to 300 nm, with the gradual addition of a calibrated amount of an acidic Fe(III) ion solution into an acidic aqueous dispersion containing the ALE-conjugated micellar nanostructures (Figure 4C) [46].

Prior to the introduction of the acidic Fe (III) ion solution, the UV-Vis absorption spectrum of the micellar nanostructures loaded with VitD3 and conjugated with ALE exhibited a band centred at 265 nm, due to the incorporation of the VitD3 in the micellar core (heavenly line, Figure 4C). As the Fe (III) ions were added, the formation of the Fe(III) ion–ALE complex occurred; the absorption band of the complex at 260 nm (Figure S4B, see Supplementary Materials) is hidden by the overlapping strong absorption signal of the VitD3 that falls in the same spectral range. When a new peak emerges at 240 nm (Figure 4C), ascribable to free Fe(III) ions in the acid solution (as shown in the UV-Vis spectrum in Figure S4A, see Supplementary Materials), this indicates that all the ALE molecules on the micellar surface have been complexed [46].

The quantitative evaluation of the amount of ALE covalently conjugated onto the micellar nanostructures resulted in an average concentration of $(5.5 \pm 0.5) \times 10^{-4}$ M.

2.3. Binding Affinity Assay

HA NPs, synthesized using the method reported in Boanini et al. [33], were used to assess their binding affinity with the ALE-conjugated micellar nanostructures. The rationale behind this evaluation was rooted in the composition of natural bone, wherein 70% of the mineral phase comprises 95% HA. Furthermore, previous studies have proved that BPs, including ALE, exhibit a robust affinity for bone mineral HA [52–56]. Consequently, given this inherent affinity, it is postulated that during the metastatic process, HA may function as a binding receptor for nanosystems conjugated with ALE [57]. The TEM and field emission scanning electron microscopy (FE-SEM) investigation proved the formation of elongated NPs that appeared as needle-like flakes; the statistical analysis based on the TEM investigation (Figure 5A,B) gave an average length of about 58 nm (σ% = 5%).

The chemical composition of the HA NPs derived from the SEM-EDX (energy-dispersive spectroscopy) analysis, reported in Figure 5(A1,A2), provides a Ca/P mole ratio of 1.67 [58], in good accordance with the expected theoretical value [59]. The binding affinity assay was carried out by incubating at 37 °C the luminescent ALE-conjugated VitD3/C-dot micellar nanostructures with the 'as synthesized' HA NPs. After 5 h, the HA NPs decorated with the luminescent nanostructures were recovered by centrifugation, re-suspended in PBS, and analyzed by PL spectroscopy (λex = 405 nm). For comparison, the same experimental procedure was used for the non-conjugated VitD3/C-dot micellar nanostructures. By examining the integrated area of the PL spectrum before and after the affinity binding assay for both non-conjugated and ALE-conjugated micellar nanostructures, (Figure 5D), the binding affinity percentages with HA NPs were estimated as approximately 56% and 19% for the ALE-conjugated and non-conjugated samples, respectively. This suggests that a slight non-specific adsorption of the micellar surface on HA NPs concurrently takes place. Nevertheless, the enhanced binding percentage calculated for the ALE-conjugated micellar nanostructures on HA NPs suggests that micellar formulations grafted with ALE could serve as promising candidates for active bone targeting, owing to their favourable affinity for the primary inorganic component of bone.

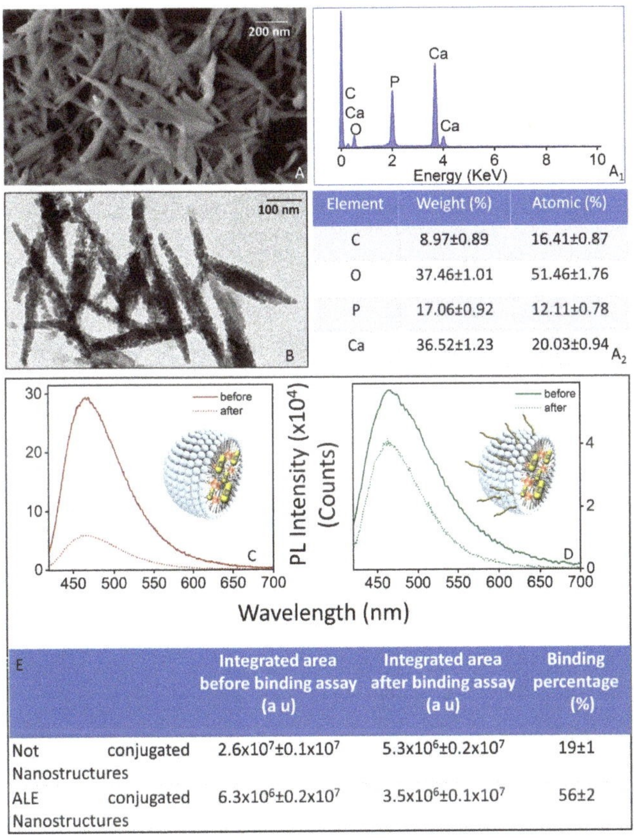

Element	Weight (%)	Atomic (%)
C	8.97±0.89	16.41±0.87
O	37.46±1.01	51.46±1.76
P	17.06±0.92	12.11±0.78
Ca	36.52±1.23	20.03±0.94

E	Integrated area before binding assay (a u)	Integrated area after binding assay (a u)	Binding percentage (%)
Not conjugated Nanostructures	$2.6x10^7 \pm 0.1x10^7$	$5.3x10^6 \pm 0.2x10^7$	19±1
ALE conjugated Nanostructures	$6.3x10^6 \pm 0.2x10^7$	$3.5x10^6 \pm 0.1x10^7$	56±2

Figure 5. Representative FE-SEM micrograph (**A**), EDX element spectrum (**A1**), element content table (**A2**), and representative TEM micrograph of the HA nanoparticles (**B**). PL spectra, before and after incubation with HA NPs, of the non-conjugated (**C**) and ALE-conjugated (**D**) VitD3/C-dot micellar nanostructures. Table reporting the binding percentage for the non-conjugated and ALE-conjugated samples obtained by estimating the integrated area under the PL spectrum, before and after the incubation of each sample with the HA NPs. The data are presented as means ± S.D (n = 3) (**E**).

3. Materials and Methods

3.1. Materials

The citric acid (anhydrous), ODE (technical grade 90%), HDA (98%), cholecalciferol (Vitamin D3, MW: 384.64 g/mol), ferric chloride hexahydrate ($FeCl_3{\cdot}6H_2O$), calcium nitrate tetrahydrate ($Ca(NO_3)_2{\cdot}4H_2O$), ammonium phosphate (($NH_4H_2PO_4$) and sodium hydroxide (NaOH), 4-aminobutyric acid, thionyl chloride ($SoCl_2$), and tris(trimethylsilyl) phosphite were purchased from Sigma (St. Louis, MO, USA). The 1,2-dipalmitoyl-sn-glycero-3-phosphoethanolamine-*N*-[methoxy (poly(ethylene glycol))-2000] (16:0 PEG2000 PE, ammonium salt) and 1,2-distearoyl-sn-glycero-3-phosphoethanolamine-*N*-[carboxy(polyethylene glycol)-2000] (DSPE-PEG(2000)–carboxylic acid, sodium salt) were purchased from Avanti Polar Lipids, while the 1-ethyl-3-(3-dimethylaminopropyl)carbodiimide hydrochloride (EDC) and *N*-hydroxylsulfosuccinimide (sulfo-NHS) were purchased from Pierce. The perchloric acid ($HClO_4$) was purchased from Fluka. All solvents (Sigma-Aldrich) were of analytical grade. The qqueous solutions were prepared using water obtained from a Milli-Q gradient A-10 system (Millipore, Burlington, MA, USA).

3.2. *Preparation of PEG–Micellar Nanostructures Loaded with C-Dots and VitD3*

The colloidal C-dots were synthesized and purified as previously described [60]. Briefly, the process involved the thermal carbonization of citric acid in the presence of ODE as a high-boiling point solvent and HDA as a surface ligand and nitrogen source. Prior to the synthesis, all reactants were thoroughly dried and degassed and the synthetic process took place under an inert nitrogen atmosphere using a Schlenk line. Here, 1.5 g of HDA was dissolved in 26 mL of ODE under vacuum conditions at 100 °C for 30 min; then, the temperature was raised above the decomposition point of citric acid (153 °C) and 1 g of citric acid was quickly added into the reaction mixture at 200 °C. The reaction proceeded for 3 h before being quenched by cooling to 25 °C. To purify the resulting C-dots, numerous cycles of non-solvent precipitation and re-dispersion in acetone were performed and then the purified C-dots were dispersed in chloroform, ready for further characterization and their encapsulation into micellar nanostructures.

For the preparation of the micellar nanostructures co-encapsulating C-dots and VitD3 (VitD3/C-382 dots/Micelles), 0.15 mL of C-dots (18 mg/mL) and calibrated amounts of VitD3 (1 mg/mL, chloroform solution) were added to the chloroform solution containing PEG-PE and DSPE-PEG-COOH (molar ratio 4:1) at a final volume of 5 mL. Depending on the final concentration of VitD3, the chloroform volumes ranged from 3.7 to 4.3 mL. After the removal of the organic solvent via evaporation, a film composed of VitD3/C-dot/PEG-modified lipids was obtained; then, it was kept under vacuum conditions for 2 h and reconstituted in phosphate-buffered solution (2 mL of 10 mM PBS, pH 7.5). Three cycles of heating (T = 80 °C) and cooling at room temperature were carried out to obtain the VitD3 and C-dot-loaded micellar nanostructures. The samples were purified firstly via centrifugation at 5000× *g* for 1 min to remove the non-encapsulated C-dots or VitD3 and then by using Centricon Plus-70 (membrane Ultracel-PL, 100 kDa, Millipore). Finally, the suspension was ultracentrifugated at 200,000× *g* for 4 h to eliminate the empty micelles that remained suspended while the pellet was recovered and dispersed in PBS. The luminescent micellar nanostructures loaded with C-dots only were prepared by following the same procedure described above, without the addition of the VitD3 to the chloroform solution and omitting the final step of ultracentrifugation.

The quantitative evaluation of the amounts of C-dots actually encapsulated in the lipid nanostructures was performed by freeze-drying the samples (1 mL, aqueous solution) for 24 h at −60 °C (α 1−4 LSC model, CHRIST freeze-dried, Osterode am Harz, Germany) and treating them with 1 mL of chloroform to induce the rupture of the micellar structures and to promote the dispersion of oil-soluble C-dots in the organic solvent. A calibration curve was plotted by performing steady state photoluminescent (PL) measurements (at an excitation wavelength of 375 nm) on the organic solutions containing the phospholipids at the fixed concentration of 7.5 mg/mL and with C-dot concentrations in the range between 21 and 324 μg/mL [38], as reported in Figure S2 (see Supplementary Materials).

3.3. *Determination of Loading and Encapsulation Efficiency Percentages of Vitamin D3 and In Vitro Release Study*

The encapsulation efficiency (EE%) and drug loading (DL%) results were obtained by evaluating the VitD3 contents in the freeze-dried samples. Each sample was treated firstly with chloroform and then, upon solvent evaporation, with methanol to extract and solubilize the VitD3. After centrifugation, the supernatants were characterized using UV-Vis absorbance spectroscopy (PerkinElmer (Waltham, NA, USA) Lambda 20 UV VIS Spectrophotometer). A calibration curve was obtained by recording the maximum absorbance value at 265 nm for standard methanol solutions containing VitD3 in the concentration range of 0.1 to 1 mg/mL, as reported in Figure S3A,B (see Supplementary Materials).

The obtained EE% was as follows:

$$EE\% = (W_t/W_i) \times 100 \quad (1)$$

where W_t is the total amount of VitD3 in the micellar nanostructures and W_i is the total amount of therapeutic compound added as a starting feed in the preparation process.

The DL% is the effective amount of drug (in weight) incorporated in the micellar system, which was calculated as follows:

$$DL\% = (W_t/W_{Mic}) \times 100 \quad (2)$$

where W_{Mic} is the weight of the micellar nanostructures.

A Franz diffusion cell was used to perform the in vitro release study of VitD3 from micellar nanostructures in PBS (10 mM, pH = 7.4) at 37 °C under magnetic stirring. A cellulose acetate membrane with an average pore size of 0.2 µm (Fisher Scientific Milano, Milan, Italy) was placed between the donor and receptor chambers. Here, a 500 µL dispersion of VitD3/C-dot micellar nanostructures in PBS was introduced into the donor chamber and 9 mL of PBS solution was added to the receptor chamber. At scheduled times, 400 µL of receptor solution was taken within 24 h and an equal volume of PBS was added to the receptor chamber. Each collected solution fraction was analyzed using UV-Vis absorbance spectroscopy to evaluate the drug content by using the calibration curve described previously. The in vitro release experiments were carried out in triplicate.

3.4. Synthesis of Alendronic Acid

The alendronic acid (4-amino-1-hydroxybutane-1,1-diyl)bis(phosphonic acid (**4** in Scheme 1) [47] was prepared starting from the commercially available 4-aminobutyric acid (**1**), which was allowed to react with phthalic anhydride in toluene under reflux conditions for 5 h, in the presence of a catalytic amount of triethylamine (Et_3N). Then, the reaction mixture was allowed to reach room temperature and the *N*-phthaloyl butyric (**2**) was extracted with EtOAc and isolated after the solvent was distilled under reduced pressure (79% yield of step (a) in Scheme 1). The *N*-phthaloyl butyric acid (**3**, 2.02 mmol) was solubilized in $SOCl_2$ (5.9 mL) and refluxed for 3 h. The solvent was evaporated under reduced pressure, affording a white solid, which in turn was dissolved in dry tetrahydrofuran (THF) (4 mL) at 0 °C before the addition of tris(trimethylsilyl)phosphite (2.02 mL, 6.06 mmol) for 40 min. Then, the mixture was stirred for 16 h at room temperature. The methanol (MeOH) (3 mL) was added and the resulting solution was stirred for 5 h at room temperature. The solvent was evaporated under vacuum conditions and the white solid was washed three times with a toluene/hexane mixture (1:1) (10 mL), then with diethyl ether and dried under vacuum, obtaining intermediate **3** (98% yield of steps (b), (c), and (d) in Scheme 1). A solution of **3** (2.01 mmol) in 12 N HCl (17 mL) was refluxed for 22 h. The solvent was removed under reduced pressure, obtaining a white solid that was washed with ethanol (70 mL) at 70 °C. The alendronic acid (**4**) solid was then isolated via filtration of the solution, washed with warm ethanol, and dried under vacuum conditions (74% yield of step (e) in Scheme 1). 1H NMR (500 MHz, D2O/NaOD, δppm): 1.32–1.36 (m, 2H), 1.47–1.50 (m, 2H), 2.22 (t, J = 7.5 Hz, 2H). 31P NMR (202 MHz, D2O/NaOD, δppm): 18.96 (s, 2P) (1H and 31P NMR spectra are reported in Figure S5 of the Supplementary Materials).

3.5. Alendronate Bioconjugation of the Micellar Nanostructures Loaded with C-Dots and Vitamin D3

The alendronate sodium trihydrate (4-amino-1-hydroxy-1-phosphonobutyl phosphonic acid, monosodium, ALE) was synthesized as previously reported [47]. The carboxylic groups on the micellar surface were activated in PBS buffer (10 mM, pH = 7.4) using sulfo-NHS/EDC at a molar ratio of 1:10 for 15 min at 25 °C. Then, after removing the sulfo-NHS/EDC excess using Centricon Plus-70 (100 kDa, 5000× *g*, 10′, Millipore), the ALE was added to the aqueous dispersion containing the amine-reactive micellar nanostructures at a final concentration of 1.4×10^{-3} M and left to react overnight (25 °C). Subsequently, the ALE-conjugated lipid nanostructures were purified using Centricon Plus-70 and washed with PBS buffer to remove unreacted cross-linking molecules. For the evaluation of the ALE content conjugated on the micellar surface, an assay based on the formation of a chromophore complex between ALE and iron (III) ions was performed, according to the procedure reported by Kuljanin et al. [46]. Briefly, an aqueous dispersion of the ALE-conjugated lipid nanostructures was diluted with an aqueous solution of perchloric acid (2 N, pH < 2). Subsequently, a solution of $FeCl_3$ 10^{-2} M in $HClO_4$ (0.2 N) was added dropwise until the formation of the complex was complete. After each addition, the formation of the ALE/iron complex with absorption at λ = 260 nm was monitored using UV-Vis spectroscopy.

3.6. Binding Assay to Synthetic Hydroxyapatite

The HA NPs were synthesized by mixing a calibrated amount of 10 mL of 100 mM $Ca(NO_3)_2{\cdot}4H_2O$ solution and 10 mL of 65 mM $NH_4H_2PO_4$ (pH = 10), as reported by Boanini et al. [33]. In particular, 10 mL of $Ca(NO_3)_2{\cdot}4H_2O$ aqueous solution was heated at 90 °C and the $NH_4H_2PO_4$ aqueous solution was added dropwise under stirring. The mixture (20 mL, final volume) was allowed to react for 5 h, then the pellet recovered via centrifugation and dispersed in PBS.

To evaluate the binding affinity of the micellar nanostructures to bone, VitD3/C-dots/micelles (11 mg/mL), used as the control, and VitD3/C-dots/ALE–micelles (11 mg/mL) were incubated with HA NPs (500 µL, 0.6 mg/mL) at 37 °C for 1 h. Then, the incubated samples were centrifugated and the pellet was dispersed in 500 µL of PBS. These solutions were analyzed via steady-state PL measurements.

3.7. DLS Investigation and ζ-Potential Measurements

A Zetasizer Nano ZS (Malvern Instruments Ltd., Worcestershires, UK) system was used to evaluate the mean hydrodynamic diameter, polydispersity index (PDI), and ζ-potential values for all of the samples, which were dispersed in PBS buffer (10 mM pH 7.4), as previously reported [61].

3.8. TEM and SEM Investigation

The TEM analysis was performed using a Jeol TEM-1011 microscope, provided with an Olympus Quemesa Camera (11 Mpx, Olympus, Tokyo, Japan). The samples were prepared by depositing on a carbon-coated Cu grid (400 mesh) a drop (5 µL) of C-dots or the micellar nanostructure solution. For sample staining, the grid was placed on the top of a drop of an aqueous phosphotungstic acid solution 2% (*w*/*v*) for 30 s, after the evaporation solvent. Then, the grid was washed with ultrapure water and left to dry. A statistical size analysis was performed on the C-dots samples using the Image J 1.53e analysis program.

Field emission scanning electron microscopy (FE-SEM) was performed using a Zeiss (Oberkochen, Germany) Sigma microscope operating in the range of 0.5–20 kV and equipped with an in-lens secondary electron detector and an INCA energy-dispersive spectroscopy (EDS) detector. The HA spray-dried samples were mounted onto stainless steel sample holders using double-sided carbon tape and grounded by silver paste.

3.9. FTIR-ATR Characterizazion

The FTIR characterization was carried out using a 670 FTIR spectrometer (Varian, Palo Alto, CA, USA) with a diamond ATR accessory measuring 2 mm and a deuterated molecules of tryglicine sulfate (DTGS) detector. Five microliters (5 µL) of each sample were placed on the internal reflection element and the solvent was allowed to evaporate. The spectra were recorded in the range of 4000–400 cm^{-1}, acquiring 16 scans with a nominal resolution of 1 cm^{-1}.

3.10. Photophysical Investigation

A Cary 5000 (Varian) UV-Vis/NIR spectrophotometer and a Fluorolog 3 (HORIBA Jobin-Yvon) spectrofluorometer, equipped with a time-correlated single photon counter (TCSPC), were used to record the UV-Vis absorption and PL emission spectra, respectively. A "Quanta-phi" (HORIBA Jobin-Yvon, Palaiseau, France) integrated sphere coated by Spectralon was used for the evaluation of the PL emission and absolute quantum yield (QY) of the C-dots dispersed in the organic solvent and of the luminescent micellar nanostructures dispersed in aqueous solution at the excitation wavelength of 360 nm.

4. Conclusions

Novel, optically traceable, PEG-stabilized micellar nanostructures were successfully designed and fabricated for the targeted delivery of VitD3. A comprehensive optical and morphological characterization process substantiated the relevant colloidal stability of these innovative nanoformulations in aqueous solutions, with an average diameter measuring less than 200 nm. The concentration of ALE conjugated on the micellar surfaces was quantified using a method reliant on the formation of a chromophoric Fe(III) ion–ALE complex. The optical emission properties of the C-dots were still preserved after their incorporation into the hydrophobic micellar core, suggesting that the obtained optically traceable nanostructures can act as luminescent probes if exploited for in vitro studies. Furthermore, the HA NPs were synthesized and characterized in terms of their morphology and chemical composition. These HA NPs were used to assess the potential ability of the ALE-conjugated nanostructures towards the primary component of the rigid bone structure. The overall findings underscore the efficacy of the mentioned nanoformulations as promising and novel optically traceable candidates for their use in in vitro studies, serving in the initial stages for validation in achieving efficient active bone targeting. Ultimately, this could pave the way for their prospective application in addressing SREs associated with cancer metastases in the future.

Supplementary Materials: The following supporting information can be downloaded at https://www.mdpi.com/article/10.3390/molecules29102367/s1. Figure S1. PL emission spectra of micellar nanostructures prepared at different starting C-dot/PEG–phospholipid weight ratio percentages. Figure S2. Calibration curve of C-dots assessed using PL spectroscopy (λex 360 nm) and the absolute QY (%) of C-dots in $CHCl_3$ dispersion and C-dots/micelles, VitD/C-dots/micelles, and VitD/C-dots/ALE–micelles nanoformulations redispersed in $CHCl_3$. Figure S3. UV-Vis absorption spectrum of the VitD3 and the calibration curve of the VitD3. Figure S4. UV-Vis absorption spectrum of Fe^{3+} and synthesized ALE-Fe^{3+} complex. Figure S5. The 1H and 31P NMR spectra of the target alendronate.

Author Contributions: Conceptualization, N.D. (Nunzio Denora) and N.D. (Nicoletta Depalo); methodology, A.P., R.C., E.F., N.D. (Nunzio Denora) and N.D. (Nicoletta Depalo); formal analysis, F.R., A.P., I.A., E.F., R.M.I. and M.G.P.; investigation, F.R., A.P., I.A., R.C., R.M.I. and M.G.P.; resources, R.C., M.S., M.L.C., A.S., N.D. (Nunzio Denora) and N.D. (Nicoletta Depalo); data curation, F.R., A.P., E.F., M.L.C., and N.D. (Nicoletta Depalo); writing—original draft preparation, F.R., A.P., E.F., M.L.C., A.S. and N.D. (Nicoletta Depalo); writing—review and editing, A.P., R.C., E.F., M.S., M.L.C., A.S., N.D. (Nunzio Denora) and N.D. (Nicoletta Depalo); supervision, N.D. (Nunzio Denora) and N.D. (Nicoletta Depalo); funding acquisition, R.C., M.S., M.L.C., A.S., N.D. (Nunzio Denora) and N.D. (Nicoletta Depalo). All authors have read and agreed to the published version of the manuscript.

Funding: This research received no external funding.

Institutional Review Board Statement: Not applicable.

Informed Consent Statement: Not applicable.

Data Availability Statement: Data are contained within the article and Supplementary Materials.

Acknowledgments: This work was funded by Project PRIN 2022 PNRR (code P2022RLFZB), Nanocrystalline Hydroxyapatite for the Local Delivery of Anticancer agents in the Treatment of Bone Tumors and Metastases (NHYLODEA); Bilateral Project CNR-RFBR Russia Joint Research Project (2021–2023); TITAN Tumor Immunotherapy by Nanotechnology, Project ID:PON ARS01_00906 I (PVO-704); Academic Horizon Europe Seeds Project BIOMAD funded by the University of Bari (Italy); the Ministry of Economic Development (MISE) "GENESI" (code 092-Prog n. F/180003/03/X43) for the development of innovative radiopharmaceuticals and biomarkers for the diagnosis of cancers of the male and female reproductive system (2021–2023); and (f) the First AIRC-MFAG2015 Grant (Project Id. 17566). We thank Morena Miciaccia, Salvatore Savino, and Anna Maria Toscano for their contribution to the synthesis of alendronic acid in the earliest phase of the work.

Conflicts of Interest: The authors declare no conflict of interest.

References

1. Coleman, R.; Hadji, P.; Body, J.J.; Santini, D.; Chow, E.; Terpos, E.; Oudard, S.; Bruland, Ø.; Flamen, P.; Kurth, A.; et al. Bone health in cancer: ESMO Clinical Practice Guidelines†. *Ann. Oncol.* **2020**, *31*, 1650–1663. [CrossRef]
2. Coleman, R. Bone-Targeted Agents and Metastasis Prevention. *Cancers* **2022**, *14*, 3640. [CrossRef] [PubMed]
3. De Rosa, G.; Misso, G.; Salzano, G.; Caraglia, M. Bisphosphonates and Cancer: What Opportunities from Nanotechnology? *J. Drug Deliv.* **2013**, *2013*, 637976. [CrossRef] [PubMed]
4. Buranrat, B.; Bootha, S. Antiproliferative and antimigratory activities of bisphosphonates in human breast cancer cell line MCF-7. *Oncol. Lett.* **2019**, *18*, 1246–1258. [CrossRef]
5. Altundag, O.; Altundag, K.; Selim Silay, Y.; Gunduz, M.; Demircan, K.; Gullu, I. Calcium and vitamin D supplementation during bisphosphonate administration may increase osteoclastic activity in patients with bone metastasis. *Med. Hypotheses* **2004**, *63*, 1010–1013. [CrossRef]
6. Asfour, M.H.; Abd El-Alim, S.H.; Kassem, A.A.; Salama, A.; Gouda, A.S.; Nazim, W.S.; Nashaat, N.H.; Hemimi, M.; Abdel Meguid, N. Vitamin D3-Loaded Nanoemulsions as a Potential Drug Delivery System for Autistic Children: Formulation Development, Safety, and Pharmacokinetic Studies. *AAPS PharmSciTech* **2023**, *24*, 58. [CrossRef]
7. Edlich, R.; Mason, S.S.; Chase, M.E.; Fisher, A.L.; Gubler, K.; Long, W.B., 3rd; Giesy, J.D.; Foley, M.L. Scientific documentation of the relationship of vitamin D deficiency and the development of cancer. *J. Environ. Pathol. Toxicol. Oncol.* **2009**, *28*, 133–141. [CrossRef] [PubMed]
8. Seraphin, G.; Rieger, S.; Hewison, M.; Capobianco, E.; Lisse, T.S. The impact of vitamin D on cancer: A mini review. *J. Steroid Biochem. Mol. Biol.* **2023**, *231*, 106308. [CrossRef]
9. Holick, M.F. Vitamin D: Importance in the prevention of cancers, type 1 diabetes, heart disease, and osteoporosis12345. *Am. J. Clin. Nutr.* **2004**, *79*, 362–371. [CrossRef]
10. Heaney, R.P.; Recker, R.R.; Grote, J.; Horst, R.L.; Armas, L.A. Vitamin D(3) is more potent than vitamin D(2) in humans. *J. Clin. Endocrinol. Metab.* **2011**, *96*, E447–E452. [CrossRef]
11. Ramalho, M.J.; Loureiro, J.A.; Gomes, B.; Frasco, M.F.; Coelho, M.A.N.; Pereira, M.C. PLGA nanoparticles as a platform for vitamin D-based cancer therapy. *Beilstein J. Nanotechnol.* **2015**, *6*, 1306–1318. [CrossRef] [PubMed]
12. Maria, J.R.; Manuel, A.N.C.; Maria, C.P. Nanoparticles for Delivery of Vitamin D: Challenges and Opportunities. In *A Critical Evaluation of Vitamin D*; Sivakumar, G., Ed.; IntechOpen: Rijeka, Croatia, 2017; Chapter 11.
13. Agwa, M.M.; Abu-Serie, M.M.; Abdelmonsif, D.A.; Moussa, N.; Elsayed, H.; Khattab, S.N.; Sabra, S. Vitamin D3/phospholipid complex decorated caseinate nanomicelles for targeted delivery of synergistic combination therapy in breast cancer. *Int. J. Pharm.* **2021**, *607*, 120965. [CrossRef] [PubMed]
14. Dałek, P.; Drabik, D.; Wołczańska, H.; Foryś, A.; Jagas, M.; Jędruchniewicz, N.; Przybyło, M.; Witkiewicz, W.; Langner, M. Bioavailability by design—Vitamin D(3) liposomal delivery vehicles. *Nanomedicine* **2022**, *43*, 102552. [CrossRef] [PubMed]
15. Nagy, N.A.; Lozano Vigario, F.; Sparrius, R.; van Capel, T.M.M.; van Ree, R.; Tas, S.W.; de Vries, I.J.M.; Geijtenbeek, T.B.H.; Slütter, B.; de Jong, E.C.; et al. Liposomes loaded with vitamin D3 induce regulatory circuits in human dendritic cells. *Front. Immunol.* **2023**, *14*, 1137538. [CrossRef] [PubMed]
16. Du, M.; Chang, C.; Zhang, X.; Zhang, Y.; Radford, M.J.; Gahler, R.J.; Kuo, Y.C.; Wood, S.; Solnier, J. Designing Vitamin D3 Formulations: An In Vitro Investigation Using a Novel Micellar Delivery System. *Nutraceuticals* **2023**, *3*, 290–305. [CrossRef]
17. Dissanayake, R.K.; Perera, K.D.C.; Perera, W.P.T.D.; Wijesinghe, W.P.S.L.; Unagolla, J.M. Enteric Coated Oral Delivery of Hydroxyapatite Nanoparticle for Modified Release Vitamin D_3 Formulation. *J. Nanomater.* **2021**, *2021*, 9972475. [CrossRef]
18. Scala, R.; Maqoud, F.; McClenaghan, C.; Harter, T.M.; Perrone, M.G.; Scilimati, A.; Nichols, C.G.; Tricarico, D. Zoledronic Acid Blocks Overactive Kir6.1/SUR2-Dependent K(ATP) Channels in Skeletal Muscle and Osteoblasts in a Murine Model of Cantú Syndrome. *Cells* **2023**, *12*, 928. [CrossRef] [PubMed]
19. Scala, R.; Maqoud, F.; Antonacci, M.; Dibenedetto, J.R.; Perrone, M.G.; Scilimati, A.; Castillo, K.; Latorre, R.; Conte, D.; Bendahhou, S.; et al. Bisphosphonates Targeting Ion Channels and Musculoskeletal Effects. *Front. Pharmacol.* **2022**, *13*, 837534. [CrossRef] [PubMed]

20. Scala, R.; Maqoud, F.; Angelelli, M.; Latorre, R.; Perrone, M.G.; Scilimati, A.; Tricarico, D. Zoledronic Acid Modulation of TRPV1 Channel Currents in Osteoblast Cell Line and Native Rat and Mouse Bone Marrow-Derived Osteoblasts: Cell Proliferation and Mineralization Effect. *Cancers* **2019**, *11*, 206. [CrossRef]
21. Shao, H.; Varamini, P. Breast Cancer Bone Metastasis: A Narrative Review of Emerging Targeted Drug Delivery Systems. *Cells* **2022**, *11*, 388. [CrossRef]
22. de Miguel, L.; Noiray, M.; Surpateanu, G.; Iorga, B.I.; Ponchel, G. Poly(γ-benzyl-l-glutamate)-PEG-alendronate multivalent nanoparticles for bone targeting. *Int. J. Pharm.* **2014**, *460*, 73–82. [CrossRef] [PubMed]
23. He, Y.; Huang, Y.; Huang, Z.; Jiang, Y.; Sun, X.; Shen, Y.; Chu, W.; Zhao, C. Bisphosphonate-functionalized coordination polymer nanoparticles for the treatment of bone metastatic breast cancer. *J. Control. Release* **2017**, *264*, 76–88. [CrossRef] [PubMed]
24. Mehnath, S.; Karthikeyan, K.; Rajan, M.; Jeyaraj, M. Fabrication of bone-targeting hyaluronic acid coupled alendronate-bioactive glass for osteosarcoma therapy. *Mater. Chem. Phys.* **2021**, *273*, 125146. [CrossRef]
25. Pham, T.T.; Nguyen, H.T.; Phung, C.D.; Pathak, S.; Regmi, S.; Ha, D.-H.; Kim, J.O.; Yong, C.S.; Kim, S.K.; Choi, J.-E.; et al. Targeted delivery of doxorubicin for the treatment of bone metastasis from breast cancer using alendronate-functionalized graphene oxide nanosheets. *J. Ind. Eng. Chem.* **2019**, *76*, 310–317. [CrossRef]
26. Sun, W.; Han, Y.; Li, Z.; Ge, K.; Zhang, J. Bone-Targeted Mesoporous Silica Nanocarrier Anchored by Zoledronate for Cancer Bone Metastasis. *Langmuir* **2016**, *32*, 9237–9244. [CrossRef] [PubMed]
27. Nieto, A.; Balas, F.; Colilla, M.; Manzano, M.; Vallet-Regí, M. Functionalization degree of SBA-15 as key factor to modulate sodium alendronate dosage. *Microporous Mesoporous Mater.* **2008**, *116*, 4–13. [CrossRef]
28. Cong, Y.; Quan, C.; Liu, M.; Liu, J.; Huang, G.; Tong, G.; Yin, Y.; Zhang, C.; Jiang, Q. Alendronate-decorated biodegradable polymeric micelles for potential bone-targeted delivery of vancomycin. *J. Biomater. Sci. Polym. Ed.* **2015**, *26*, 629–643. [CrossRef] [PubMed]
29. Kadu, K.; Hemmadi, V.; Biswas, M.; Kowshik, M.; Ramanan, S.R. Novel hydroxyapatite nanoparticle-based antibiotic alternative to combat methicillin-resistant S. aureus: A mechanism by targeting the structural and functional stability of MRSA membrane protein. *J. Mater. Res.* **2023**, *38*, 1609–1619. [CrossRef]
30. Farrell, K.B.; Karpeisky, A.; Thamm, D.H.; Zinnen, S. Bisphosphonate conjugation for bone specific drug targeting. *Bone Rep.* **2018**, *9*, 47–60. [CrossRef]
31. Stapleton, M.; Sawamoto, K.; Alméciga-Díaz, C.J.; Mackenzie, W.G.; Mason, R.W.; Orii, T.; Tomatsu, S. Development of Bone Targeting Drugs. *Int. J. Mol. Sci.* **2017**, *18*, 1345. [CrossRef]
32. Pascaud, P.; Gras, P.; Coppel, Y.; Rey, C.; Sarda, S. Interaction between a Bisphosphonate, Tiludronate, and Biomimetic Nanocrystalline Apatites. *Langmuir* **2013**, *29*, 2224–2232. [CrossRef] [PubMed]
33. Boanini, E.; Gazzano, M.; Rubini, K.; Bigi, A. Composite Nanocrystals Provide New Insight on Alendronate Interaction with Hydroxyapatite Structure. *Adv. Mater.* **2007**, *19*, 2499–2502. [CrossRef]
34. Wang, B.; Cai, H.; Waterhouse, G.I.N.; Qu, X.; Yang, B.; Lu, S. Carbon Dots in Bioimaging, Biosensing and Therapeutics: A Comprehensive Review. *Small Sci.* **2022**, *2*, 2200012. [CrossRef]
35. Depalo, N.; Iacobazzi, R.M.; Valente, G.; Arduino, I.; Villa, S.; Canepa, F.; Laquintana, V.; Fanizza, E.; Striccoli, M.; Cutrignelli, A.; et al. Sorafenib delivery nanoplatform based on superparamagnetic iron oxide nanoparticles magnetically targets hepatocellular carcinoma. *Nano Res.* **2017**, *10*, 2431–2448. [CrossRef]
36. Depalo, N.; Carrieri, P.; Comparelli, R.; Striccoli, M.; Agostiano, A.; Bertinetti, L.; Innocenti, C.; Sangregorio, C.; Curri, M.L. Biofunctionalization of Anisotropic Nanocrystalline Semiconductor–Magnetic Heterostructures. *Langmuir* **2011**, *27*, 6962–6970. [CrossRef] [PubMed]
37. Valente, G.; Depalo, N.; de Paola, I.; Iacobazzi, R.M.; Denora, N.; Laquintana, V.; Comparelli, R.; Altamura, E.; Latronico, T.; Altomare, M.; et al. Integrin-targeting with peptide-bioconjugated semiconductor-magnetic nanocrystalline heterostructures. *Nano Res.* **2016**, *9*, 644–662. [CrossRef]
38. Depalo, N.; Mallardi, A.; Comparelli, R.; Striccoli, M.; Agostiano, A.; Curri, M.L. Luminescent nanocrystals in phospholipid micelles for bioconjugation: An optical and structural investigation. *J. Colloid Interface Sci.* **2008**, *325*, 558–566. [CrossRef]
39. Depalo, N.; De Leo, V.; Corricelli, M.; Gristina, R.; Valente, G.; Casamassima, E.; Comparelli, R.; Laquintana, V.; Denora, N.; Fanizza, E.; et al. Lipid-based systems loaded with PbS nanocrystals: Near infrared emitting trackable nanovectors. *J. Mater. Chem. B* **2017**, *5*, 1471–1481. [CrossRef] [PubMed]
40. Latronico, T.; Depalo, N.; Valente, G.; Fanizza, E.; Laquintana, V.; Denora, N.; Fasano, A.; Striccoli, M.; Colella, M.; Agostiano, A.; et al. Cytotoxicity Study on Luminescent Nanocrystals Containing Phospholipid Micelles in Primary Cultures of Rat Astrocytes. *PLoS ONE* **2016**, *11*, e0153451. [CrossRef]
41. Panniello, A.; Di Mauro, A.E.; Fanizza, E.; Depalo, N.; Agostiano, A.; Curri, M.L.; Striccoli, M. Luminescent Oil-Soluble Carbon Dots toward White Light Emission: A Spectroscopic Study. *J. Phys. Chem. C* **2018**, *122*, 839–849. [CrossRef]
42. Wang, J.; Fang, X.; Liang, W. Pegylated Phospholipid Micelles Induce Endoplasmic Reticulum-Dependent Apoptosis of Cancer Cells but not Normal Cells. *ACS Nano* **2012**, *6*, 5018–5030. [CrossRef]
43. Cheng, X.; Wei, J.; Ge, Q.; Xing, D.; Zhou, X.; Qian, Y.; Jiang, G. The optimized drug delivery systems of treating cancer bone metastatic osteolysis with nanomaterials. *Drug Deliv.* **2021**, *28*, 37–53. [CrossRef]
44. Giordano, F.; Lenna, S.; Rampado, R.; Brozovich, A.; Hirase, T.; Tognon, M.G.; Martini, F.; Agostini, M.; Yustein, J.T.; Taraballi, F. Nanodelivery Systems Face Challenges and Limitations in Bone Diseases Management. *Adv. Ther.* **2021**, *4*, 2100152. [CrossRef]

45. Di Nunno, L.; Di Nunno, L.; Scilimati, A. Synthesis of 3-aryl-4, 5-dihydro-5-hydroxy-1,2-oxazoles by reaction of substituted benzonitrile oxides with the enolate ion of acetaldehyde. *Tetrahedron* **1987**, *43*, 2181–2189. [CrossRef]
46. Kuljanin, J.; Janković, I.; Nedeljković, J.; Prstojević, D.; Marinković, V. Spectrophotometric determination of alendronate in pharmaceutical formulations via complex formation with Fe(III) ions. *J. Pharm. Biomed. Anal.* **2002**, *28*, 1215–1220. [CrossRef]
47. Savino, S.; Toscano, A.; Purgatorio, R.; Profilo, E.; Laghezza, A.; Tortorella, P.; Angelelli, M.; Cellamare, S.; Scala, R.; Tricarico, D.; et al. Novel bisphosphonates with antiresorptive effect in bone mineralization and osteoclastogenesis. *Eur. J. Med. Chem.* **2018**, *158*, 184–200. [CrossRef]
48. Wang, S.; Mamedova, N.; Kotov, N.A.; Chen, W.; Studer, J. Antigen/Antibody Immunocomplex from CdTe Nanoparticle Bioconjugates. *Nano Lett.* **2002**, *2*, 817–822. [CrossRef]
49. Reissig, F.; Hübner, R.; Steinbach, J.; Pietzsch, H.-J.; Mamat, C. Facile preparation of radium-doped, functionalized nanoparticles as carriers for targeted alpha therapy. *Inorg. Chem. Front.* **2019**, *6*, 1341–1349. [CrossRef]
50. Liu, X.; Qu, S.; Lu, X.; Ge, X.; Leng, Y. Time-of-flight secondary ion mass spectrometry study on the distribution of alendronate sodium in drug-loaded ultra-high molecular weight polyethylene. *Biomed. Mater.* **2009**, *4*, 065008. [CrossRef]
51. Turhanen, P.A.; Vepsäläinen, J.J.; Peräniemi, S. Advanced material and approach for metal ions removal from aqueous solutions. *Sci. Rep.* **2015**, *5*, 8992. [CrossRef]
52. Ke, J.; Dou, H.; Zhang, X.; Uhagaze, D.S.; Ding, X.; Dong, Y. Determination of pKa values of alendronate sodium in aqueous solution by piecewise linear regression based on acid-base potentiometric titration. *J. Pharm. Anal.* **2016**, *6*, 404–409. [CrossRef]
53. Hengst, V.; Oussoren, C.; Kissel, T.; Storm, G. Bone targeting potential of bisphosphonate-targeted liposomes. Preparation, characterization and hydroxyapatite binding in vitro. *Int. J. Pharm.* **2007**, *331*, 224–227. [CrossRef]
54. Miller, K.; Eldar-Boock, A.; Polyak, D.; Segal, E.; Benayoun, L.; Shaked, Y.; Satchi-Fainaro, R. Antiangiogenic Antitumor Activity of HPMA Copolymer–Paclitaxel–Alendronate Conjugate on Breast Cancer Bone Metastasis Mouse Model. *Mol. Pharm.* **2011**, *8*, 1052–1062. [CrossRef]
55. Ozcan, I.; Bouchemal, K.; Segura-Sánchez, F.; Ozer, O.; Güneri, T.; Ponchel, G. Synthesis and characterization of surface-modified PBLG nanoparticles for bone targeting: In vitro and in vivo evaluations. *J. Pharm. Sci.* **2011**, *100*, 4877–4887. [CrossRef]
56. Torres Martin de Rosales, R.; Finucane, C.; Mather, S.J.; Blower, P.J. Bifunctional bisphosphonate complexes for the diagnosis and therapy of bone metastases. *Chem. Commun.* **2009**, *32*, 4847–4849. [CrossRef]
57. Uludag, H.; Kousinioris, N.; Gao, T.; Kantoci, D. Bisphosphonate Conjugation to Proteins as a Means to Impart Bone Affinity. *Biotechnol. Prog.* **2000**, *16*, 258–267. [CrossRef]
58. Chen, H.; Li, G.; Chi, H.; Wang, D.; Tu, C.; Pan, L.; Zhu, L.; Qiu, F.; Guo, F.; Zhu, X. Alendronate-conjugated amphiphilic hyperbranched polymer based on Boltorn H40 and poly(ethylene glycol) for bone-targeted drug delivery. *Bioconjug. Chem.* **2012**, *23*, 1915–1924. [CrossRef]
59. Habibah, T.U.; Salisbury, H.G. Hydroxyapatite Dental Material. In *StatPearls*; StatPearls Publishing: Treasure Island, FL, USA, 2019.
60. Beaufils, S.; Rouillon, T.; Millet, P.; Le Bideau, J.; Weiss, P.; Chopart, J.-P.; Daltin, A.-L. Synthesis of calcium-deficient hydroxyapatite nanowires and nanotubes performed by template-assisted electrodeposition. *Mater. Sci. Eng. C* **2019**, *98*, 333–346. [CrossRef]
61. Latronico, T.; Rizzi, F.; Panniello, A.; Laquintana, V.; Arduino, I.; Denora, N.; Fanizza, E.; Milella, S.; Mastroianni, C.M.; Striccoli, M.; et al. Luminescent PLGA Nanoparticles for Delivery of Darunavir to the Brain and Inhibition of Matrix Metalloproteinase-9, a Relevant Therapeutic Target of HIV-Associated Neurological Disorders. *ACS Chem. Neurosci.* **2021**, *12*, 4286–4301. [CrossRef]

molecules

MDPI

Article

Pioglitazone Phases and Metabolic Effects in Nanoparticle-Treated Cells Analyzed via Rapid Visualization of FLIM Images

Biagio Todaro [1,*], Luca Pesce [1], Francesco Cardarelli [1] and Stefano Luin [1,2,*]

1 NEST Laboratory, Scuola Normale Superiore, Piazza San Silvestro 12, 56127 Pisa, Italy; luca.pesce1@sns.it (L.P.); francesco.cardarelli@sns.it (F.C.)
2 NEST Laboratory, Istituto Nanoscienze-CNR, Piazza San Silvestro 12, 56127 Pisa, Italy
* Correspondence: biagio.todaro@sns.it (B.T.); s.luin@sns.it (S.L.)

Abstract: Fluorescence lifetime imaging microscopy (FLIM) has proven to be a useful method for analyzing various aspects of material science and biology, like the supramolecular organization of (slightly) fluorescent compounds or the metabolic activity in non-labeled cells; in particular, FLIM phasor analysis (phasor-FLIM) has the potential for an intuitive representation of complex fluorescence decays and therefore of the analyzed properties. Here we present and make available tools to fully exploit this potential, in particular by coding via hue, saturation, and intensity the phasor positions and their weights both in the phasor plot and in the microscope image. We apply these tools to analyze FLIM data acquired via two-photon microscopy to visualize: (i) different phases of the drug pioglitazone (PGZ) in solutions and/or crystals, (ii) the position in the phasor plot of non-labelled poly(lactic-co-glycolic acid) (PLGA) nanoparticles (NPs), and (iii) the effect of PGZ or PGZ-containing NPs on the metabolism of insulinoma (INS-1 E) model cells. PGZ is recognized for its efficacy in addressing insulin resistance and hyperglycemia in type 2 diabetes mellitus, and polymeric nanoparticles offer versatile platforms for drug delivery due to their biocompatibility and controlled release kinetics. This study lays the foundation for a better understanding via phasor-FLIM of the organization and effects of drugs, in particular, PGZ, within NPs, aiming at better control of encapsulation and pharmacokinetics, and potentially at novel anti-diabetics theragnostic nanotools.

Keywords: fluorescence lifetime imaging microscopy (FLIM); pioglitazone characterization; insulinoma (INS-1) cells; PLGA nanoparticles; phasor-FLIM analysis; MATLAB tool; drug delivery

1. Introduction

Fluorescence lifetime analysis (FLA) has demonstrated significant potential for non-invasive, real-time analysis across a diverse range of compounds and materials. Specifically within biomedicine, it has been applied in several key areas, like (i) measurement of intracellular biochemical parameters [1–7], (ii) resolving the physical state of encapsulated fluorescent drugs [8–18]; and (iii) biomedical diagnostics and neuroscience research [19–27].

Fluorescence lifetime imaging microscopy (FLIM), unlike traditional fluorescence microscopy where the contrast is given by emission intensity, delves into the time dimension of fluorescence decay. In the simplest implementation, the contrast is given by fluorescence lifetime, the average time a fluorophore remains in the excited state before emitting a photon. This temporal information can unveil valuable insights into the microenvironment, molecular interactions, and biochemical properties of fluorophores since fluorophores exhibit characteristic fluorescence decay patterns influenced by their surroundings. These decay patterns provide a quantitative means to assess molecular processes, such as energy transfer, molecular binding, and changes in local pH. In particular, FLIM has been widely used to analyze cells' metabolic states, starting with the pioneering work of Ragan et al. (1969) focused on the oxidation–reduction changes in flavin and pyridine nucleotides in perfused rat liver [28]. Lakowicz et al. (1992) conducted work on imaging the short-lived fluorescence of both free and protein-bound NADH, determining the changes in their ratio, a critical parameter for assessing cellular metabolism [29]. Ferri et al. (2020) recently exploited this parameter for investigating the metabolic response of Insulinoma 1E cells to glucose stimulation, and Azzarello et al. (2022) used it to examine the metabolic response of α and β cells to glucose in living human Langerhans islets [30,31].

However, the average lifetime is not always enough to characterize the decay patterns; one can study the complete decay curves, fitting them with multiexponential decays, in order to dissect various contributions in each pixel of an image. However, fit parameters often have too big uncertainties, especially if the single component lifetimes are too close (closer than a factor of 2 or 3) and if the measurements are noisy, as it happens especially in the case of fast measurements. Moreover, each component is characterized by an amplitude and a lifetime, and all these parameters are not always easy to represent in an image. A valid alternative for representing FLIM data is given by the phasor approach (phasor-FLIM): this involves transforming fluorescence decay data into points on a phasor plot, essentially a two-dimensional representation in the complex plane of the Fourier transform of the decay curve at a fixed frequency, with real component G on the x-axis and imaginary component S on the y-axis. Each pixel in a FLIM "image" is mapped to a position in the phasor plot, creating clusters of data points that represent various fluorescence decay characteristics. In the case of a monoexponential decay, expected for a simple pure compound in solution, the phasor falls along the universal semicircle (centered on (1/2, 1/2) and with radius 1/2, for positive S), with shorter lifetimes more on the right; for bi- or multi-exponential decays, the phasor falls within this semicircle. When more than a compound is present in a pixel, the phasor falls in a position given by the average of the phasors of each compound weighted by the contribution of the compound to the total intensity of fluorescence in that pixel; in simpler terms, the phasor position in such cases is given by the linear combination of the ones of pure compounds. This aspect provides valuable and intuitive insights into the compounds composition within a pixel of an image, allowing for a more comprehensive understanding of complex molecular environments.

For example, Stringari et al. (2011) utilized the phasor approach to distinguish various metabolic states of germ cells in live tissue, providing crucial insights into cellular metabolic function [2]. A recent study by Tentori et al. (2022) demonstrated the utility of phasor-FLIM in unveiling the supramolecular organization of doxorubicin (DOX) in the standard Doxoves® liposomal formulation (DOX®), underscoring its potential in elucidating the complex interplay between nanoparticles and biological systems. They determined that DOX® includes three different fractions: crystallized DOX (98%), free DOX (1.4%), and an unexpected liposomal-membrane-bound DOX (0.7%); relative concentrations were determined through phasor-FLIM and spectroscopy on pure standards, demonstrating applicability for studying the state of encapsulated drugs from the production to within living matter [15]. A bottleneck that still affects FLIM adoption by a broader audience is the lack of a facile tool for presenting in an intuitive way the large amount of data generated, particularly for researchers without extensive expertise in data analysis [32]. There are some pieces of software developed to this aim: commercial ones such as those provided by Becker & Hickl GmbH (Berlin, Germany), PicoQuant (Berlin, Germany), or Leica Microsystems (now part of Danaher, Washington, DC, USA), and a few freely distributed ones such as SimFCS, FLUTE, PAM and one developed by some of us [33–36]. However, they are still limited in representing the whole two-dimensional phasor plane in the FLIM image, using a color scale changing mostly in one direction within the phasor plot or just highlighting in the image a subset of the phasor plot.

From a biomedical point of view, polymeric nanoparticles (NPs), and in particular poly(lactic-co-glycolic acid) (PLGA), have garnered significant interest as versatile drug delivery platforms due to their biocompatibility, controlled release kinetics, and tunable physicochemical properties [37–39]. Recent advancements in nanoparticle engineering, including surface modification and functionalization, offer opportunities to enhance drug encapsulation efficiency, target-specific delivery, and cellular uptake [40–51]. In particular, a drug that would benefit from an NP formulation is pioglitazone (PGZ), a thiazolidinedione derivative, which is a well-known pharmacological agent for addressing insulin resistance and hyperglycemia in type 2 diabetes mellitus (T2DM) patients. Metabolic disorders, such as T2DM, present a significant global health challenge, driving the exploration of innovative monitoring devices for diabetes management and therapeutic approaches to mitigate associated complications and improve patient outcomes [52,53]. In this context, the PGZ mechanism of action involves the activation of peroxisome proliferator-activated receptor gamma (PPARγ), a nuclear receptor pivotal in regulating glucose and lipid metabolism, adipogenesis, and inflammation. Despite PGZ's clinical efficacy, challenges related to its pharmacokinetic properties, including low solubility and bioavailability, underscore the importance of exploring innovative drug delivery strategies to optimize therapeutic outcomes. A recent study from Todaro et al. (2022) elucidated the most reliable synthesis method for PGZ-loaded PLGA nanoparticles, highlighting the potential of PLGA as a suitable nanocarrier material and demonstrating controlled release capabilities for PGZ [54]. The nanoprecipitation method employed for these formulations has proven effective, showcasing favorable attributes such as size, polydispersity index, encapsulation efficiency, drug loading, cost-effectiveness, and processing time [54]. The successful synthesis and characterization of PGZ-loaded PLGA NPs set the stage for a deeper investigation into the drug's intrinsic fluorescence signals. Among all the methods available for the polymeric NPs characterization [55–62], FLIM can play an important role in terms of manufacturing process control, and also explain drug pharmacokinetics properties.

Here, we present and make available a tool (coded in MATLAB) that maps the whole phasor plot to different hue and saturation values and represents the distribution in the phasor plot with an intensity that considers each pixel intensity in the image. The color map can be chosen in different ways, in order to characterize more than two possible coexisting decays characteristics of possibly different fluorescent molecules.

As a proof of concept, we apply this tool to the study of different phases of PGZ, and we analyze its effects (both when free and encapsulated within NPs) on the metabolism of INS-1E cells, an insulinoma cell line. Indeed, the investigation presented in this article exploits PGZ intrinsic fluorescence to collect information regarding its physical state through the application of FLIM, by analyzing the differences in the fluorescence decay of PGZ when existing in various states, such as dry crystalline, solvated, or dissolved forms. Furthermore, we present the observed phasor distributions for PLGA nanoparticles, empty or encapsulating PGZ. Finally, we investigate cellular NAD(P)H autofluorescence variations between its free and bound form in the presence of PGZ-loaded PLGA nanoparticles.

2. Results

We developed an algorithm, implemented in MATLAB R2017B (and tested in version R2023B), which allows determining at a glance the position in the phasor plot of the phasor corresponding to each pixel in the image; in the phasor plot, the phasors distribution is weighted with the intensity in each pixel, and is shown with colors corresponding to the ones in the image. The colors are determined in order to highlight the position of the phasors with respect to chosen "principal" points in the phasor plot, ideally corresponding to the position for pure fluorophores, and in particular with respect to the segments joining them. The first examples of this representation are reported in Figure 1, using the same color coding in every image, with a light gray triangle superimposed on the phasor plots that highlights the considered principal points at its vertices; the choice of these principal points will be explained in the following section. Intensities are shown in a linear but also in a logarithmic scale, in order to appreciate the shape of the observed features, but also the less intense "tails" of the phasor distribution and the less intense pixels in the image, respectively.

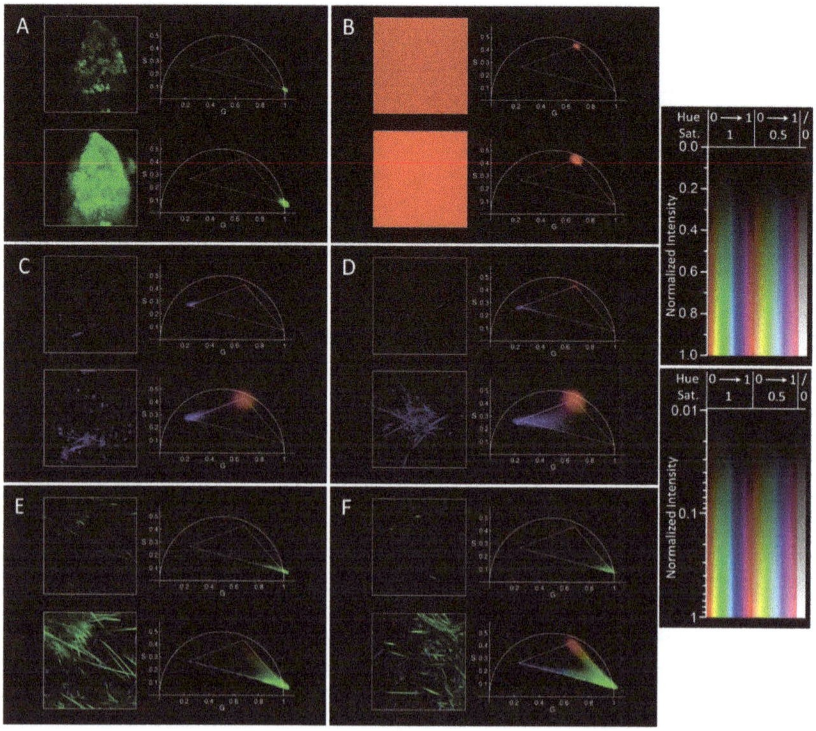

Figure 1. Characterization of free PGZ using FLIM. For each panel, on the left are reported the FLIM images and on the right the phasor plots (with corresponding colors): (**A**) PGZ solid, (**B**) PGZ in DMF at 37 °C at time 0, (**C**) PGZ in DMF at 37 °C at 20 min, (**D**) at 30 min, (**E**) at 50 min, and (**F**) at 55 min in a different position; in the phasor plot, vertices of the triangle correspond to the "principal" points, and the "center" point, where the saturation is 0 (see Sections 3 and 4.5) is shown in cyan. For all the panels: on top, figures with a linear intensity scale (normalized to maximum); on the bottom, the same figures with a logarithmic intensity scale starting from a 0.01 fraction of the maximum intensity in the image; on the right these intensity scales are shown in corresponding positions for various values of hue and saturation. Note how the evaporation of DMF with time causes the formation of PGZ crystals, and that the used color coding based on the position of the phasor plot for each pixel allows appreciating at a glance the different forms of PGZ and their position within the images. The side of the square microscopy image is 106 μm here and in all the following figures.

2.1. *Phases of Pioglitazone (PGZ)*

The data reported in Figure 1 derive from a detailed examination, employing FLIM, of free PGZ in different conditions.

Initially, solid PGZ was examined on a glass slide, revealing a monoexponential decay characterized by a very short lifetime (phasor on the universal semicircle at high S and low G; Figure 1A); to this point, we assigned a hue of 1/3, corresponding to green. In parallel with what was observed on doxorubicin [5], we consider the observed short lifetime indicative of the crystalline nature of solid PGZ; the shortness of the lifetime is most probably caused by self-quenching of PGZ molecules strongly interacting with each other in the close packing of the crystal. We then analyzed PGZ dissolved in dimethylformamide (DMF), a solvent where it is highly soluble, differently than in water (we did not observe enough fluorescence intensity from a saturated solution of PGZ in water to determine its decay characteristics with our setup). DMF-solved PGZ presents an almost monoexponential decay at a longer, intermediate lifetime (Figure 1B, time 0 from the positioning of a drop of DMF with solved PGZ on the microscope cover glass). We assigned to this phasor position a hue of 0 (and 1), corresponding to red. Notice that we also measured a pure DMF solution, finding no autofluorescence (and therefore positions in the phasor plot close to the origin of axes, as expected for noise or for light uncorrelated with the pulsed laser reaching the detector). Leaving the drop at 37 °C, the DMF started to evaporate, the PGZ reached saturation, and crystals started to grow within the solution (Figure 1C,D). Unexpectedly, the phasor position in the pixels corresponding to these observed crystals did not fall close (or tended towards) the "green" point mentioned above; instead, they tended towards a different point in the phasor plot, corresponding to a longer multiexponential lifetime, and to which we assigned a hue of 2/3 corresponding to blue. We consider this a sign of a different crystal form, a "solvated crystal", where many DMF molecules (or possibly water impurities, since we did not use anhydrous DMF and all the experiments were performed in air, containing some humidity) enter in the composition of the crystal and influence the interactions amongst PGZ molecules. Note that in Figure 1C, with intensities represented with a linear scale, the two populations of the bright but less abundant pixels with solvated crystal and the dim but much more numerous pixels with solved PGZ are both visible in the phasor plot (while the last population would overwhelm the first one employing standard representations of the phasor plot), but this last population red color is not appreciable in the image on the left. Instead, using a logarithmic intensity scale, the "red" part of the image is evident, and the crystals can be seen in their entirety; in the phasor plot, a "smear" connecting the "blue" and "red" principal points is visible, and this corresponds to pixels where the point spread function contained both part of a crystal and part of the solution. In Figure 1D, a shift of the average phasor towards the crystalline region is observable, indicating the progression of crystallization, evident also from the higher number of bigger crystals in the image on the left. Moreover, some low-saturation points, also towards a green color, start to appear (visible especially in the figure with logarithmic intensity scale), indicative of the fact that some crystals more similar to the original ones begin to form. Subsequent analysis at 50 and 55 min revealed fluorescence arising predominantly from a crystalline sample, evidenced by a significant shift towards very short lifetimes in the phasor analysis (Figure 1E,F). These observations underscore the dynamics of PGZ dissolution and crystallization over time, allowing for the conceptualization of a triangle, with the three reference species (the solid form, the solved form, and the "solvated crystal" form of PGZ) at its vertices.

2.2. *Phasors of PGZ-Loaded PLGA NPs*

Subsequently, empty PLGA nanoparticles and PGZ-loaded PLGA NPs were synthesized and analyzed. The synthesis of these samples was carried out as previously described, with slight modifications [54]. The characterization of three independent formulations is shown in Table 1, demonstrating reproducibility over size, PDI, Z potential, and encapsulation efficiency.

The samples were analyzed at the microscope using FLIM. Unfortunately, repeating the experiments on different batches we observed very different values of fluorescence intensities and phasor positions. For both types of samples, phasors fell approximately along a line connecting the origin (phasor position of noise) and a point shown in the top right graph of panels A–E of Figure 2 as a light gray cross; this line passes very close to the vertex of the triangle corresponding to the solvated phase of PGZ. Moreover, for both samples, the phasors in case of high enough fluorescence were close to the point cited above. Some examples of these measurements are reported in panels A–D of Figure 2, on top of each panel with the same color coding and linear intensity scale used for the top half of each panel in Figure 1. Being a dispersion, in the images reported on the left part we can see a quite uniform field, with some possible aggregates (possibly moving during the measurements) visible especially for the experiments with the lowest fluorescence. These behaviors did not depend on the buffer where the NPs were dispersed (we used PBS and RPMI, the last for comparison with experiments in cells reported below). In order to understand the origin of these fluorescence decay characteristics, we measured the lifetime characteristic of solid PLGA, discovering an unexpected fluorescence, whose characteristic phasor fell on the point cited above (see Figure 2E). In this case, the observed image reported on the left is not optimal, most probably because we used the standard setup, and in particular an objective with silicon oil as immersion medium, to visualize a piece of mostly transparent solid placed on a cover glass in the air; in any case, the fluorescence decay characteristics do not depend on the quality of the image.

Table 1. Size distributions measured using a Zetasizer Nano ZS equipment (Malvern Instruments Ltd., Worcestershire, UK), and encapsulation efficiency (EE) % measured using an analytical RP-HPLC (Shimadzu Nexera UHPLC, equipped with a Shimadzu SPD-M20A UV/visible detector) instrument. The hydrodynamic radius ± SEM (standard error of the mean), polydispersity PDI ± SEM, ζ potential ± SEM, and PGZ encapsulation efficiency % ± SEM are indicated. Results from n = 3 repetitions of measures on each of the N = 3 independently manufactured nanoparticle batches (total of 9 measurements).

		Size (nm)	PDI	ζ Potential (mV)	EE %
PGZ-loaded PLGA NPs	Average	143.32	0.25	−11.27	27.37
	SEM	2.61	0.02	0.21	0.67
Empty NPs	Average	131.92	0.12	−13.76	/
	SEM	3.76	0.01	2.11	/

These experiments demonstrate the possibility of measuring PLGA nanoparticles with phasor-FLIM; however, the too high noise, the autofluorescence of the used PLGA most probably overwhelming the one of the encapsulated PGZ, and the closeness of the PLGA phasor to possible ones characterizing the PGZ do not allow for understanding the state of PGZ within the PLGA. One could check if different batches of PLGA present lower autofluorescence, and try to obtain more concentrated NPs colloids, but this is going beyond the scope of this work. We wanted to explore all the possible positions for the phasors linked to fluorescence arising from our NPs and to understand if there would be some fluorescence arising from them in the measurements presented in the following section.

In the images discussed above (top part of each panel A–E in Figure 2), all the phasors result in being blue/violet, even if they are in different positions. For the purpose of highlighting even more the potential of our algorithm in presenting phasor-FLIM data, we show in the bottom part of panels A–E of Figure 2 the same data, but using more and different "principal points" (in a clockwise order: the origin, the average phasor measured in a RPMI solution as shown in Figure 3A below, the point for solvated PGZ, and the average phasor position for solid PLGA, for dissolved PGZ, and for dry crystalline PGZ). This representation allows for easily visualizing the different observed decay characteristics for the NPs colloids. In particular, in panels A and B of Figure 2 we observe the same cyan color of PLGA, as shown in panel E. In panel C, we see a phasor distribution elongated along the line connecting the origin (or the RPMI typical phasor) with the PLGA phasor, intermediate between these points, with a green color. In panel D, we observe a phasor distribution closer to the "noise zone", and the different red to yellowish-green colors are quite mixed in the image on the left, demonstrating that the distribution is mostly caused by noise in the measurements, with just some possible aggregates with a more yellowish-green color, more towards the PLGA/NP typical phasor.

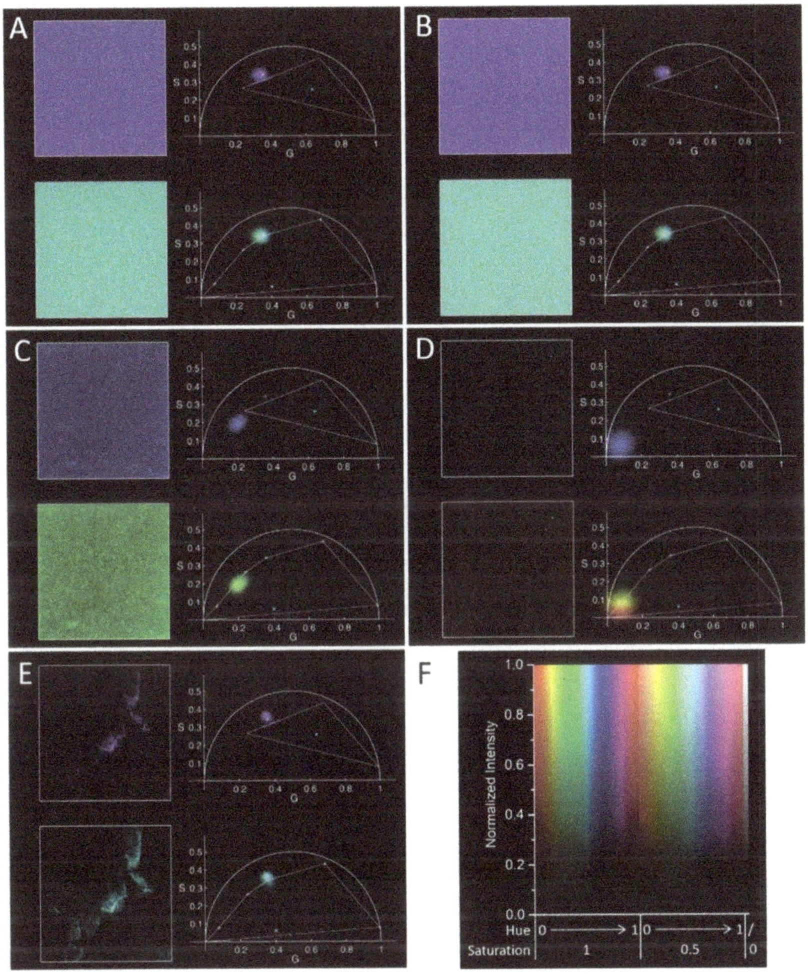

Figure 2. Characterization of empty PLGA nanoparticles and PGZ-loaded PLGA NPs using FLIM. For each panel, on the left are reported the FLIM images and on the right the phasor plots (with corresponding colors) for exemplary cases for NPs (**A**–**D**) and for solid PLGA (**E**): (**A**) empty PLGA NPs in RPMI, (**B**) PGZ-loaded PLGA NPs in RPMI, (**C**) empty PLGA NPs in PBS, (**D**) PGZ-loaded PLGA NPs in PBS, (**E**) solid PLGA. A linear scale was used for the intensity normalized to the maximum in each picture (like on top in Figure 1; color scale reported in panel (**F**)). Two color codes were used, one like in Figure 1 (top figures in each panel), one with additional principal points (see main text), as shown in the right bottom figure in each panel (vertices of the polygon and light gray crosses), with hue of 0/1 at (0,0) and increasing clockwise, and a "center" point (cyan ×) inside but towards the bottom of the polygon.

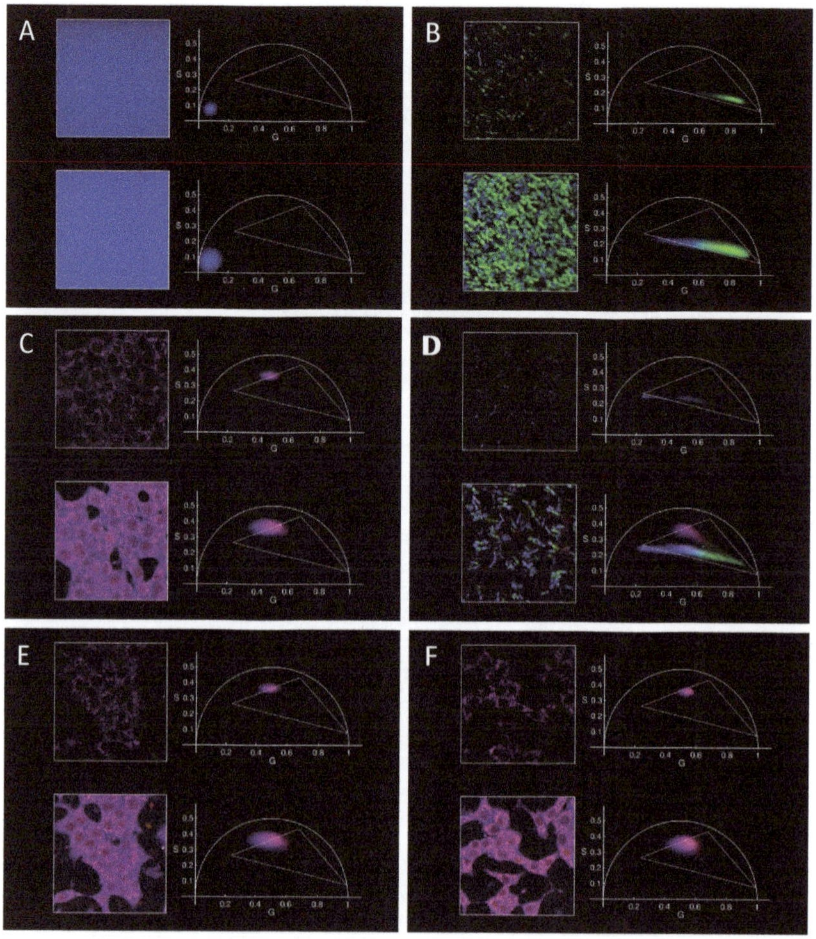

Figure 3. FLIM of PGZ and of INS-1E cells in RPMI medium, also upon co-incubation and incubation with nanoparticles for 24 h at 37 °C. (**A**) RPMI, (**B**) PGZ in RPMI, (**C**) INS-1E in RPMI, (**D**) INS-1E in RPMI in the presence of 0.1 mg/mL PGZ, (**E**) INS-1E in RPMI in presence of empty PLGA NPs, (**F**) INS-1E in RPMI in presence of PGZ-loaded PLGA NPs. Each panel has the same composition, color coding, and intensity scales as in Figure 1 (and in the top parts of the panels in Figure 2 for the linear intensity scale), in order to compare more easily the results and to show at-a-glance possible signals arising from the species observed in the previous cases.

2.3. *Autofluorescence Characteristics Changes in INS-1E Cell in the Presence of PGZ-Loaded PLGA NPs*

In the final experiments, we incubated INS-1E cell lines with the previously analyzed samples at 37 °C for 24 h and measured them in our two-photon FLIM microscope. First, we checked that the used RPMI medium was negligibly fluorescent, resulting in a phasor falling very close to the origin, the zone where noise falls (Figure 3A). As a control, 20 μL of 10 mg/mL PGZ was incubated in 1980 μL of RPMI at 37 °C (final nominal PGZ concentration of 0.1 mg/mL or ~280 μM), both alone (Figure 3B) and in the presence of cells (Figure 3C). In both cases, we observed a precipitation of PGZ, as expected for a maximum reported PGZ solubility in water around 0.07 mg/mL or 200 μM at 37 °C [63]. We observed microscopic solids characterized by a complex fluorescence decay, illustrated by a phasor distribution ranging within points very close to the ones characterizing the solvated crystal in DMF and the anhydrous crystal species (Figure 3B). The differences between this case and the one in DMF can be easily rationalized considering the different impact of included water (and not DMF) on the interactions between the PGZ molecules within the solid. The slightly curved line formed by the local maxima in the distribution points more towards the possible presence of a continuum of species with different quenching rather than just a mixture of two species [64].

The presence of precipitated crystals in Figure 3D ensures that the solved drug is at saturation, and therefore at its maximum possible concentration; we will show that it does not make it more difficult to understand the observed fluorescence decays from within the cells thanks to the way we are presenting the data. We also report the FLIM results on control cells without anything added in the medium (Figure 3C). The fluorescence of cells with the used channel characteristics (two-photon excitation at 740 nm, emission around 440 nm) arises mostly from NAD(P)H, and indeed the cell phasor positions are in agreement with previously observed ones [7]. Subsequently, the cells were incubated with PGZ-loaded nanoparticles and empty nanoparticles (as negative control), and the corresponding phasor-FLIM results are reported in Figure 3E,F with the same color coding. Again, the fluorescence from the cells is the only one noticeable, while no fluorescence arising from NPs can be identified in the phasor plot. Note that, although the cell autofluorescence was not considered in deciding the color coding used in Figure 3 (the same used in Figure 1), the phasor corresponding to cell-containing pixels fall in a zone characterized by a violet color, therefore they are clearly discernible from the PGZ precipitate in Figure 3D.

As hinted in the introduction, free and bound NAD(P)H, more abundant when oxidative metabolism is slower and faster, respectively, have different fluorescence decay characteristics and therefore different positions in the phasor plot [7,29–31]. By looking carefully at the data reported in Figure 3C–F, even if the color encoding is not ideal for this purpose, it seems that the negative control (Figure 3E) and the cells alone (Figure 3C) present a very similar phasor distribution, while in the case of cells in the presence of PGZ-loaded NPs, the phasor distribution is shifted from slightly at the left (Figure 3C,E) to the right (Figure 3F) of the top left side of the drawn triangle (as clearer in the top images in the panels, with the linear intensity scale). This could also be the case for the cells in the presence of free PGZ, but the analysis is hindered in such cases by the presence of the more fluorescent PGZ precipitate.

To facilitate grasping these fluorescence decay characteristics changes (and to show the versatility and potential of our methods for FLIM data presentation), we changed the color encoding. We considered three principal points (Figure 4, vertices of the triangles): two based on the position of the phasors for cells in RPMI only and in the presence of PGZ-loaded PLGA NPs (examples in Figure 3C,F), and a third one in the middle of the smear corresponding to the PGZ precipitate. It is again easy to discern the cells from the precipitated solids (Figure 4B); moreover, in this case, it is much easier to appreciate the average shift from a situation with the NAD(P)H phasor distribution characterizing more bound NADH (at a relatively longer lifetime, red zones in Figure 4) to one characterized by more free NADH (green in Figure 4), widely accepted to be linked to a decrease in oxidative metabolism (mitochondrial respiration) or to an increase in glycolytic metabolism [7,30,65]. Moreover, with this color coding, it is possible to check the possible heterogeneity amongst different cells (see, e.g., the redder ones, especially in Figure 4B, bottom left panel) or even the modulation of NAD(P)H status within single cells.

The shift observed in the phasor related to free and bound NAD(P)H in response to PGZ can be attributed to its impact on cellular metabolism. PGZ, a member of the thiazolidinedione class of antidiabetic drugs, exerts its effects primarily by activating peroxisome proliferator-activated receptor gamma (PPARγ), a nuclear receptor involved in the regulation of glucose and lipid metabolism. Activation of PPARγ by PGZ leads to transcriptional regulation of genes involved in insulin sensitivity, glucose uptake, and lipid metabolism. Furthermore, PGZ has been shown to enhance mitochondrial function and biogenesis, leading to increased oxidative phosphorylation and ATP production in insulin-sensitive cells, but to have an opposite effect on beta cells in pancreatic islets, from which INS-1E cells are derived and of which they are a model, with a decrease in aerobic metabolism and in insulin secretion [66–68]. This metabolic shift towards decreased aerobic metabolism in beta cells is reflected in changes to the cellular redox state and is therefore in agreement with our observed alterations in the free and bound NAD(P)H ratio.

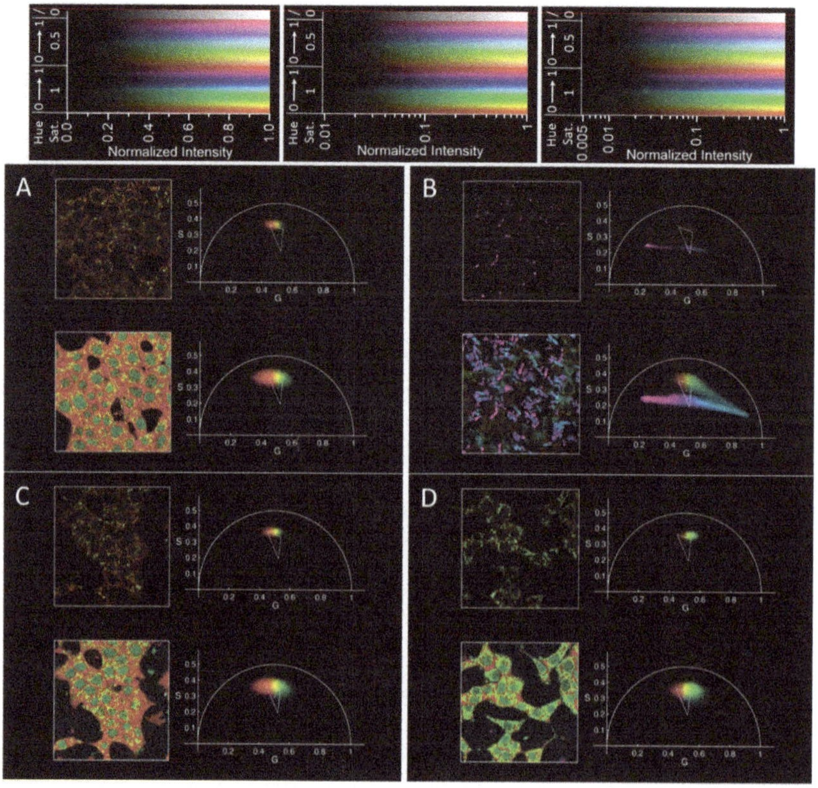

Figure 4. FLIM characterization of INS-1E cells interacting with PGZ and with the nanoparticles considered in this work. The same data of Figure 3C–F are here reported with a different color encoding for phasor position (principal points at the vertices of the triangle and center point in cyan in the right part of each panel), in order to better appreciate the position of phasors characterizing fluorescence arising from within the cells. (**A**) INS-1E in RPMI, (**B**) INS-1E in RPMI in the presence of PGZ, (**C**) INS-1E in RPMI in the presence of empty PLGA NPs, (**D**) INS-1E in RPMI in the presence of PGZ-loaded PLGA NPs. For each panel: on the left, FLIM images; on the right, phasor plots with corresponding colors; on the top, a linear intensity scale is used (the most on the left on the top of the figure), on the bottom a logarithmic one starting from 1% (panels (**A**,**C**,**D**), center color scale on top of the figure) or from 0.5% (panel (**B**), rightmost color scale on the top of the figure) of the maximum intensity in each image. Note that, on average, the apparent intensities of cells in the bottom image of panel (**B**) are similar to the ones on the top images in the other panels.

3. Discussion and Conclusions

The applications of fluorescence-based techniques have transcended conventional limits, offering profound insights into the molecular complexities of various pharmaceutical agents. For instance, the drug organization within a polymeric or biologic matrix can be studied using phasor-FLIM approaches [11,15]; by leveraging the capabilities of FLIM, researchers can gain insights into drug release kinetics, intracellular trafficking, and metabolic responses, thereby facilitating the rational design of drug delivery systems with enhanced efficacy and safety profiles. However, the widespread adoption of FLIM in scientific, industrial, and clinical fields is hindered by the complexity of the needed instrumentation and data analysis and presentation. Some steps have been taken towards the mitigation of the first point [69], and this work represents another step towards a more intuitive presentation of the results of fluorescence lifetime microscopy, in cases where the impact of three or more species present in a sample needs to be easily recognized and mapped.

The MATLAB scripts and functions used in this manuscript (and made freely available) allow defining interactively the "principal" positions in the phasor plots, i.e., the ones considered important in the data presentation (e.g., the ones of pure species or the same species in different environments), to which particular hue values and high saturations are assigned. Moreover, it is possible to define a "center" point where the saturation becomes zero (else, it is considered to be in the middle of the principal points). It is also possible to consider these points as constant and to apply the same color coding to a big number of files containing phasor-encoded images. Importantly, the correspondence between the phasor plot position and (hue, saturation) pair is in principle bijective, so that it can be reversed. In the phasor plot, the intensity follows a distribution where each pixel in the image is weighted by its intensity so that the phasor regions with the highest contributions in the observed field can be noticed at a glance without the need to define an arbitrary threshold (even if the user can impose low and high thresholds, also interactively, if needed). More details are contained in the comments at the beginning of each file.

We applied our algorithms in order to study different phases of PGZ, visualize PLGA nanoparticles, and observe cells and the metabolic shift within them. An interesting observation, which could be neglected in studies involving the effect of non-perfectly soluble drugs on adherent cells, is the one of precipitated 0.1 mg/mL PGZ in various solid phases. This precipitation would largely increase the local concentration of the drug in the proximity of the cells and therefore can lead to an overestimation of the drug effect at the nominal concentration (probably, unreachable by the free form of the drug). Instead, we did not observe any precipitate with the empty or PGZ-loaded NPs, while we could reach the nominal concentration of 0.1 mg/mL of PGZ contained within them. Indeed, an important conclusion arising from our label-free fluorescence lifetime measurements on the NADH-linked metabolism of living cells, is that the effect of PGZ-loaded NPs is higher than the one of dissolved PGZ, even if in this last case crystals of precipitated PGZ were very close to the adherent cells. This points towards a higher effectiveness of the NP-encapsulated drug versus the free-form one.

We could not observe a clear signal from PGZ phases within NPs, probably because of an unexpected too high autofluorescence of the used batch of PLGA or a too low final equivalent concentration of PGZ. However, we believe that the results presented here prove the usefulness of our method for presenting FLIM data in complicated samples, especially when autofluorescence (of drugs, cells, or other components) can be exploited. Indeed, any material can be studied with a setup similar to the one presented here if it is fluorescent, in our case upon two-photon excitation. Depending on the fluorescence properties of other biocompatible polymers (batches) for the synthesis of NPs, they could behave as shown here, could have higher fluorescence intensity and therefore more reproducible phasors, or might be fluorescence-free and therefore make easier studying the drug organization within them, as it happens for liposomes [11,15]. Regarding the drug, if fluorescent, we expect its fluorescent decay to be different in crystalline or solved form in most if not all cases (because of the completely different environment that should change at least the fluorescence quantum yield). However, it is difficult to predict if there could be other phases with different fluorescence decays as it happens for the "solvated" PGZ crystals. In any case, the system presented here is potentially applicable to other drug-nanoparticle conjugates.

Finally, the results reported here represent a step forward in understanding the effect of PGZ on beta-type cells and in developing drug-embedded NPs with more controlled pharmacokinetics, and they can be useful to suggest different characterizations of autofluorescent materials, e.g., various drugs, and of cell response to drugs and/or to changes in their environment.

4. Materials and Methods

4.1. Materials

Pioglitazone (PGZ), Resomer® RG 503 H, PLGA acid terminated (lactide:glycolide 50:50, Mw 24,000–38,000, referred to as PLGA), D-(+)-Trehalose dihydrate, 4-Morpholineethanesulfonic acid (MES), polyvinyl alcohol (87–89% hydrolyzed, Mw approx. 18,000, PVA) and all other chemicals were purchased from Merck KgaA (Darmstadt, Germany) and were used without further purification. INS-1E cells were kindly provided by Prof. C. Wollheim, University of Geneva, Medical Center [70]. Ultrapure water was generated in-house using a MilliQ plus System (Merck KgaA, Darmstadt, Germany), while all the other solvents, including acetone and dimethyl sulfoxide (DMSO), were purchased from Merck KgaA (Darmstadt, Germany). All other chemical reagents were purchased from Aldrich (Saint Quentin Fallavier, France) or Acros (Noisy-Le-Grand, France).

4.2. Synthesis and Characterization of PGZ-Loaded PLGA Nanoparticles

PGZ-loaded PLGA NPs were synthesized using the nanoprecipitation method, with some modifications based on our previous publication [15]. In brief, 400 μL of PLGA (24–32 kDa) dissolved in acetone (10 mg/mL) and 50 μL of PGZ dissolved in DMF (10 mg/mL) were combined and added dropwise to 1600 μL of an aqueous phase comprising 1:1 MES buffer (0.1 M, pH 6.2) and PVA (4%, 18 kDa) under continuous stirring. The resulting suspension was stirred for a minimum of 3 h to facilitate solvent evaporation and nanoparticle formation. Subsequently, the nanoparticles were collected via dialysis (1 kDa cutoff) against 2 L of 1:1 MES buffer (0.1 M, pH 6.2) and PVA (4%, 18 kDa) solution at 4 °C overnight. The physicochemical properties of NPs (including hydrodynamic radius, polydispersity and ζ-potential) were characterized using a Zetasizer Nano ZS equipment (Malvern Instruments Ltd., Worcestershire, UK) at 25 °C, while the entrapment efficiency (EE%) was characterized using a Shimadzu Nexera UHPLC, equipped with a Shimadzu SPD-M20A UV/visible detector, as already reported in our last publication [15]. Finally, the nanoparticles were stored in a 10 mg/mL trehalose solution until use.

4.3. INS-1E Cell Culture

Insulinoma 1E (INS-1E) cells [70] were cultured in a climate-controlled incubator maintained at 37 °C with 5% CO_2. The cells were cultured in RPMI 1640 medium supplemented with 11.1 mmol/L D-glucose, 10 mmol/L HEPES, 2 mmol/L L-glutamine, 100 U/mL penicillin–streptomycin, 1 mmol/L sodium pyruvate, and 50 μmol/L β-mercaptoethanol. For lifetime experiments, cells were grown in sterilized microscopy-compatible dishes (IbiTreat μ-Dish 35-mm, Ibidi) until they reached 70% confluence (24–48 h).

4.4. FLIM Setup

Fluorescence Lifetime Imaging Microscopy (FLIM) was conducted using an Olympus (now Evident, Tokyo, Japan) FVMPE-RS microscope coupled with a two-photon Ti:sapphire laser (MaiTai HP, Newport SpectraPhysics, Santa Clara, CA, USA) operating at a repetition rate of 80 MHz. The FLIM data were acquired with the FLIMbox system for lifetime acquisition (ISS, Champaign, IL, USA). Calibration of the ISS Flimbox system was performed using the known mono-exponential lifetime decay of Fluorescein at pH = 11.0 (4.0 ns upon two-photon excitation at 740 nm, collection range: 400–570 nm). The calibration sample consisted of a stock solution of 100 mmol/L Fluorescein in EtOH, prepared and diluted 1:1000 in NaOH water solution at pH 11.0 for each calibration measurement. Excitation was performed at a wavelength λ = 740 nm, fluorescence collection range was 400–570 nm, laser power was 0.6%, and acquisition was made by a GaAsP photomultiplier tube (PMT) detector with voltage at 850 V; image sampling was set at 512 × 512 pixels with 10 μs/pixel.

For FLIM measurements of PGZ and PGZ-loaded PLGA NPs, experimental conditions included λ = 740 nm and a specific filter for the NADH metabolism range (420–460 nm). Used laser power ranged from 2.0 to 10.0%, and the voltage on the GaAsP PMT was set at 850 V, with image sampling maintained at 512 × 512 pixels, frame size: 106 × 106 μm^2, with a pixel size of 0.207 × 0.207 μm^2 and scanning at 10 μs/pixel.

4.5. Phasor Visualization

The pixel colors in the microscopy image and in the phasor plot have a hue/saturation/value encoding, with hue and saturation depending on the position of the phasor in the phasor plot, and intensity value given by the pixel intensity in the image, and by the sum of the intensities of points within a 2D bin ("pixel") in the phasor plot. The intensities are always normalized to the maximum one (separately for the image and for the phasor plot) and are shown in a linear or in a logarithmic scale (actually, the scale is linear between 0 and x% of the maximum intensity, then it is logarithmic, with x = 1 unless specified otherwise). The phasor plot pixels have standard dimensions of 0.02 × 0.02 but can be specified otherwise.

Hue and saturation are calculated starting from a certain number of "principal" points (minimum two, better if at least three) in the phasor plots, ideally the positions in the phasor plot of the pure fluorescent species present in the sample, plus a "center" point. If not given when calling the function calculating hue and saturation, the user can choose them on a binned scatter plot for all the phasors in the image; ideally, most of the phasors should be included in the region having them as vertices, and this region should be (but does not have to be) convex. If the center point is not given, it is calculated as the average position of the principal points. The hue is calculated from the angle between the segments from the center point to the desired spot and from the center point to the principal points and is always increasing going clockwise or anticlockwise (depending on the order of the given principal points, eventually corrected to be always increasing in the chosen orientation if they are more than three). The principal points have equidistant values (with 0 and 1 both corresponding to the first principal point); the hue of a phasor with an angle included within the ones of two principal points is the average of the hues of these two points weighted with the angular distance from the opposite one. The saturation is zero on the central point and increases radially. Considering the intercept of the half line from the center point to the considered phasor with the line between two central points and with the borders of the universal semicircles, the hue increases (with a function proportional to sin(x) for x from 0 to 1) between 0 and a certain first value up to the first encountered intersection point, then linearly between this value and a second one between the two intersection points, then it tends exponentially to 1 for higher distances. The second value is fixed; the first one is corrected starting from a given value so that it is closer to the second one the closer the two intersection points are. In the plots shown in this work, these values were 0.95 and 0.85 (uncorrected value). The decay constant for the exponential function is the average of the distances from the center points to the two intersection points. The algorithm considers different increasing functions for nonstandard situations, possible, e.g., if the center point is chosen outside the universal semicircle and/or the region having the "principal points" as vertices.

Before calculating the phasors distribution and for the representation in the images, the values of intensities and of the G and S coordinates have been smoothed starting from their dependence on the pixel positions in the image. The intensities are treated with a 2D Gaussian filter with a given standard deviation (1 pixel in the cases shown here). The values for G and S are transformed in each pixel considering a weighted average with weights given by a Gaussian centered in the considered pixel with the same standard deviation used for the intensities, multiplied by the intensity values of the corresponding pixels.

OriginPro 8.0 was used for preliminary visualization of average phasor positions within the universal circle. MATLAB R2017B was employed for advanced mathematical modeling enabling the derivation of quantitative information on phasors, for calculating the color coding mapping, and preparing all images shown in this work. Additionally, Fiji, a free image-processing package, was used for preliminary spatial analysis of microscopy and FLIM data.

Author Contributions: Conceptualization, B.T., L.P. and S.L.; methodology, B.T., L.P., F.C. and S.L.; software, S.L.; validation, F.C. and S.L.; formal analysis, B.T. and S.L.; investigation, B.T., L.P. and S.L.; resources, F.C. and S.L.; writing—original draft preparation, B.T. and S.L.; writing—review and editing, B.T. and S.L.; visualization, B.T. and S.L.; supervision, S.L.; project administration, S.L.; funding acquisition, F.C. and S.L. All authors have read and agreed to the published version of the manuscript.

Funding: This research received funding from Scuola Normale Superiore (RICBASE_2022_LUIN, RICBASE_2023_LUIN, RICBASE_2024_LUIN), from the European Union Next-Generation EU through the PIANO NAZIONALE DI RIPRESA E RESILIENZA (PNRR—MISSIONE 4 COMPONENTE 2) within the National Quantum Science and Technology Institute (NQSTI—INVESTIMENTO 1.3; PE_00000023) and the Tuscany Health Ecosystem (THE—INVESTIMENTO 1.5; ECS_00000017; Spoke 4: Nanotechnologies for diagnosis and therapy), and from the European Research Council (ERC) under the European Union's Horizon 2020 research and innovation program (grant agreement No 866127, project CAPTUR3D).

Institutional Review Board Statement: Not applicable.

Informed Consent Statement: Not applicable.

Data Availability Statement: MATLAB codes for functions and scripts used to produce the images and the results presented in the manuscript are available at https://github.com/Stefano-Luin/phasor_plots (accessed on 3 April 2024), and can be used if this paper is properly cited in any obtained result. Datasets are available on request from the authors.

Acknowledgments: The authors thank Mario Bernardi (Scuola Normale Superiore, Italy) for his precious assistance with FLIM data analysis.

Conflicts of Interest: The authors declare no conflicts of interest. The funders had no role in the design of the study; in the collection, analyses, or interpretation of data; in the writing of the manuscript; or in the decision to publish the results.

References

1. Vitali, M.; Picazo, F.; Prokazov, Y.; Duci, A.; Turbin, E.; Götze, C.; Llopis, J.; Hartig, R.; Visser, A.J.W.G.; Zuschratter, W. Wide-Field Multi-Parameter FLIM: Long-Term Minimal Invasive Observation of Proteins in Living Cells. *PLoS ONE* **2011**, *6*, e15820. [CrossRef] [PubMed]
2. Stringari, C.; Cinquin, A.; Cinquin, O.; Digman, M.A.; Donovan, P.J.; Gratton, E. Phasor Approach to Fluorescence Lifetime Microscopy Distinguishes Different Metabolic States of Germ Cells in a Live Tissue. *Proc. Natl. Acad. Sci. USA* **2011**, *108*, 13582–13587. [CrossRef]
3. Sameni, S.; Syed, A.; Marsh, J.L.; Digman, M.A. The Phasor-FLIM Fingerprints Reveal Shifts from OXPHOS to Enhanced Glycolysis in Huntington Disease. *Sci. Rep.* **2016**, *6*, 34755. [CrossRef] [PubMed]
4. Lakner, P.H.; Monaghan, M.G.; Möller, Y.; Olayioye, M.A.; Schenke-Layland, K. Applying Phasor Approach Analysis of Multiphoton FLIM Measurements to Probe the Metabolic Activity of Three-Dimensional in Vitro Cell Culture Models. *Sci. Rep.* **2017**, *7*, 42730. [CrossRef] [PubMed]
5. Bec, J.; Vela, D.; Phipps, J.E.; Agung, M.; Unger, J.; Margulies, K.B.; Southard, J.A.; Buja, L.M.; Marcu, L. Label-Free Visualization and Quantification of Biochemical Markers of Atherosclerotic Plaque Progression Using Intravascular Fluorescence Lifetime. *JACC Cardiovasc. Imaging* **2021**, *14*, 1832–1842. [CrossRef]
6. Goryashchenko, A.S.; Pakhomov, A.A.; Ryabova, A.V.; Romanishkin, I.D.; Maksimov, E.G.; Orsa, A.N.; Serova, O.V.; Mozhaev, A.A.; Maksimova, M.A.; Martynov, V.I.; et al. FLIM-Based Intracellular and Extracellular pH Measurements Using Genetically Encoded pH Sensor. *Biosensors* **2021**, *11*, 340. [CrossRef] [PubMed]
7. Pugliese, L.A.; De Lorenzi, V.; Bernardi, M.; Ghignoli, S.; Tesi, M.; Marchetti, P.; Pesce, L.; Cardarelli, F. Unveiling Nanoscale Optical Signatures of Cytokine-Induced β-Cell Dysfunction. *Sci. Rep.* **2023**, *13*, 13342. [CrossRef]
8. Dai, X.; Yue, Z.; Eccleston, M.E.; Swartling, J.; Slater, N.K.H.; Kaminski, C.F. Fluorescence Intensity and Lifetime Imaging of Free and Micellar-Encapsulated Doxorubicin in Living Cells. *Nanomed. Nanotechnol. Biol. Med.* **2008**, *4*, 49–56. [CrossRef] [PubMed]
9. Saxl, T.; Khan, F.; Matthews, D.R.; Zhi, Z.-L.; Rolinski, O.; Ameer-Beg, S.; Pickup, J. Fluorescence Lifetime Spectroscopy and Imaging of Nano-Engineered Glucose Sensor Microcapsules Based on Glucose/Galactose-Binding Protein. *Biosens. Bioelectron.* **2009**, *24*, 3229–3234. [CrossRef]

10. Duong, H.T.T.; Hughes, F.; Sagnella, S.; Kavallaris, M.; Macmillan, A.; Whan, R.; Hook, J.; Davis, T.P.; Boyer, C. Functionalizing Biodegradable Dextran Scaffolds Using Living Radical Polymerization: New Versatile Nanoparticles for the Delivery of Therapeutic Molecules. *Mol. Pharm.* **2012**, *9*, 3046–3061. [CrossRef]
11. Cardarelli, F.; Beltram, F.; Tentori, P.; Caracciolo, G.; Pozzi, D. Determination of the Supramolecular Organization of Encapsulated Molecules by Luminescence Lifetime Analysis. US Patent 11,913,882, 8 November 2021.
12. Zhang, X.; Shastry, S.; Bradforth, S.E.; Nadeau, J.L. Nuclear Uptake of Ultrasmall Gold-Doxorubicin Conjugates Imaged by Fluorescence Lifetime Imaging Microscopy (FLIM) and Electron Microscopy. *Nanoscale* **2015**, *7*, 240–251. [CrossRef]
13. Piccirillo, G.; Bochicchio, B.; Pepe, A.; Schenke-Layland, K.; Hinderer, S. Electrospun Poly-l-Lactide Scaffold for the Controlled and Targeted Delivery of a Synthetically Obtained Diclofenac Prodrug to Treat Actinic Keratosis. *Acta Biomater.* **2017**, *52*, 187–196. [CrossRef] [PubMed]
14. Saari, H.; Lisitsyna, E.; Rautaniemi, K.; Rojalin, T.; Niemi, L.; Nivaro, O.; Laaksonen, T.; Yliperttula, M.; Vuorimaa-Laukkanen, E. FLIM Reveals Alternative EV-Mediated Cellular up-Take Pathways of Paclitaxel. *J. Control. Release* **2018**, *284*, 133–143. [CrossRef]
15. Tentori, P.; Signore, G.; Camposeo, A.; Carretta, A.; Ferri, G.; Pingue, P.; Luin, S.; Pozzi, D.; Gratton, E.; Beltram, F.; et al. Fluorescence Lifetime Microscopy Unveils the Supramolecular Organization of Liposomal Doxorubicin. *Nanoscale* **2022**, *14*, 8901–8905. [CrossRef] [PubMed]
16. Angiolini, L.; Cohen, B.; Douhal, A. Single Crystal FLIM Characterization of Clofazimine Loaded in Silica-Based Mesoporous Materials and Zeolites. *Int. J. Mol. Sci.* **2019**, *20*, 2859. [CrossRef]
17. Bruun, K.; Hille, C. Study on Intracellular Delivery of Liposome Encapsulated Quantum Dots Using Advanced Fluorescence Microscopy. *Sci. Rep.* **2019**, *9*, 10504. [CrossRef]
18. Bernardi, M.; Signore, G.; Moscardini, A.; Pugliese, L.A.; Pesce, L.; Beltram, F.; Cardarelli, F. Fluorescence Lifetime Nanoscopy of Liposomal Irinotecan Onivyde: From Manufacturing to Intracellular Processing. *ACS Appl. Bio Mater.* **2023**, *6*, 4277–4289. [CrossRef]
19. Bowman, A.J.; Huang, C.; Schnitzer, M.J.; Kasevich, M.A. Wide-Field Fluorescence Lifetime Imaging of Neuron Spiking and Subthreshold Activity In Vivo. *Science* **2023**, *380*, 1270–1275. [CrossRef] [PubMed]
20. Liput, D.J.; Nguyen, T.A.; Augustin, S.M.; Lee, J.O.; Vogel, S.S. A Guide to Fluorescence Lifetime Microscopy and Förster's Resonance Energy Transfer in Neuroscience. *Curr. Protoc. Neurosci.* **2020**, *94*, e108. [CrossRef]
21. Alfonso-Garcia, A.; Bec, J.; Weyers, B.; Marsden, M.; Zhou, X.; Li, C.; Marcu, L. Mesoscopic Fluorescence Lifetime Imaging: Fundamental Principles, Clinical Applications and Future Directions. *J. Biophotonics* **2021**, *14*, e202000472. [CrossRef]
22. Gouzou, D.; Taimori, A.; Haloubi, T.; Finlayson, N.; Wang, Q.; Hopgood, J.R.; Vallejo, M. Applications of Machine Learning in Time-Domain Fluorescence Lifetime Imaging: A Review. *Methods Appl. Fluoresc.* **2024**, *12*, 022001. [CrossRef] [PubMed]
23. Stringari, C.; Nourse, J.L.; Flanagan, L.A.; Gratton, E. Phasor Fluorescence Lifetime Microscopy of Free and Protein-Bound NADH Reveals Neural Stem Cell Differentiation Potential. *PLoS ONE* **2012**, *7*, e48014. [CrossRef] [PubMed]
24. Theurey, P.; Connolly, N.M.C.; Fortunati, I.; Basso, E.; Lauwen, S.; Ferrante, C.; Moreira Pinho, C.; Joselin, A.; Gioran, A.; Bano, D.; et al. Systems Biology Identifies Preserved Integrity but Impaired Metabolism of Mitochondria Due to a Glycolytic Defect in Alzheimer's Disease Neurons. *Aging Cell* **2019**, *18*, e12924. [CrossRef] [PubMed]
25. Smith, J.T.; Yao, R.; Sinsuebphon, N.; Rudkouskaya, A.; Un, N.; Mazurkiewicz, J.; Barroso, M.; Yan, P.; Intes, X. Fast Fit-Free Analysis of Fluorescence Lifetime Imaging via Deep Learning. *Proc. Natl. Acad. Sci. USA* **2019**, *116*, 24019–24030. [CrossRef] [PubMed]
26. Oasa, S.; Krmpot, A.J.; Nikolić, S.N.; Clayton, A.H.A.; Tsigelny, I.F.; Changeux, J.-P.; Terenius, L.; Rigler, R.; Vukojević, V. Dynamic Cellular Cartography: Mapping the Local Determinants of Oligodendrocyte Transcription Factor 2 (OLIG2) Function in Live Cells Using Massively Parallel Fluorescence Correlation Spectroscopy Integrated with Fluorescence Lifetime Imaging Microscopy (mpFCS/FLIM). *Anal. Chem.* **2021**, *93*, 12011–12021. [CrossRef] [PubMed]
27. Chen, Y.-I.; Chang, Y.-J.; Liao, S.-C.; Nguyen, T.D.; Yang, J.; Kuo, Y.-A.; Hong, S.; Liu, Y.-L.; Rylander, H.G.; Santacruz, S.R.; et al. Generative Adversarial Network Enables Rapid and Robust Fluorescence Lifetime Image Analysis in Live Cells. *Commun. Biol.* **2022**, *5*, 18. [CrossRef] [PubMed]
28. Ragan, C.I.; Garland, P.B. The Intra-Mitochondrial Localization of Flavoproteins Previously Assigned to the Respiratory Chain. *Eur. J. Biochem.* **1969**, *10*, 399–410. [CrossRef] [PubMed]
29. Lakowicz, J.R.; Szmacinski, H.; Nowaczyk, K.; Johnson, M.L. Fluorescence Lifetime Imaging of Free and Protein-Bound NADH. *Proc. Natl. Acad. Sci. USA* **1992**, *89*, 1271–1275. [CrossRef]
30. Ferri, G.; Tesi, M.; Massarelli, F.; Marselli, L.; Marchetti, P.; Cardarelli, F. Metabolic Response of Insulinoma 1E Cells to Glucose Stimulation Studied by Fluorescence Lifetime Imaging. *FASEB BioAdv.* **2020**, *2*, 409–418. [CrossRef]
31. Azzarello, F.; Pesce, L.; De Lorenzi, V.; Ferri, G.; Tesi, M.; Del Guerra, S.; Marchetti, P.; Cardarelli, F. Single-Cell Imaging of α and β Cell Metabolic Response to Glucose in Living Human Langerhans Islets. *Commun. Biol.* **2022**, *5*, 1232. [CrossRef]
32. Malacrida, L. Phasor Plots and the Future of Spectral and Lifetime Imaging. *Nat. Methods* **2023**, *20*, 965–967. [CrossRef] [PubMed]
33. SIMFCS. Available online: https://Www.Lfd.Uci.Edu/Globals/ (accessed on 30 April 2024).
34. Gottlieb, D.; Asadipour, B.; Kostina, P.; Ung, T.P.L.; Stringari, C. FLUTE: A Python GUI for Interactive Phasor Analysis of FLIM Data. *Biol. Imaging* **2023**, *3*, e21. [CrossRef] [PubMed]
35. Hanley, Q.S.; Lidke, K.A.; Heintzmann, R.; Arndt-Jovin, D.J.; Jovin, T.M. Fluorescence Lifetime Imaging in an Optically Sectioning Programmable Array Microscope (PAM). *Cytometry A* **2005**, *67*, 112–118. [CrossRef] [PubMed]

36. Bernardi, M.; Cardarelli, F. Phasor Identifier: A Cloud-Based Analysis of Phasor-FLIM Data on Python Notebooks. *Biophys. Rep.* **2023**, *3*, 100135. [CrossRef] [PubMed]
37. Makadia, H.K.; Siegel, S.J. Poly Lactic-Co-Glycolic Acid (PLGA) as Biodegradable Controlled Drug Delivery Carrier. *Polymers* **2011**, *3*, 1377–1397. [CrossRef] [PubMed]
38. Alsaab, H.O.; Alharbi, F.D.; Alhibs, A.S.; Alanazi, N.B.; Alshehri, B.Y.; Saleh, M.A.; Alshehri, F.S.; Algarni, M.A.; Almugaiteeb, T.; Uddin, M.N.; et al. PLGA-Based Nanomedicine: History of Advancement and Development in Clinical Applications of Multiple Diseases. *Pharmaceutics* **2022**, *14*, 2728. [CrossRef] [PubMed]
39. Lu, Y.; Cheng, D.; Niu, B.; Wang, X.; Wu, X.; Wang, A. Properties of Poly (Lactic-Co-Glycolic Acid) and Progress of Poly (Lactic-Co-Glycolic Acid)-Based Biodegradable Materials in Biomedical Research. *Pharmaceuticals* **2023**, *16*, 454. [CrossRef] [PubMed]
40. Patil, Y.B.; Toti, U.S.; Khdair, A.; Ma, L.; Panyam, J. Single-Step Surface Functionalization of Polymeric Nanoparticles for Targeted Drug Delivery. *Biomaterials* **2009**, *30*, 859–866. [CrossRef] [PubMed]
41. Todaro, B.; Ottalagana, E.; Luin, S.; Santi, M. Targeting Peptides: The New Generation of Targeted Drug Delivery Systems. *Pharmaceutics* **2023**, *15*, 1648. [CrossRef]
42. Abd Ellah, N.H.; Abouelmagd, S.A. Surface Functionalization of Polymeric Nanoparticles for Tumor Drug Delivery: Approaches and Challenges. *Expert Opin. Drug Deliv.* **2017**, *14*, 201–214. [CrossRef]
43. Hickey, J.W.; Santos, J.L.; Williford, J.-M.; Mao, H.-Q. Control of Polymeric Nanoparticle Size to Improve Therapeutic Delivery. *J. Control. Release* **2015**, *219*, 536–547. [CrossRef] [PubMed]
44. Danhier, F.; Ansorena, E.; Silva, J.M.; Coco, R.; Le Breton, A.; Préat, V. PLGA-Based Nanoparticles: An Overview of Biomedical Applications. *J. Control. Release* **2012**, *161*, 505–522. [CrossRef] [PubMed]
45. Ghitman, J.; Biru, E.I.; Stan, R.; Iovu, H. Review of Hybrid PLGA Nanoparticles: Future of Smart Drug Delivery and Theranostics Medicine. *Mater. Des.* **2020**, *193*, 108805. [CrossRef]
46. Ding, D.; Zhu, Q. Recent Advances of PLGA Micro/Nanoparticles for the Delivery of Biomacromolecular Therapeutics. *Mater. Sci. Eng. C* **2018**, *92*, 1041–1060. [CrossRef] [PubMed]
47. Cai, Q.; Wang, L.; Deng, G.; Liu, J.; Chen, Q.; Chen, Z. Systemic Delivery to Central Nervous System by Engineered PLGA Nanoparticles. *Am. J. Transl. Res.* **2016**, *8*, 749–764.
48. Patra, J.K.; Das, G.; Fraceto, L.F.; Campos, E.V.R.; Rodriguez-Torres, M.D.P.; Acosta-Torres, L.S.; Diaz-Torres, L.A.; Grillo, R.; Swamy, M.K.; Sharma, S.; et al. Nano Based Drug Delivery Systems: Recent Developments and Future Prospects. *J. Nanobiotechnol.* **2018**, *16*, 71. [CrossRef] [PubMed]
49. Li, M.; Sun, X.; Yin, M.; Shen, J.; Yan, S. Recent Advances in Nanoparticle-Mediated Co-Delivery System: A Promising Strategy in Medical and Agricultural Field. *Int. J. Mol. Sci.* **2023**, *24*, 5121. [CrossRef] [PubMed]
50. Taghavizadeh Yazdi, M.E.; Qayoomian, M.; Beigoli, S.; Boskabady, M.H. Recent Advances in Nanoparticle Applications in Respiratory Disorders: A Review. *Front. Pharmacol.* **2023**, *14*, 1059343. [CrossRef] [PubMed]
51. Rahman, M.M.; Islam, M.R.; Akash, S.; Harun-Or-Rashid, M.; Ray, T.K.; Rahaman, M.S.; Islam, M.; Anika, F.; Hosain, M.K.; Aovi, F.I.; et al. Recent Advancements of Nanoparticles Application in Cancer and Neurodegenerative Disorders: At a Glance. *Biomed. Pharmacother.* **2022**, *153*, 113305. [CrossRef]
52. Todaro, B.; Begarani, F.; Sartori, F.; Luin, S. Is Raman the Best Strategy towards the Development of Non-Invasive Continuous Glucose Monitoring Devices for Diabetes Management? *Front. Chem.* **2022**, *10*, 994272. [CrossRef]
53. Marín-Peñalver, J.J.; Martín-Timón, I.; Sevillano-Collantes, C.; Cañizo-Gómez, F.J.D. Update on the Treatment of Type 2 Diabetes Mellitus. *World J. Diabetes* **2016**, *7*, 354. [CrossRef] [PubMed]
54. Todaro, B.; Moscardini, A.; Luin, S. Pioglitazone-Loaded PLGA Nanoparticles: Towards the Most Reliable Synthesis Method. *Int. J. Mol. Sci.* **2022**, *23*, 2522. [CrossRef] [PubMed]
55. Modena, M.M.; Rühle, B.; Burg, T.P.; Wuttke, S. Nanoparticle Characterization: What to Measure? *Adv. Mater.* **2019**, *31*, 1901556. [CrossRef] [PubMed]
56. Zielińska, A.; Carreiró, F.; Oliveira, A.M.; Neves, A.; Pires, B.; Venkatesh, D.N.; Durazzo, A.; Lucarini, M.; Eder, P.; Silva, A.M.; et al. Polymeric Nanoparticles: Production, Characterization, Toxicology and Ecotoxicology. *Molecules* **2020**, *25*, 3731. [CrossRef] [PubMed]
57. Tehrani, S.F.; Bharadwaj, P.; Leblond Chain, J.; Roullin, V.G. Purification Processes of Polymeric Nanoparticles: How to Improve Their Clinical Translation? *J. Control. Release* **2023**, *360*, 591–612. [CrossRef] [PubMed]
58. Liu, Y.; Wu, X.; Mi, Y.; Zhang, B.; Gu, S.; Liu, G.; Li, X. PLGA Nanoparticles for the Oral Delivery of Nuciferine: Preparation, Physicochemical Characterization and in Vitro/in Vivo Studies. *Drug Deliv.* **2017**, *24*, 443–451. [CrossRef] [PubMed]
59. Ibarra, J.; Melendres, J.; Almada, M.; Burboa, M.G.; Taboada, P.; Juárez, J.; Valdez, M.A. Synthesis and Characterization of Magnetite/PLGA/Chitosan Nanoparticles. *Mater. Res. Express* **2015**, *2*, 095010. [CrossRef]
60. Mourdikoudis, S.; Pallares, R.M.; Thanh, N.T.K. Characterization Techniques for Nanoparticles: Comparison and Complementarity upon Studying Nanoparticle Properties. *Nanoscale* **2018**, *10*, 12871–12934. [CrossRef] [PubMed]
61. Todaro, B.; Santi, M. Characterization and Functionalization Approaches for the Study of Polymeric Nanoparticles: The State of the Art in Italian Research. *Micro* **2022**, *3*, 9–21. [CrossRef]
62. Cho, E.J.; Holback, H.; Liu, K.C.; Abouelmagd, S.A.; Park, J.; Yeo, Y. Nanoparticle Characterization: State of the Art, Challenges, and Emerging Technologies. *Mol. Pharm.* **2013**, *10*, 2093–2110. [CrossRef]

63. Pandit, V.; Gorantla, R.; Devi, K.; Pai, R.; Sarasija, S. Preparation and Characterization of Pioglitazone Cyclodextrin Inclusion Complexes. *J. Young Pharm. JYP* **2011**, *3*, 267–274. [CrossRef] [PubMed]
64. Ranjit, S.; Malacrida, L.; Jameson, D.M.; Gratton, E. Fit-Free Analysis of Fluorescence Lifetime Imaging Data Using the Phasor Approach. *Nat. Protoc.* **2018**, *13*, 1979–2004. [CrossRef] [PubMed]
65. Gómez, C.A.; Sutin, J.; Wu, W.; Fu, B.; Uhlirova, H.; Devor, A.; Boas, D.A.; Sakadžić, S.; Yaseen, M.A. Phasor Analysis of NADH FLIM Identifies Pharmacological Disruptions to Mitochondrial Metabolic Processes in the Rodent Cerebral Cortex. *PLoS ONE* **2018**, *13*, e0194578. [CrossRef] [PubMed]
66. Lamontagne, J.; Pepin, É.; Peyot, M.-L.; Joly, É.; Ruderman, N.B.; Poitout, V.; Madiraju, S.R.M.; Nolan, C.J.; Prentki, M. Pioglitazone Acutely Reduces Insulin Secretion and Causes Metabolic Deceleration of the Pancreatic β-Cell at Submaximal Glucose Concentrations. *Endocrinology* **2009**, *150*, 3465–3474. [CrossRef] [PubMed]
67. Lamontagne, J.; Jalbert-Arsenault, É.; Pepin, É.; Peyot, M.-L.; Ruderman, N.B.; Nolan, C.J.; Joly, E.; Madiraju, S.R.M.; Poitout, V.; Prentki, M. Pioglitazone Acutely Reduces Energy Metabolism and Insulin Secretion in Rats. *Diabetes* **2013**, *62*, 2122–2129. [CrossRef] [PubMed]
68. Karunakaran, U.; Elumalai, S.; Moon, J.S.; Won, K.C. Pioglitazone-Induced AMPK-Glutaminase-1 Prevents High Glucose-Induced Pancreatic β-Cell Dysfunction by Glutathione Antioxidant System. *Redox Biol.* **2021**, *45*, 102029. [CrossRef]
69. Rossetta, A.; Bernardi, M.; Cardarelli, F. Fluorescence Lifetime Analysis (FLA) for the Screening of Healthcare Nanoformulations: Towards a Compact and Versatile Device. In Proceedings of the Reporters, Markers, Dyes, Nanoparticles, and Molecular Probes for Biomedical Applications XVI, San Francisco, CA, USA, 30–31 January 2024; Volume 12862, pp. 37–40.
70. Merglen, A.; Theander, S.; Rubi, B.; Chaffard, G.; Wollheim, C.B.; Maechler, P. Glucose Sensitivity and Metabolism-Secretion Coupling Studied during Two-Year Continuous Culture in INS-1E Insulinoma Cells. *Endocrinology* **2004**, *145*, 667–678. [CrossRef]

molecules

MDPI

Article

A Rapid Self−Assembling Peptide Hydrogel for Delivery of TFF3 to Promote Gastric Mucosal Injury Repair

Jialei Chen [1], Jing Luo [2], Di Su [1], Na Lu [1], Jiawei Zhao [1] and Zhongli Luo [1,*]

[1] Molecular Medicine and Cancer Research Center, College of Basic Medical Sciences, Chongqing Medical University, Chongqing 400016, China; chenjialei0917@163.com (J.C.); sd199877@163.com (D.S.); lunar@stu.cqmu.edu.cn (N.L.); zjw980312@163.com (J.Z.)

[2] Department of Pathology and Pathophysiology, Chongqing Medical University, Chongqing 400016, China; luojing668yeah@163.com

* Correspondence: zhongliluo@163.com

Abstract: Self-assembled peptide-based nanobiomaterials exhibit promising prospects for drug delivery applications owing to their commendable biocompatibility and biodegradability, facile tissue uptake and utilization, and minimal or negligible unexpected toxicity. TFF3 is an active peptide autonomously secreted by gastric mucosal cells, possessing multiple biological functions. It acts on the surface of the gastric mucosa, facilitating the repair process of gastric mucosal damage. However, when used as a drug, TFF3 faces significant challenges, including short retention time in the gastric mucosal cavity and deactivation due to degradation by stomach acid. In response to this challenge, we developed a self−assembled short peptide hydrogel, Rqdl10, designed as a delivery vehicle for TFF3. Our investigation encompasses an assessment of its properties, biocompatibility, controlled release of TFF3, and the mechanism underlying the promotion of gastric mucosal injury repair. Congo red/aniline blue staining revealed that Rqdl10 promptly self-assembled in PBS, forming hydrogels. Circular dichroism spectra indicated the presence of a stable β-sheet secondary structure in the Rqdl10 hydrogel. Cryo-scanning electron microscopy and atomic force microscopy observations demonstrated that the Rqdl10 formed vesicle-like structures in the PBS, which were interconnected to construct a three-dimensional nanostructure. Moreover, the Rqdl10 hydrogel exhibited outstanding biocompatibility and could sustainably and slowly release TFF3. The utilization of the Rqdl10 hydrogel as a carrier for TFF3 substantially augmented its proliferative and migratory capabilities, while concurrently bolstering its anti-inflammatory and anti-apoptotic attributes following gastric mucosal injury. Our findings underscore the immense potential of the self-assembled peptide hydrogel Rqdl10 for biomedical applications, promising significant contributions to healthcare science.

Keywords: self−assembly peptide; TFF3; gastric mucosal injury; gastric mucosal repair; drug delivery

1. Introduction

Hydrogels, composed of hydrophilic polymers, possess a distinctive three-dimensional structure and retain substantial water content [1]. Over recent decades, molecular hydrogels have garnered significant interest as promising biomaterials with diverse applications in biomedicine and nanomedicine, including but not limited to cell culture [2], tissue engineering [3], cancer therapy [4], drug delivery [5], and regenerative medicine [6]. Peptides consist of short sequences of amino acids, and their self-assembly refers to the process whereby peptide molecules spontaneously form specific nanostructures [7]. The amino acid residues carried by self-assembling peptides can drive the self-assembly of peptides into stable, low-energy structures through non−covalent interactions, including hydrogen bonding, electrostatic forces, hydrophobic/hydrophilic interactions, π-π stacking, and van der Waals forces. Peptide molecules, when rationally designed, can self-assemble into specific nanostructures with rich hierarchical levels under varying conditions such as pH, temperature, and ionic strength, including vesicles [8], nanotubes [9], nanofibers [10], and hydrogels [7]. Peptide-based nanogel systems, owing to their exceptional biocompatibility and biodegradability, have been widely utilized as ideal delivery vehicles for various drugs [11]. Self-assembling peptide hydrogel carriers can effectively address issues such as low water solubility, instability, uneven biological distribution, high degradation rates, and lack of targeted functionality of drugs, thereby enhancing the bioavailability and therapeutic efficacy of the medications [12]. Currently, self-assembling peptide hydrogel delivery systems have successfully achieved precise delivery and controlled release of a variety of peptide-based active pharmaceuticals. For instance, the RAD16-II self-assembling peptide nanogel has been employed for the intramyocardial delivery of platelet-derived growth factor (PDGF) and vascular endothelial growth factor (VEGF), aimed at promoting revascularization in the myocardial infarction areas of rats and pigs, while effectively avoiding issues such as pulmonary hypertension caused by the systemic administration of PDGF [13,14]. Similarly, employing RADA16 self-assembling peptide hydrogel to encapsulate recombinant Bone Morphogenetic Protein-2 (BMP-2) not only effectively stores and releases BMP-2 but also preserves its biological activity, significantly enhancing the stability of BMP-2. This strategy has been successfully applied to the healing of bone defects [15].

Gastric mucosal injury is common in daily life [16]. Typically, the damaged gastric mucosa does not always heal quickly within a short period, and the damage may even be accompanied by potential serious complications such as bleeding or perforation [17]. Due to its diverse etiology, achieving the treatment and complete cure of gastric mucosal injury poses significant challenges. Currently, the primary approaches to promoting the repair of gastric mucosal injury involve inhibiting gastric acid secretion, administering anti-Helicobacter pylori therapy, and utilizing gastric mucosal protectants [18]. However, these medications may induce various side effects, including drug resistance, allergic reactions, and abnormal heart rhythms [19]. Hence, identifying a natural active ingredient with high safety, minimal side effects, and enhanced efficacy is imperative for promoting the repair of gastric mucosal injury.

The maintenance of gastric mucosa integrity is reliant on the concerted action of numerous secreted factors, among which the secretion of trefoil factor 3 (TFF3) plays a crucial role [20]. TFF3 is a small peptide rich in cysteine, comprising 59 amino acids. Upon maturation, TFF3 is secreted and folded into a characteristic cloverleaf-like compact tricyclic structure, formed by six conserved cysteine residues linked by three disulfide bonds [21]. While TFF3 expression is typically challenging to detect in normal gastric mucosa, the robust expression of TFF3 can be observed in the periulcer tissues of gastric ulcer patients and rats [22,23]. Animal studies have demonstrated that TFF3 administration mitigates gastric mucosal injury induced by various factors including alcohol [24], NSAIDs [25], stress [26], and lipopolysaccharide [27]. The potential roles of TFF3 encompass the maintenance of gastric pH, stimulation of gastric mucosal healing, and enhancement of gastric mucosal defense [25,28]. Notably, unlike many gastroprotective agents, the gastric mucosal protective effect of TFF3 operates independently of prostaglandins and is realized at the surface of the gastric mucosal lumen [28]. Different routes of administration can markedly influence the efficacy of TFF3 in disease treatment. In a rat model of colitis, the intestinal administration of TFF3 has demonstrated greater efficacy compared to systemic administration. Conversely, the subcutaneous injection of TFF3 monomer has been shown to exacerbate colitis induced by mitomycin C or dextran sulfate sodium salt [29]. Previous investigations have highlighted the characteristic cloverleaf structure of TFF3, which imparts stability against digestion by protein hydrolases, thereby facilitating its role in the luminal environment of the digestive tract [20,21,30,31]. However, recent findings indicate that TFF3, along with its homodimeric and cloverleaf domains, are susceptible to degradation and inactivation in an acidic environment containing pepsin [32–34]. In response to this formidable challenge, Nayara and collaborators utilized chemical synthesis methodologies to generate TFF3 analogs, notably TFF3 (C57Acm), TFF310-50, and TFF37-54, exhibiting TFF3 activity and distinctive trilobal architectures tailored to fortify stability in the gastrointestinal tract [35]. Nevertheless, drug modification encounters multifarious obstacles, including subtle structural alterations capable of eliciting profound discrepancies in drug efficacy, pharmacokinetics, and toxicity profiles. Another auspicious strategy involves the development of apt drug delivery systems aimed at augmenting stability, solubility, and targeting precision, thereby amplifying therapeutic efficacy while curtailing adverse effects [36].

TFF3 is an active peptide with various biological functions, acting on the gastric mucosal surface to facilitate the repair process of gastric mucosal damage. However, when used as a drug, TFF3 faces significant challenges, including short retention time in the gastric mucosal cavity and deactivation due to degradation by stomach acid. To address these issues, our research team innovatively synthesized a new chiral self-assembling peptide hydrogel, Rqdl10, for the delivery of TFF3. Furthermore, the involvement and underlying mechanism of TFF3@Rqdl10 in the repair of gastric mucosal injury were elucidated through a combination of in vivo and in vitro experiments. Our findings offer novel perspectives and insights into advancing the repair of gastric mucosal injury.

2. Results

2.1. Characteristics of Rqdl10 Hydrogel

The amino acid sequence of Rqdl10, RQDLKTEIRYDFKADE-NH2, is a linear peptide from the N-terminus to the C-terminus. The relative molecular mass of Rqdl10 was determined to be 2026.2 (Figure 1A), with a purity of 97.40% (Figure 1B). The Rqdl10 solution can self-assemble into a hydrogel upon ion triggering through hydrogen bonding, van der Waals forces, aromatic stacking, charge–charge interactions, and hydrophobic–hydrophilic interactions [7] (Figure 2A). Circular dichroism spectroscopy revealed that the Rqdl10, after 24 h of self-assembly, exhibited a positive peak at 192.5 nm and a negative peak at 211.5 nm, indicative of the formation of a typical β-sheet structure (Figure 2B). Atomic force microscopy (AFM) analysis demonstrated the formation of vesicle-like structures by the Rqdl10 after 24 h of self-assembly, with diameters ranging from 100 to 150 nm and an average diameter of 127 nm. The vesicles were interlaced with each other to form vesicle-like three-dimensional nanostructures (Figure 2C). The cryo-scanning electron microscopy results revealed that the Rqdl10 hydrogel exhibited a vesicular morphology whose nanostructures connected to each other in the field of view of 200 nm and 500 nm. Upon expanding the field of view to 1 μm and 5 μm, it was observed that the vesicular nanostructures intertwined to form a three-dimensional network structure (Figure 2D). Additionally, the Congo red/aniline blue staining of the Rqdl10 hydrogel indicated the presence of an evacuation film structure at 0 h of self-assembly. However, with an extension of self-assembly time to 12, 24, and 48 h, this structure transformed into a denser, lamellar, and more stable configuration (Figure 2E,F).

2.2. Rqdl10 Hydrogel Delivery of TFF3

To assess the controlled release efficacy of the Rqdl10 hydrogel, we investigated its effect on the release of TFF3. Our findings indicate that while there were slight variations in the controlled release of TFF3 among different concentrations of the Rqdl10 hydrogel, the TFF3@Rqdl10 solution achieved a near-complete release of TFF3 after 24 h. Specifically, the controlled release of TFF3 by the Rqdl10 hydrogel was determined to be 92.3%, 87.2%, and 81.1% at concentrations of 5 mg/mL, 7.5 mg/mL, and 10 mg/mL, respectively (Figure 3A). Given the optimal stability observed with 10 mg/mL Rqdl10 hydrogel for the controlled release of TFF3, we selected this concentration as the delivery vehicle for TFF3. Similarly, in vitro imaging of TFF3 within the Rqdl10 hydrogel demonstrated that TFF3 could be retained in Rqdl10 hydrogels for more than 36 h (Figure 3B). Given that the concentration of pepsin in the stomach fluctuates between 0.5 and 1.0 mg/mL, we utilized a 2 mg/mL pepsin solution (dissolved in pH = 3 buffer) to simulate the intragastric environment. Our results revealed that the Rqdl10 hydrogel significantly attenuated the diffusion of pepsin from the upper chamber to the lower chamber within 32 h compared to the no hydrogel group (Figure 3C). In the in vivo experiments, both FITC−Rqdl10 and Cy5.5−TFF3 in Cy5.5−TFF3@Rqdl10 can be detected and kept in the stomach from 0 h to 36 h after injection, while no detectable signal of Cy5.5−TFF3 was observed at 12 h after injection (Figure 3D,E). This indicates that TFF3@Rqdl10 can effectively adhere to the surface of the gastric mucosa, efficiently sequestering pepsin while sustainably and slowly releasing TFF3.

A

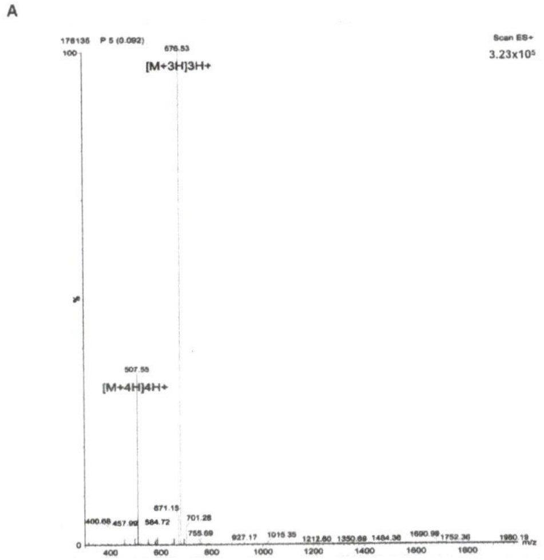

B

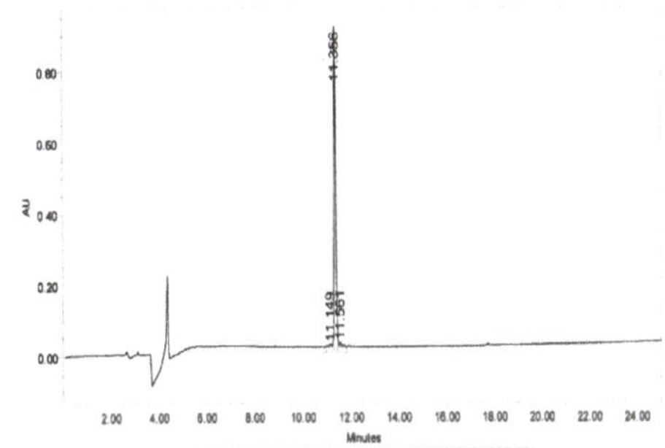

	RT	Area	%Area	Height
1	11.149	44,630	1.00	5593
2	11.359	4,346,302	97.40	894,785
3	11.561	71,244	1.60	11,292

Figure 1. Mass spectrometry and HPLC analysis of peptide Rqdl10. (**A**) Mass spectrometry analysis of peptide Rqdl10; (**B**) HPLC analysis of peptide Rqdl10.

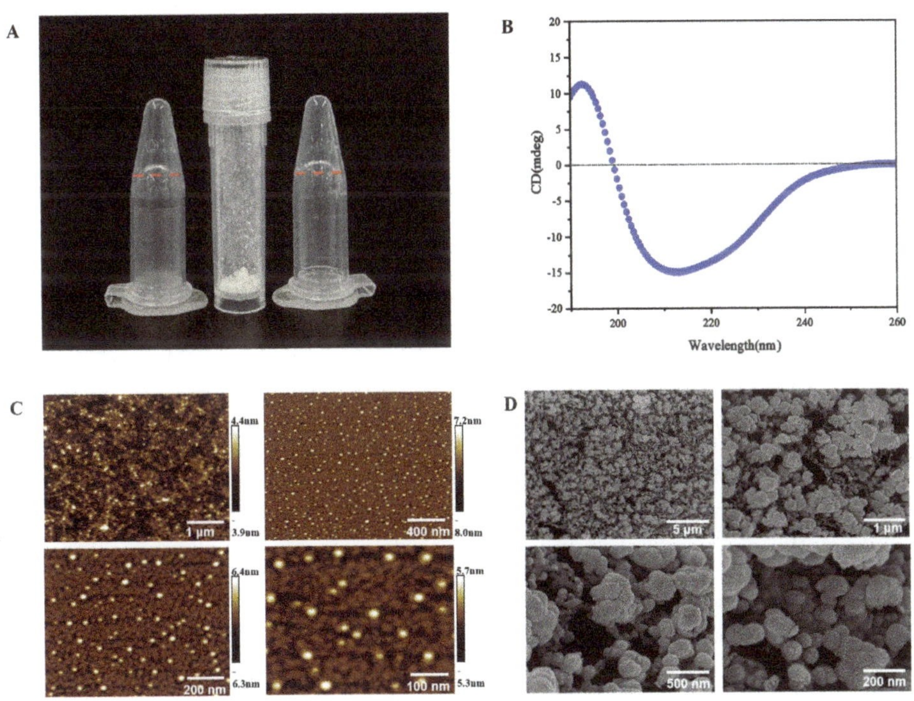

Figure 2. *Cont.*

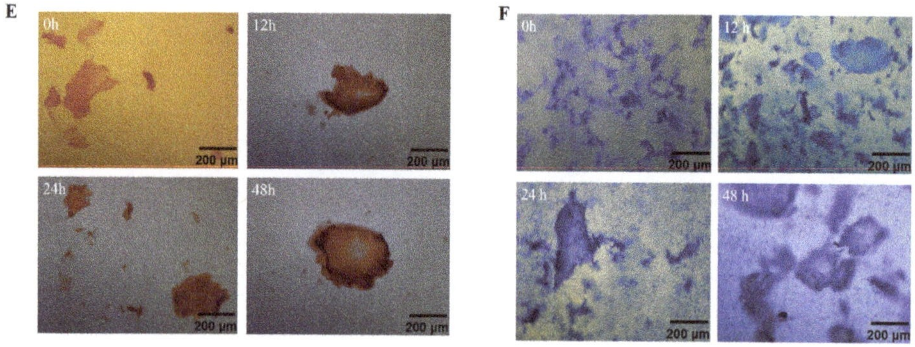

Figure 2. Characterization of Rqdl10 hydrogel. (**A**) Hydrogel formed by self−assembling peptide Rqdl10,The red line represents the lower edge of Rqdl10 hydrogel; (**B**) Circular dichroic analysis of Rqdl10 hydrogel; (**C**) Atomic force microscopy (AFM) analysis of Rqdl10 hydrogel; (**D**) Cryogenic scanning electron microscopy (cryo-SEM) analysis of Rqdl10 hydrogel; (**E**) Congo red staining results of Rqdl10 hydrogel at 0 h, 12 h, 24 h and 48 h; (**F**) aniline blue staining results of Rqdl10 hydrogel at 0 h, 12 h, 24 h and 48 h.

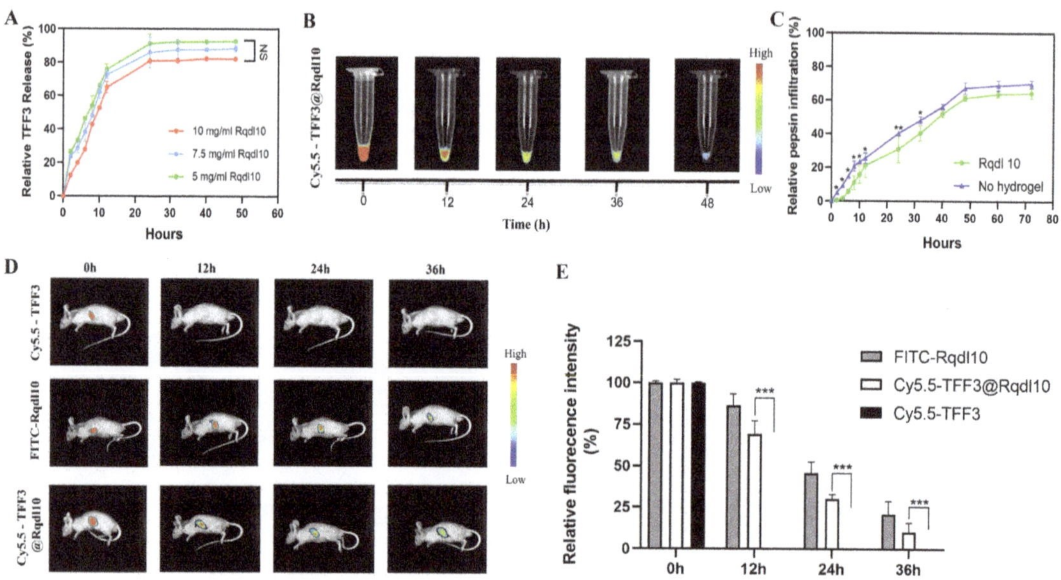

Figure 3. Rqdl10 hydrogel delivery of TFF3. (**A**) In vitro release curve of TFF3 from different concentrations of Rqdl10 hydrogel in PBS; (**B**) In vitro imaging of TFF3 in Rqdl10 hydrogel; (**C**) Sequestration effect of Rqdl10 hydrogel on pepsin. * $p < 0.05$, ** $p < 0.01$,Comparison between Rqdl10 hydrogel group and no hydrogel group; (**D**) Representative images of optical in vivo imaging; (**E**) Quantification analysis of the fluorescence intensity retention in stomach. *** $p < 0.001$. Statistics for each group are expressed as mean ± SD ($n = 4$).

2.3. Biocompatibility of Rqdl10

The assessment of biocompatibility is pivotal in determining the suitability of hydrogels for biomedical applications. To ascertain the biocompatibility of the Rqdl10 hydrogel, the cell viability of GES1 cells was evaluated using a cell proliferation toxicity assay employing the CCK8 method. The results of the cell proliferation assay revealed that the

GES1 cells in the control group exhibited continuous growth over the initial 3 days. In contrast, the proliferation of GES1 cells within the Rqdl10 hydrogel matrix was slower; however, they remained in a state of slow proliferation, with no discernible decline in cell activity observed (Figure 4A). Furthermore, cytotoxicity assessments demonstrated that the GES1 cells in the control group exhibited the highest cell activity on day one, followed by a gradual decrease thereafter. Conversely, the activity of GES1 cells within the Rqdl10 hydrogel matrix remained relatively stable, displaying a slight increasing trend (Figure 4B). These findings collectively suggest that the Rqdl10 hydrogel exhibits favorable biocompatibility.

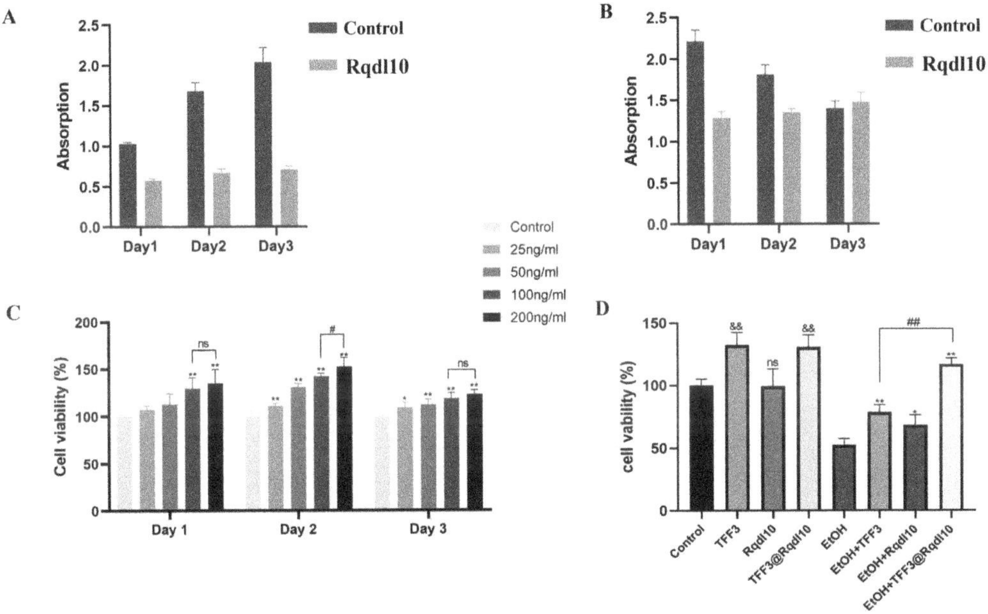

Figure 4. Determination of cell viability of GES−1 under different treatments. (**A**) Proliferation assay of GES-1 cells in Rqdl10 hydrogel matrix; (**B**) Cytotoxicity assay of GES-1 cells in Rqdl10 hydrogel matrix; (**C**) Optimal concentration of TFF3 to promote GES-1 proliferation,* $p < 0.05$,** $p < 0.01$ (vs. control group), # $p < 0.05$, ns means no statistical significance; (**D**) Effect of TFF3, Rqdl10 hydrogel, and TFF3@Rqdl10 treatment on GES-1 cell viability in the presence or absence of ethanol. && $p < 0.01$ (vs. control group), * $p < 0.05$, ** $p < 0.01$ (vs. EtOH Group), ## $p < 0.01$. Statistics for each group are expressed as mean ± SD ($n = 6$).

2.4. TFF3@Rqdl10 Promoted Cell Proliferation and Migration

The GES-1 cells were exposed to various concentration gradients of TFF3 for 24 h to determine the optimal environment. Cell viability was assessed using the CCK8 assay after 24 h of treatment. The results revealed that a concentration of 200 ng/mL of TFF3 was optimal for promoting the proliferation of GES-1 cells (Figure 4C). Based on these findings, we selected a concentration of 200 ng/mL of TFF3 for subsequent experiments. In an ethanol-free environment, treatment with TFF3 and TFF3@Rqdl10 significantly enhanced GES-1 cell proliferation, whereas treatment with Rqdl10 hydrogel alone showed no such effect. Conversely, in the presence of ethanol, the viability of the GES-1 cells in the EtOH group decreased to 52.45% of the control group. However, pre-treatment with TFF3, Rqdl10 hydrogel, and TFF3@Rqdl10 increased cell viability to 78.57%, 68.17%, and 116.71%, respectively (Figure 4D). In Figure 5A, both the TFF3 and TFF3@Rqdl10 treatments demonstrated significant enhancement in promoting GES-1 cell migration, whereas the Rqdl10 hydrogel treatment did not exhibit a similar effect (Figure 5B). Furthermore, we assessed cell migration under ethanol-stimulated conditions. The results revealed that following treatment with TFF3, Rqdl10 hydrogel, and TFF3@Rqdl10, the rate of the scratch closure of the GES-1 cells was notably faster compared to the EtOH group within 48 h (Figure 5C). Notably, the TFF3@Rqdl10 treatment significantly facilitated GES-1 migration after ethanol-induced damage more effectively than TFF3 alone ($p < 0.01$) (Figure 5D). These findings suggest that while the Rqdl10 hydrogel treatment mitigated ethanol-induced injury to the GES-1 cells, it did not promote their proliferation and migration. Conversely, the TFF3 treatment promoted both the proliferation and migration of the GES-1 cells, while the TFF3@Rqdl10 treatment not only reduced the ethanol-induced injury to the GES-1 cells but also enhanced their proliferation and migration.

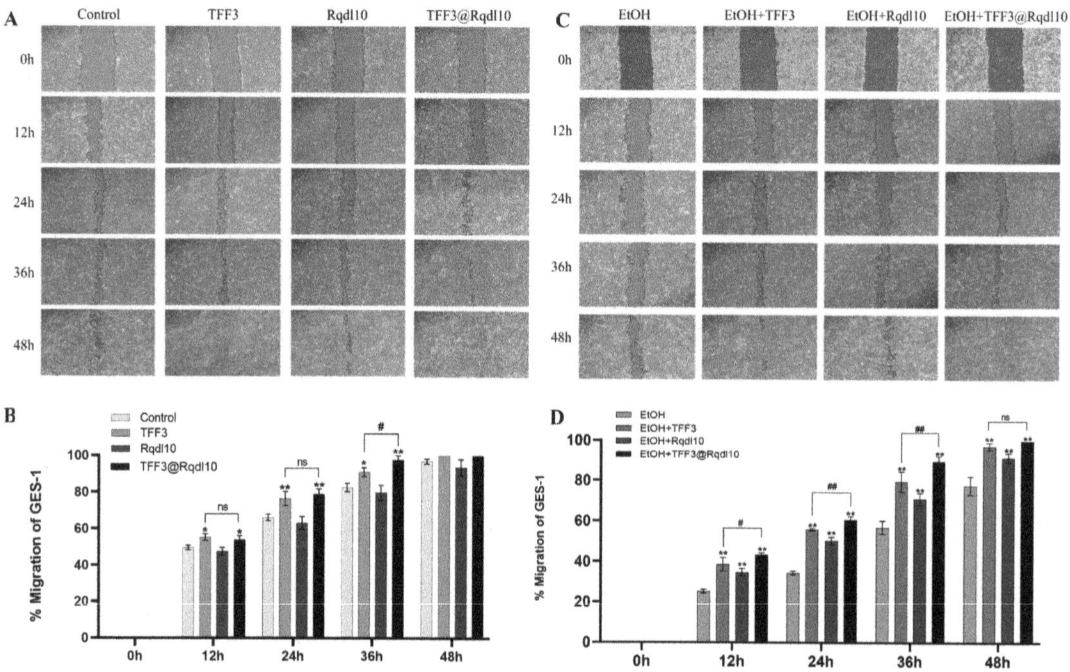

Figure 5. Effect of TFF3, Rqdl10 hydrogel, and TFF3@Rqdl10 treatment on GES−1 cell migration in the presence or absence of ethanol. (**A**) The scratch assay on GES−1 cell migration in treatment with TFF3, Rqdl10 hydrogel, and TFF3@Rqdl10 at different incubation times; (**B**) Migration rate of GES-1 cells after treatment with TFF3, Rqdl10 hydrogel, and TFF3@Rqdl10, * $p < 0.05$, ** $p < 0.01$ (vs. control group), # $p < 0.05$, ns means no statistical significance; (**C**) The scratch assay on GES−1 cell migration in treatment with TFF3, Rqdl10 hydrogel, and TFF3@Rqdl10 at different incubation times in ethanol environment; (**D**) Migration rate of GES−1 cells after treatment with TFF3, Rqdl10 hydrogel, and TFF3@Rqdl10 in ethanol environment. ** $p < 0.01$ (vs. EtOH Group), # $p < 0.05$, ## $p < 0.01$, ns means no statistical significance. Statistics for each group are expressed as mean ± SD ($n = 4$).

2.5. In Vitro Anti-Apoptosis and Anti-Inflammatory Activity of TFF3@Rqdl10

Calcein-AM stains live cells green, while PI stains dead cells red. As shown in Figure 6A, under ethanol-free conditions, GES-1 cells exhibit a spindle-shaped and flattened morphology with no overlap or aggregation between cells. In the TFF3 group, the cell density increases compared to the control group. After ethanol treatment, the GES-1 cells change from spindle-shaped to spherical and aggregate, with numerous red-stained dead cells scattered throughout. In the EtOH + TFF3 and EtOH + Rqdl10 groups, a small number of GES-1 cells with normal morphology and a large number with irregular morphology are observed, with a slightly higher density of green-stained live cells than the EtOH group, and fewer red-stained dead cells than the EtOH group. The EtOH+TFF3@Rqdl10 group demonstrates the most potent anti-apoptotic ability, with the GES-1 cells exhibiting a predominantly normal morphology and only scattered red-stained dead cells. Flow cytometry was employed to assess the apoptosis of the GES-1 cells following ethanol injury (Figure 6B). Under normal conditions, the number of apoptotic GES-1 cells is minimal. The ethanol treatment significantly increased the apoptosis rate, reaching 24.58% for the GES-1 cells in the EtOH group. However, after pretreatment with TFF3, Rqdl10 hydrogel, and TFF3@Rqdl10, the apoptosis rate of the GES-1 cells decreased to 15.23%, 18.96%, and 11.9%, respectively (Figure 6C). Notably, the TFF3@Rqdl10 treatment exhibited a significant inhibitory effect on apoptosis, whereas the effect of the Rqdl10 hydrogel treatment was primarily observed in delaying the onset of apoptosis. Furthermore, Western Blotting results (Figure 7A–C) demonstrated that TFF3 did not alter the expression of Bax and Bcl2 in normal GES-1 cells ($p > 0.05$). In the ethanol injury model, ethanol induces the upregulation of Bax and downregulation of Bcl2 expression in the GES-1 cells. The expression levels of Bax and Bcl2 in the GES-1 cells treated with TFF3, Rqdl10 hydrogel, and TFF3@Rqdl10 significantly differed from those in the EtOH group ($p < 0.01$), indicating that all the treatments effectively inhibit the apoptosis of GES-1 cells. Additionally, there was a significant difference in the ability of the TFF3@Rqdl10 treatment to downregulate Bax and upregulate Bcl2 compared to TFF3 alone ($p < 0.01$). Next, we will shift our focus to the expression of intracellular inflammation-related proteins. Inflammation is an inevitable response when cells or tissues are injured. TNF-α and IL-6, as biomarkers of acute inflammatory response, are actively involved in several inflammatory processes and are closely associated with the severity of gastric mucosal injury [37]. On the other hand, NF-κB, as a major regulator of inflammatory response, plays an important role in promoting the transcription of TNF-α and IL-6. Therefore, we selected TNF-α, IL-6 and NF-κB to elucidate the mechanisms associated with the alleviation by TFF3@Rqdl10 of ethanol-induced acute gastric mucosal injury. The ethanol treatment resulted in the increased expression of pro-inflammatory factors such as TNF-α, IL-6, and NF-κB in the GES-1 cells (Figure 7D–G). However, the inflammatory state of the GES-1 cells was significantly ameliorated following the treatment with TFF3, Rqdl10 hydrogel, and TFF3@Rqdl10 compared to the ethanol group. Moreover, the anti-inflammatory and anti-apoptotic capacities of the GES-1 cells after the TFF3 treatment were found to be significantly weaker than those of the TFF3@Rqdl10 treatment ($p < 0.01$).

2.6. *In Vivo Anti-Apoptosis and Anti-Inflammatory Activity of TFF3@Rqdl10*

TFF3, an active peptide secreted by gastric mucosal cells, possesses a variety of biological functions, and its action on the surface of the gastric mucosa helps to promote the repair process of gastric mucosal damage. However, when used as a drug, TFF3 faces significant challenges, including short retention time in the gastric mucosal cavity and deactivation due to degradation by stomach acid. To further investigate, we explored the effects of TFF3, Rqdl10 hydrogel, and TFF3@Rqdl10 treatment on the expression of inflammation and apoptosis-related proteins by establishing a rat acetic acid gastric mucosal injury model. As depicted in the Western Blotting results (Figure 8A–G), the TFF3, Rqdl10 hydrogel, and TFF3@Rqdl10 treatments all effectively suppressed the expression of TNF-α, IL-6, and NF-κB, while also inhibiting Bax expression and promoting Bcl2 expression. Interestingly, the Rqdl10 hydrogel treatment exhibited a significantly stronger inhibition of inflammatory and apoptotic responses compared to the TFF3 treatment in the in vivo experiments ($p < 0.01$). This difference may be due to the fact that TFF3 is easily lost and susceptible to degradation by stomach acid when locally applied to the site of gastric mucosal injury. In contrast, the Rqdl10 hydrogel can adhere to the surface of damaged gastric mucosa for an extended duration, reducing the continuous stimulation of gastric acid on the damaged mucosa and creating a favorable environment for gastric mucosal healing. In addition, treatment with TFF3@Rqdl10 demonstrated superior suppression of inflammatory and apoptotic responses compared to treatment with TFF3 alone. This implies that TFF3@Rqdl10 not only shields the damaged gastric mucosa from continuous gastric acid stimulation but also gradually releases TFF3 to facilitate the repair of gastric mucosal injury. These findings suggest that the Rqdl10 hydrogel can serve as an optimal vehicle for TFF3, thereby promoting the mending of gastric mucosal injury.

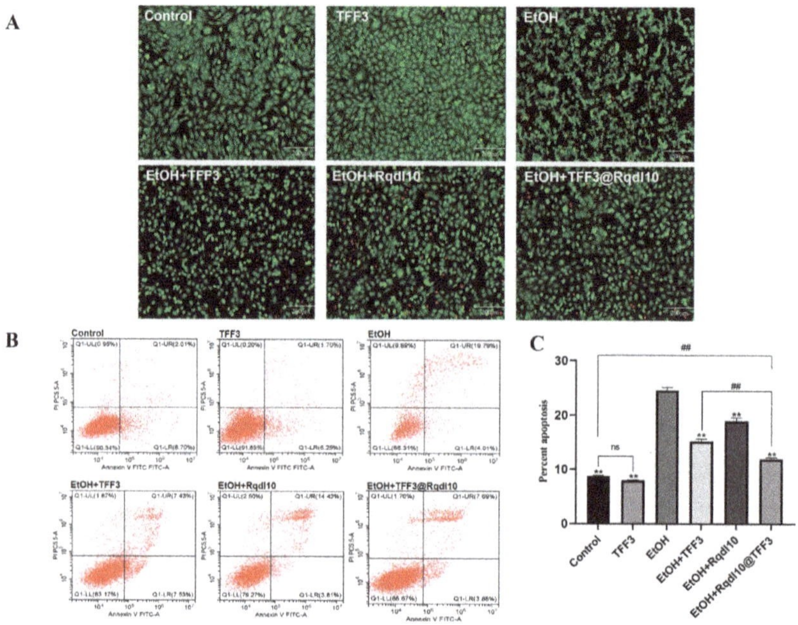

Figure 6. Apoptosis detection in GES-1 cells. (**A**) The live/dead staining of GES-1 cell treatment with TFF3, Rqdl10 hydrogel, and TFF3@Rqdl10; (**B**) Flow cytometric analysis for quantification of apoptotic cells; (**C**) Percentage of apoptotic GES−1 cells. ** $p < 0.01$ (vs. EtOH Group); ## $p < 0.01$; ns means no statistical significance. Statistics for each group are expressed as mean ± SD ($n = 4$).

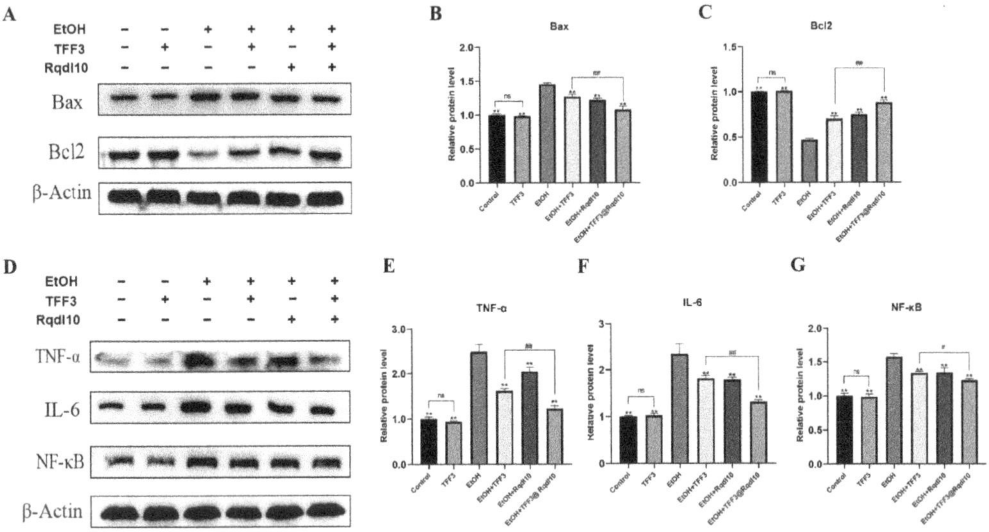

Figure 7. The impact of TFF3@Rqdl10 on apoptosis and inflammation-related protein expression in GES−1 cells after ethanol-induced injury. (**A**) WB analysis of Bax and Bcl2 in GES-1 cells after ethanol injury. Relative protein level of Bax (**B**) and Bcl2 (**C**), ** $p < 0.01$ (vs. EtOH group), ## $p < 0.01$, ns means no statistical significance; (**D**) WB analysis of TNF-α, IL-6, and NF-κB in GES-1 cells after ethanol injury; Relative protein level of TNF-α (**E**), IL-6 (**F**), and NF-κB (**G**), ** $p < 0.01$ (vs. EtOH group), # $p < 0.05$, ## $p < 0.01$, ns means no statistical significance. Statistics for each group are expressed as mean ± SD ($n = 6$).

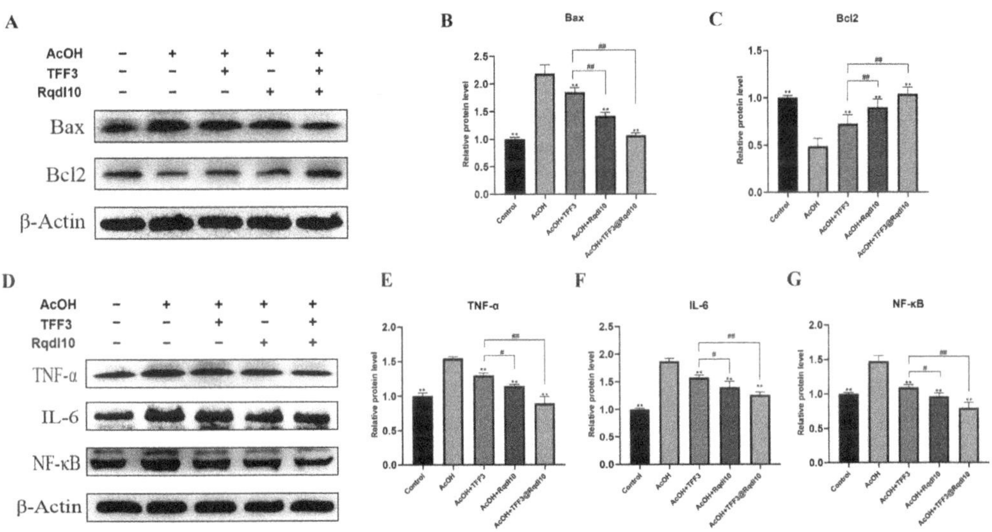

Figure 8. The impact of TFF3@Rqdl10 on apoptosis and inflammation−related protein expression after acetic acid injury in rat gastric mucosa. (**A**) WB analysis of Bax and Bcl2 in gastric tissue after acetic acid injury. Relative protein level of Bax (**B**) and Bcl2 (**C**), ** $p < 0.01$ (vs. EtOH group), ## $p < 0.01$, ns means no statistical significance; (**D**) WB analysis of TNF-α, IL-6, and NF-κB in gastric tissue after acetic acid injury; Relative protein level of TNF-α (**E**), IL-6 (**F**), and NF-κB (**G**), ** $p < 0.01$ (vs. AcOH group), # $p < 0.05$, ## $p < 0.01$, ns means no statistical significance. Statistics for each group are expressed as mean ± SD ($n = 6$).

3. Discussion

Numerous drugs suffer from limited bioavailability and inadequate therapeutic effectiveness, primarily attributed to factors such as low water solubility, instability, suboptimal biodistribution, rapid degradation, and a lack of targeting specificity [38]. Presently, conventional drug delivery platforms encompass viruses, liposomes, polymers, and synthetic inorganic materials [39–42]. Self-assembled peptides emerge as promising candidates for drug delivery vehicles owing to their remarkable biocompatibility, biodegradability, facile tissue absorption and utilization, and minimal or absent unexpected toxicities [11]. Self-assembled short peptides utilize various molecular forces including hydrogen bonding, electrostatic interactions, hydrophilic–hydrophobic interactions, π-π interactions, and van der Waals forces generated by self−contained amino acid residues to encapsulate or adsorb drugs, thereby forming a stable drug delivery system [43]. These self-assembled peptide vehicles can enhance drug pharmacokinetics and therapeutic efficacy by facilitating the controlled release and precise delivery of drugs [44]. Additionally, they can improve drug bioavailability by responding to environmental cues for drug release and minimizing drug degradation during circulation [45]. Currently, the self−assembled short peptide delivery system has achieved the precise delivery and controlled release of various substances including hydrophobic drugs, peptides, nucleic acids, vaccines, and more [46].

The repair of gastric mucosal injury constitutes a complex and coordinated biological process, encompassing multiple critical steps to ensure the effective repair and functional restoration of damaged tissue [47]. Throughout this process, the proliferation and migration of injured mucosal cells, along with apoptosis and inflammatory responses, play pivotal roles. Proliferation and migration facilitate the formation of new cells, filling the damaged areas and establishing a complete cellular architecture, thus accelerating the healing of the injury site [48]. Following gastric mucosal damage, there is a rapid increase in cell apoptosis, leading to further tissue destruction [49]. By inhibiting apoptosis, excessive cell death can be prevented, aiding in the maintenance of tissue integrity and providing favorable conditions for repair [50]. The inflammatory response that follows closely typically dictates the outcomes of healing [51]. Inflammation subsequent to gastric mucosal injury unfolds in distinct phases to facilitate the restoration of tissue architecture. Initially, an early pro-inflammatory response orchestrates the recruitment of key inflammatory cells to initiate the repair cascade. Subsequently, this pro-inflammatory cascade begins to subside, concomitant with a phenotypic transition of macrophages to a reparative state. Finally, as inflammatory cells vacate the injury site or undergo apoptosis, tissue homeostasis is restored [52,53]. The microenvironment of chronic wounds is typically characterized by the accumulation of many pro-inflammatory macrophages, along with the upregulation of inflammatory mediators such as NF-κB, TNF-α, and IL-6 [54]. Chronic inflammation can lead to sustained tissue damage and even the formation of ulcers. By inhibiting the inflammatory response, the release of inflammatory mediators can be reduced, decelerating the process of tissue destruction and facilitating the creation of a conducive environment for repair [54]. Precisely regulating these responses and their interactions during the gastric mucosal injury repair process is an effective therapeutic strategy for enhancing the healing of gastric mucosal damage. TFF3 is an active peptide with multiple biological functions, playing roles not only in promoting the proliferation and migration of GES-1 cells but also exhibiting significant anti-inflammatory and anti-apoptotic properties. As a chiral self-assembling peptide hydrogel, Rqdl10 hydrogel has not yet been observed as having a definitive biological function. However, the Rqdl10 can self−assemble into a hydrogel, and through a physical barrier function similarly to gastric mucus, it effectively protects the gastric mucosa and diminishes the damage induced by ethanol and acetic acid. Our research also discovered that the therapeutic effect of the Rqdl10 hydrogel on the repair of gastric mucosal damage in in vivo models surpasses that of TFF3. The in vitro models reveal that TFF3's protective effect against ethanol-induced gastric mucosal injury is superior to that of the Rqdl10 hydrogel. This phenomenon might be related to the fact that TFF3, when co-cultured with GES-1 cells under in vitro conditions, has its bioactivity and duration of action fully ensured. In contrast, when TFF3 is directly applied as a drug to the gastric mucosal cavity, its retention time and bioactivity in the stomach may not be guaranteed to the same extent. TFF3@Rqdl10 adheres to the gastric mucosa and prolongs the retention time of TFF3 in the stomach by slowly releasing TFF3. It also enhances the stability of TFF3 in the gastric mucosal cavity through the sequestration of pepsin. Compared to the use of TFF3 or Rqdl10 hydrogel alone, TFF3@Rqdl10 significantly enhances the reparative effects on gastric mucosal damage, more effectively facilitating the proliferation and migration of gastric mucosal cells, and inhibiting inflammation and apoptotic responses, thus offering multi-layered support for the repair of gastric mucosal injuries. These results indicate that TFF3@Rqdl10 is an effective strategy for treating gastric mucosal injuries.

4. Materials and Methods

4.1. Synthesis of Rqdl10

Rqdl10 was designed by our research team and synthesized by Chengdu Sciobio Surgery Institute (Chengdu, China). The amino acid sequence of Rqdl10 is RQDLK-TEIRYDF KADE-NH2, constituting a linear polypeptide from the N-terminus to the C-terminus. The peptide's molecular weight and purity were determined using mass spectrometry (LC3000, SHIMADZU, Kyoto, Japan) and HPLC (Nexera UHPLC, SHIMADZU, Kyoto, Japan), respectively.

4.2. Hydrogel Preparation

A peptide solution was prepared by dissolving 20 mg of Rqdl10 in 1 mL of sterile water. Subsequently, 1 mL of PBS was added to the peptide solution to induce self-assembly of the hydrogel at room temperature for 24 h, denoted as Rqdl10 hydrogel. Rqdl10 was dissolved in a sterile aqueous solution of TFF3 and then added to PBS to self-assemble into a drug-loaded hydrogel at room temperature, denoted as TFF3@Rqdl10.

4.3. Characterization of Rqdl10 Hydrogel

To investigate the secondary structure of the Rqdl10 hydrogel, a JASCO J-815 Spectrometer (JASCO, Kyoto, Japan) was utilized for detection. AFM (multimode8, Bruker, Massachusetts, USA) was employed to acquire the surface topography and structural information for the Rqdl10 hydrogel. The three-dimensional structure of the Rqdl10 hydrogel was captured using cryo-SEM (SU8010, Hitachi, Kyoto, Japan). The gel formation was observed through Congo red/aniline blue staining at 0 h, 12 h, 24 h, and 48 h following Rqdl10 self-assembly.

4.4. Controlled Release of TFF3 by Rqdl10 Hydrogel In Vitro

TFF3@Rqdl10 was prepared following previously described methods. Briefly, 100 μL of TFF3@Rqdl10 (1 ug/mL TFF3) was dispensed into the bottom of a 96-well plate, followed by the addition of 100 μL of PBS to each well. The plate was then incubated at 37 °C and continuously agitated on a shaker. To ensure consistent initial conditions, all the drug-containing wells for various time points were prepared simultaneously. At specified time intervals (0 h, 2 h, 4 h, 6 h, 8 h, 10 h, 12 h, 24 h, 32 h, 40 h, 48 h), supernatants were collected from selected wells (n = 3), while others remained undisturbed. TFF3 concentrations were quantified using a commercial ELISA kit (Cusabio, Wuhan, China) as per the manufacturer's protocol, and the release profile of Rqdl10 for TFF3 was determined.

4.5. Analysis of Pepsin Sequestration by Rqdl10 Hydrogel In Vitro

We prepared a 24-well plate in advance by adding 1100 μL of buffer (pH = 3.0). Then, we took 100 μL of the Rqdl10 hydrogel (10 mg/mL) and placed it at the bottom of the upper chamber of the transwell, gently shaking to ensure it lay flat. Next, we added 200 μL of pepsin solution (2 mg/mL, pH = 3.0) to the upper chamber and placed the smaller chamber in the buffer. We collected and replenished the buffer at 0 h, 2 h, 4 h, 6 h, 8 h, 10 h, 12 h, 24 h, 36 h, 48 h, 60 h, and 72 h time points. We measured the absorbance at 562 nm using the CBA method and calculated the percentage of pepsin that had infiltrated into the lower chamber using a standard curve.

4.6. In Vitro Imaging of Cy5.5−TFF3 in Rqdl10 Hydrogel

Cy5.5 dye was dissolved in DMF at a concentration of 12.56 mM. TFF3 (5 μg/μL) solution was prepared in pure water; then, Cy5.5 dye was added to the TFF3 solution at a molar ratio of 3:1 (Cy5.5:TFF3) and incubated for 30 min at 37 °C in a thermostat protected from light. Free dye was removed using 3KD ultrafiltration tubes. Cy5.5-TFF3@Rqdl10 (Rqdl10 10 mg/mL) was prepared as previously described. Next, 50 μL of Cy5.5-TFF3@Rqdl10 was placed in a 1.5 mL EP tube, and 200 μL of PBS was then added. At the indicated time points (0 h, 12 h, 24 h, 36 h, 48 h), the supernatant was removed and Cy5.5-TFF3@Rqdl10 in the EP tube was visualized using an in vivo imaging system (VILBER, Collégien, France).

4.7. In Vivo Imaging of Cy5.5−TFF3, FITC−Rqdl10 Hydrogel, and Cy5.5−TFF3@Rqdl10 in Mice

BALB/c nude mice were fasted for 24 h and abstained from drinking for 12 h. They were then anesthetized with sodium pentobarbital (intraperitoneally, 50 mg/kg), and a midline epigastric incision was made to fully expose the gastric tissue. Sequentially, 100 μL of Cy5.5-TFF3, FITC-Rqdl10 hydrogel (10 mg/mL), and Cy5.5-TFF3@Rqdl10 were injected into the gastric lumen to adhere to the gastric mucosa as much as possible, after which the incision was sutured. The nude mice were anesthetized at the indicated time points (0 h, 12 h, 24 h, and 36 h) after the injections, and the measurements were performed using the in vivo imaging system (VILBER, France).

4.8. Cell Culture and Treatment

Human gastric mucosal epithelial cells (GES-1 cells) were procured from Saibekang Biotechnology (Shanghai, China). GES-1 cells were cultured routinely in DMEM supplemented with 10% FBS and 1% penicillin and streptomycin, maintaining them in a humidified incubator at 37 °C with 5% CO_2. The cytocompatibility of the Rqdl10 hydrogel was assessed using the CCK8 method. A 100 μL cell suspension was inoculated into a 96-well plate, followed by the addition of 25 μL of Rqdl10 solution and 25 μL of PBS. The mixture was gently mixed to ensure encapsulation of GES-1 cells into the Rqdl10 hydrogel. The proliferation and toxicity test were conducted at cell densities of 5×10^3 cells/well and 2×10^4 cells/well. After 1, 2, and 3 days, 10 μL of CCK8 was added and incubated for 2 h, followed by absorbance measurement at 450 nm to calculate cell viability. GES-1 cells were seeded in 96-well plates at a density of 5×10^3 cells/well and pretreated with TFF3, Rqdl10 hydrogel, or TFF3@Rqdl10 for 24 h. Subsequently, acute injury was induced in GES-1 cells by co-incubation with 6% ethanol DMEM medium for 4 h. Changes in inflammation and apoptosis−related proteins in GES-1 were analyzed using Western Blotting.

4.9. Cell Scratch Assay

Assessment of potential cell migration capacity was conducted using the cell scratch method. In the absence of ethanol stimulation, GES-1 cells were cultured with TFF3, Rqdl10 hydrogel, or TFF3@Rqdl10 for 24 h, and cell scratches were created on the cell layer using a cell scraper. The cell debris was washed with PBS, and photographs were captured at 0 h, 12 h, 24 h, 36 h, and 48 h to measure the size of the scratches. Under ethanol exposure, GES-1 cells were treated with TFF3, Rqdl10 hydrogel, or TFF3@Rqdl10 for 24 h, followed by treatment with 6% ethanol DMEM medium for 4 h. Subsequently, cell migration was observed under a microscope at 0 h, 12 h, 24 h, 36 h, and 48 h, and the scratch area was assessed using ImageJ.

4.10. Evaluation of Anti-Apoptosis Effects In Vitro

Detection of apoptosis levels in GES-1 cells was performed using the Calcein-AM/PI Apoptosis Detection Kit (Beyotime, China). Briefly, GES-1 cells were seeded into 96-well plates at a density of 5×10^3 cells per well. After treatment with various experimental conditions, the cells were washed once with PBS, and then 100 μL of the prepared Calcein-AM/PI fluorescent staining solution was added to each well. The plates were then incubated at 37 °C for 30 min in the dark. Subsequently, the cells were examined under a fluorescence microscope. For flow cytometry analysis, GES-1 cells were seeded into 6-well plates at a density of 1×10^6 cells per well. After treatment with different experimental conditions, the cells were collected into centrifuge tubes according to their respective groups. A 1 mL cell suspension (1×10^6 cells/mL) was centrifuged at 1000 rpm for 5 min, and then 1 mL of Calcein-AM/PI assay working solution was added. After resuspending the cells as a single-cell suspension, they were incubated at 37 °C in the dark for 30 min. Finally, the cells were analyzed using a flow cytometer (CytoFLEX, Beckman, Brea, CA, USA).

4.11. Acetic Acid-Induced Gastric Injury in Rats

Adult healthy SD rats weighing 200–250 g were selected and included in the experiment. The animals were housed under standardized conditions, including controlled temperature, humidity, and a 12 h light–dark cycle, and were provided with standard feed and tap water ad libitum. All procedures related to animal experiments were approved by the Experimental Animal Ethics Committee of Chongqing Medical University. Acetic acid (AcOH) was used to induce gastric mucosal injury in rats, following the method reported by Kang [55]. Briefly, SD rats were randomly divided into the control group, AcOH group, AcOH + TFF3 group, AcOH + Rqdl10 group, and AcOH + TFF3@Rqdl10 group. The rats were fasted for 24 h before surgery, and then anesthetized with sodium pentobarbital (50 mg/kg) by intraperitoneal injection to fully expose the gastric tissue. A circular EP tube with a diameter of approximately 10 mm was positioned adjacent to the serosa of the gastric antrum. Subsequently, 0.1 mL of 100% glacial acetic acid was injected into the tube, where it was allowed to remain for 60 s. Following this, the acetic acid was aspirated, and the serosa was rinsed twice with PBS. Each of the anterior and posterior walls of the gastric antrum underwent modeling once, resulting in the formation of two ulcers with symmetrical size and location. The posterior wall served as the AcOH group, while the anterior wall was designated as the experimental group. In the AcOH group, 100 μL of PBS was injected into the ulcer, whereas in the AcOH+TFF3 group, 100 μL of TFF3 solution was injected into the ulcer. Similarly, the AcOH + Rqdl10 group received an injection of 100 μL of Rqdl10 hydrogel into the ulcer, and the AcOH + TFF3@Rqdl10 group received 100 μL of TFF3@Rqdl10 into the ulcer. Following the procedure, the omentum was covered, and the peritoneal, abdominal wall tissues, and skin were intermittently sutured. The rats were then housed individually. After a period of 5 days, the rats were sacrificed under anesthesia.

4.12. Western Blotting

Proteins were extracted from gastric tissues or GES-1 cells using radioimmunoprecipitation assay (RIPA) lysis buffer (Beyotime, Shanghai, China), and protein quantification was conducted using the BCA method (Beyotime, China). Equal amounts of proteins were then separated on a 10% SDS-PAGE gel and subsequently transferred to a polyvinylidene difluoride (PVDF) membrane. Following blocking for 10 min at room temperature using rapid blocking solution (Ncmbio, Suzhou, China), PVDF membranes were incubated with primary antibodies overnight at 4 °C. Afterward, the PVDF membrane was washed three times using tris−buffered saline (TBST) and incubated with secondary antibody for 1 h at room temperature. Finally, emitter-coupled logic (ECL) substrate (Ncmbio, China) was added dropwise, and the membrane was observed using a chemiluminescent detection system (Bio-Rad, Hercules, CA, USA). Quantification of protein bands was performed using Image J software (1.53K). The antibodies used were as follows: β-actin (AB0035, 1:5000, Abways, Beijing, China), Bax (A20227, 1:2000, ABclonal, Wuhan, China), Bcl2 (A20777,

1:1000, ABclonal, China), TNF−α (ER1919-22, 1:500, HuaBio, Hangzhou, China), IL−6 (R1412-2, 1:500, HuaBio, China), and NF−κB (PSH0−27, 1:1000, HuaBio, China).

4.13. Statistical Analysis

All data were presented as mean ± SD (n = 3) and analyzed using a one-way ANOVA test followed by the Tukey honest significant difference (HSD) test using SPSS software (version 22, Chicago, IL, USA), and $p < 0.05$ was considered a significant difference.

5. Conclusions

In this study, we engineered an optimal drug delivery vehicle, Rqdl10 hydrogel, for TFF3. The Rqdl10 hydrogel exhibits excellent biocompatibility, enabling the sustainable and slow release of TFF3. Moreover, the Rqdl10 hydrogel effectively protects the gastric mucosa through a physical barrier action similar to that of gastric mucus, mitigating damage caused by ethanol or gastric acid, thereby providing an optimal healing microenvironment for gastric mucosal repair. Compared to the treatment with TFF3 or Rqdl10 hydrogel alone, the TFF3@Rqdl10 system combines the physical barrier function of the Rqdl10 hydrogel and the biological activity advantages of TFF3, promoting the repair of gastric mucosal damage through multi−level and multifaceted actions, including the promotion of the proliferation and migration of gastric mucosal epithelial cells, and the inhibition of inflammation and apoptotic responses. These findings underscore the promising therapeutic potential of self−assembled peptide Rqdl10 hydrogels in biomedical applications, potentially revolutionizing healthcare science.

Author Contributions: Conceptualization: J.C. and Z.L. Methodology: J.C. and J.L. Investigation: J.C., J.L. and D.S. Data curation: J.C., D.S., N.L. and J.Z. Visualization: J.C., J.L. and Z.L. Resources: J.C., J.L. and Z.L. Writing—original draft: J.C. and Z.L. Writing—review & editing: J.L., D.S., N.L., J.Z., J.L. and Z.L. Project administration: Z.L. Funding acquisition: Z.L. All authors have read and agreed to the published version of the manuscript.

Funding: This program is supported by the Chengdu Sciobio Surgery Institute, China (Project Number: CSSI−JZ20211021-0002). Zhongli Luo was supported by a grant from the National Natural Science Foundation of China (Project Number: NSFC 31771101).

Institutional Review Board Statement: The animal study protocol was approved by by the Experimental Animal Ethics Committee of Chongqing Medical University (protocol code IACUC-CQMU-2024-0134).

Informed Consent Statement: Not applicable.

Data Availability Statement: The data presented in this study are available in the article.

Conflicts of Interest: The authors declare no conflicts of interest.

References

1. Van Vlierberghe, S.; Dubruel, P.; Schacht, E. Biopolymer-based hydrogels as scaffolds for tissue engineering applications: A review. *Biomacromolecules* **2011**, *12*, 1387–1408. [CrossRef] [PubMed]
2. Mañas-Torres, M.C.; Gila-Vilchez, C.; Vazquez-Perez, F.J.; Kuzhir, P.; Momier, D.; Scimeca, J.C.; Borderie, A.; Goracci, M.; Burel-Vandenbos, F.; Blanco-Elices, C.; et al. Injectable Magnetic-Responsive Short-Peptide Supramolecular Hydrogels: Ex Vivo and In Vivo Evaluation. *ACS Appl. Mater. Interfaces* **2021**, *13*, 49692–49704. [CrossRef] [PubMed]
3. Bidarra, S.J.; Barrias, C.C.; Granja, P.L. Injectable alginate hydrogels for cell delivery in tissue engineering. *Acta Biomater.* **2014**, *10*, 1646–1662. [CrossRef] [PubMed]
4. Tian, R.; Chen, J.; Niu, R. The development of low-molecular weight hydrogels for applications in cancer therapy. *Nanoscale* **2014**, *6*, 3474–3482. [CrossRef] [PubMed]
5. Vashist, A.; Vashist, A.; Gupta, Y.K.; Ahmad, S. Recent advances in hydrogel based drug delivery systems for the human body. *J. Mater. Chem. B* **2014**, *2*, 147–166. [CrossRef]
6. Lin, C.C.; Anseth, K.S. PEG hydrogels for the controlled release of biomolecules in regenerative medicine. *Pharm. Res.* **2009**, *26*, 631–643. [CrossRef] [PubMed]
7. Gelain, F.; Luo, Z.; Zhang, S. Self-Assembling Peptide EAK16 and RADA16 Nanofiber Scaffold Hydrogel. *Chem. Rev.* **2020**, *120*, 13434–13460. [CrossRef] [PubMed]

8. Lomander, A.; Hwang, W.; Zhang, S. Hierarchical self-assembly of a coiled-coil peptide into fractal structure. *Nano Lett.* **2005**, *5*, 1255–1260. [CrossRef] [PubMed]
9. Chen, C.; Gu, Y.; Deng, L.; Han, S.; Sun, X.; Chen, Y.; Lu, J.R.; Xu, H. Tuning gelation kinetics and mechanical rigidity of β-hairpin peptide hydrogels via hydrophobic amino acid substitutions. *ACS Appl. Mater. Interfaces* **2014**, *6*, 14360–14368. [CrossRef]
10. Mazza, M.; Patel, A.; Pons, R.; Bussy, C.; Kostarelos, K. Peptide nanofibres as molecular transporters: From self-assembly to in vivo degradation. *Faraday Discuss.* **2013**, *166*, 181–194. [CrossRef]
11. Cui, H.; Xu, B. Supramolecular medicine. *Chem. Soc. Rev.* **2017**, *46*, 6430–6432. [CrossRef]
12. Zhao, C.; Chen, H.; Wang, F.; Zhang, X. Amphiphilic self-assembly peptides: Rational strategies to design and delivery for drugs in biomedical applications. *Colloids Surf. B Biointerfaces* **2021**, *208*, 112040. [CrossRef] [PubMed]
13. Hsieh, P.C.; MacGillivray, C.; Gannon, J.; Cruz, F.U.; Lee, R.T. Local controlled intramyocardial delivery of platelet-derived growth factor improves postinfarction ventricular function without pulmonary toxicity. *Circulation* **2006**, *114*, 637–644. [CrossRef] [PubMed]
14. Lin, Y.D.; Luo, C.Y.; Hu, Y.N.; Yeh, M.L.; Hsueh, Y.C.; Chang, M.Y.; Tsai, D.C.; Wang, J.N.; Tang, M.J.; Wei, E.I.; et al. Instructive nanofiber scaffolds with VEGF create a microenvironment for arteriogenesis and cardiac repair. *Sci. Transl. Med.* **2012**, *4*, 146ra109. [CrossRef] [PubMed]
15. Phipps, M.C.; Monte, F.; Mehta, M.; Kim, H.K. Intraosseous Delivery of Bone Morphogenic Protein-2 Using a Self-Assembling Peptide Hydrogel. *Biomacromolecules* **2016**, *17*, 2329–2336. [CrossRef] [PubMed]
16. Lanas, A.; Chan, F.K.L. Peptic ulcer disease. *Lancet* **2017**, *390*, 613–624. [CrossRef] [PubMed]
17. Sverdén, E.; Agréus, L.; Dunn, J.M.; Lagergren, J. Peptic ulcer disease. *BMJ* **2019**, *367*, l5495. [CrossRef] [PubMed]
18. Kamada, T.; Satoh, K.; Itoh, T.; Ito, M.; Iwamoto, J.; Okimoto, T.; Kanno, T.; Sugimoto, M.; Chiba, T.; Nomura, S.; et al. Evidence-based clinical practice guidelines for peptic ulcer disease 2020. *J. Gastroenterol.* **2021**, *56*, 303–322. [CrossRef]
19. Duan, Z.; Yu, S.; Wang, S.; Deng, H.; Guo, L.; Yang, H.; Xie, H. Protective Effects of Piperine on Ethanol-Induced Gastric Mucosa Injury by Oxidative Stress Inhibition. *Nutrients* **2022**, *14*, 4744. [CrossRef]
20. Sands, B.E.; Podolsky, D.K. The trefoil peptide family. *Annu. Rev. Physiol.* **1996**, *58*, 253–273. [CrossRef]
21. Thim, L.; May, F.E. Structure of mammalian trefoil factors and functional insights. *Cell. Mol. Life Sci.* **2005**, *62*, 2956–2973. [CrossRef]
22. Kouznetsova, I.; Peitz, U.; Vieth, M.; Meyer, F.; Vestergaard, E.M.; Malfertheiner, P.; Roessner, A.; Lippert, H.; Hoffmann, W. A gradient of TFF3 (trefoil factor family 3) peptide synthesis within the normal human gastric mucosa. *Cell Tissue Res.* **2004**, *316*, 155–165. [CrossRef]
23. Alison, M.R.; Chinery, R.; Poulsom, R.; Ashwood, P.; Longcroft, J.M.; Wright, N.A. Experimental ulceration leads to sequential expression of spasmolytic polypeptide, intestinal trefoil factor, epidermal growth factor and transforming growth factor alpha mRNAs in rat stomach. *J. Pathol.* **1995**, *175*, 405–414. [CrossRef] [PubMed]
24. Yu, K.; Jiang, S.F.; Lin, M.F.; Wu, J.B.; Lin, J. Extraction and purification of biologically active intestinal trefoil factor from human meconium. *Lab. Investig.* **2004**, *84*, 390–392. [CrossRef]
25. Chinery, R.; Playford, R.J. Combined intestinal trefoil factor and epidermal growth factor is prophylactic against indomethacin-induced gastric damage in the rat. *Clin. Sci.* **1995**, *88*, 401–403. [CrossRef]
26. Huang, Y.; Wang, M.M.; Yang, Z.Z.; Ren, Y.; Zhang, W.; Sun, Z.R.; Nie, S.N. Pretreatment with intestinal trefoil factor alleviates stress-induced gastric mucosal damage via Akt signaling. *World J. Gastroenterol.* **2020**, *26*, 7619–7632. [CrossRef]
27. Sun, Z.; Liu, H.; Yang, Z.; Shao, D.; Zhang, W.; Ren, Y.; Sun, B.; Lin, J.; Xu, M.; Nie, S. Intestinal trefoil factor activates the PI3K/Akt signaling pathway to protect gastric mucosal epithelium from damage. *Int. J. Oncol.* **2014**, *45*, 1123–1132. [CrossRef]
28. Babyatsky, M.W.; deBeaumont, M.; Thim, L.; Podolsky, D.K. Oral trefoil peptides protect against ethanol- and indomethacin-induced gastric injury in rats. *Gastroenterology* **1996**, *110*, 489–497. [CrossRef] [PubMed]
29. Poulsen, S.S.; Kissow, H.; Hare, K.; Hartmann, B.; Thim, L. Luminal and parenteral TFF2 and TFF3 dimer and monomer in two models of experimental colitis in the rat. *Regul. Pept.* **2005**, *126*, 163–171. [CrossRef]
30. Lemercinier, X.; Muskett, F.W.; Cheeseman, B.; McIntosh, P.B.; Thim, L.; Carr, M.D. High-resolution solution structure of human intestinal trefoil factor and functional insights from detailed structural comparisons with the other members of the trefoil family of mammalian cell motility factors. *Biochemistry* **2001**, *40*, 9552–9559. [CrossRef]
31. Taupin, D.; Podolsky, D.K. Trefoil factors: Initiators of mucosal healing. *Nat. Rev. Mol. Cell Biol.* **2003**, *4*, 721–732. [CrossRef] [PubMed]
32. Poulsen, S.S.; Thulesen, J.; Hartmann, B.; Kissow, H.L.; Nexø, E.; Thim, L. Injected TFF1 and TFF3 bind to TFF2-immunoreactive cells in the gastrointestinal tract in rats. *Regul. Pept.* **2003**, *115*, 91–99. [CrossRef]
33. Kjellev, S.; Vestergaard, E.M.; Nexø, E.; Thygesen, P.; Eghøj, M.S.; Jeppesen, P.B.; Thim, L.; Pedersen, N.B.; Poulsen, S.S. Pharmacokinetics of trefoil peptides and their stability in gastrointestinal contents. *Peptides* **2007**, *28*, 1197–1206. [CrossRef] [PubMed]
34. Houben, T.; Harder, S.; Schlüter, H.; Kalbacher, H.; Hoffmann, W. Different Forms of TFF3 in the Human Saliva: Heterodimerization with IgG Fc Binding Protein (FCGBP). *Int. J. Mol. Sci.* **2019**, *20*, 5000. [CrossRef] [PubMed]
35. Braga Emidio, N.; Meli, R.; Tran, H.N.T.; Baik, H.; Morisset-Lopez, S.; Elliott, A.G.; Blaskovich, M.A.T.; Spiller, S.; Beck-Sickinger, A.G.; Schroeder, C.I.; et al. Chemical Synthesis of TFF3 Reveals Novel Mechanistic Insights and a Gut-Stable Metabolite. *J. Med. Chem.* **2021**, *64*, 9484–9495. [CrossRef]

36. Karavasili, C.; Fatouros, D.G. Self-assembling peptides as vectors for local drug delivery and tissue engineering applications. *Adv. Drug Deliv. Rev.* **2021**, *174*, 387–405. [CrossRef] [PubMed]
37. Choi, J.I.; Raghavendran, H.R.; Sung, N.Y.; Kim, J.H.; Chun, B.S.; Ahn, D.H.; Choi, H.S.; Kang, K.W.; Lee, J.W. Effect of fucoidan on aspirin-induced stomach ulceration in rats. *Chem. Biol. Interact.* **2010**, *183*, 249–254. [CrossRef]
38. Qi, X.; Wei, W.; Li, J.; Su, T.; Pan, X.; Zuo, G.; Zhang, J.; Dong, W. Design of Salecan-containing semi-IPN hydrogel for amoxicillin delivery. *Mater. Sci. Eng. C Mater. Biol. Appl.* **2017**, *75*, 487–494. [CrossRef] [PubMed]
39. Chen, S.; Hao, X.; Liang, X.; Zhang, Q.; Zhang, C.; Zhou, G.; Shen, S.; Jia, G.; Zhang, J. Inorganic Nanomaterials as Carriers for Drug Delivery. *J. Biomed. Nanotechnol.* **2016**, *12*, 1–27. [CrossRef]
40. Kotrchová, L.; Kostka, L.; Etrych, T. Drug carriers with star polymer structures. *Physiol. Res.* **2018**, *67* (Suppl. S2), S293–S303. [CrossRef]
41. Almeida, B.; Nag, O.K.; Rogers, K.E.; Delehanty, J.B. Recent Progress in Bioconjugation Strategies for Liposome-Mediated Drug Delivery. *Molecules* **2020**, *25*, 5672. [CrossRef]
42. Ertl, H.C. Viral vectors as vaccine carriers. *Curr. Opin. Virol.* **2016**, *21*, 1–8. [CrossRef] [PubMed]
43. Eskandari, S.; Guerin, T.; Toth, I.; Stephenson, R.J. Recent advances in self-assembled peptides: Implications for targeted drug delivery and vaccine engineering. *Adv. Drug Deliv. Rev.* **2017**, *110–111*, 169–187. [CrossRef] [PubMed]
44. Zhou, X.R.; Cao, Y.; Zhang, Q.; Tian, X.B.; Dong, H.; Chen, L.; Luo, S.Z. Self-assembly nanostructure controlled sustained release, activity and stability of peptide drugs. *Int. J. Pharm.* **2017**, *528*, 723–731. [CrossRef] [PubMed]
45. Qu, J.; Peng, S.; Wang, R.; Yang, S.T.; Zhou, Q.H.; Lin, J. Stepwise pH-sensitive and biodegradable polypeptide hybrid micelles for enhanced cellular internalization and efficient nuclear drug delivery. *Colloids Surf. B Biointerfaces* **2019**, *181*, 315–324. [CrossRef] [PubMed]
46. Yu, Z.; Xu, Q.; Dong, C.; Lee, S.S.; Gao, L.; Li, Y.; D'Ortenzio, M.; Wu, J. Self-Assembling Peptide Nanofibrous Hydrogel as a Versatile Drug Delivery Platform. *Curr. Pharm. Des.* **2015**, *21*, 4342–4354. [CrossRef] [PubMed]
47. Hagen, S.J. Mucosal defense: Gastroduodenal injury and repair mechanisms. *Curr. Opin. Gastroenterol.* **2021**, *37*, 609–614. [CrossRef] [PubMed]
48. Von Herbay, A.; Rudi, J. Role of apoptosis in gastric epithelial turnover. *Microsc. Res. Tech.* **2000**, *48*, 303–311. [CrossRef]
49. Szabó, I.; Tarnawski, A.S. Apoptosis in the gastric mucosa: Molecular mechanisms, basic and clinical implications. *J. Physiol. Pharmacol.* **2000**, *51*, 3–15.
50. Shi, G.Y.; Zhao, L.L.; Zhang, K.; Zhou, H.X.; Liu, A.H.; Li, J.; Li, G.; Zhu, L.H. Effects of BCL2 transfection on the cell cycle and proliferation of human GES-1 cells. *Genet. Mol. Res.* **2015**, *14*, 12022–12029. [CrossRef]
51. Zhang, Y.; Yuan, Z.; Chai, J.; Zhu, D.; Miao, X.; Zhou, J.; Gu, X. ALDH2 ameliorates ethanol−induced gastric ulcer through suppressing NLPR3 inflammasome activation and ferroptosis. *Arch. Biochem. Biophys.* **2023**, *743*, 109621. [CrossRef] [PubMed]
52. Oishi, Y.; Manabe, I. Macrophages in inflammation, repair and regeneration. *Int. Immunol.* **2018**, *30*, 511–528. [CrossRef] [PubMed]
53. Eming, S.A.; Wynn, T.A.; Martin, P. Inflammation and metabolism in tissue repair and regeneration. *Science* **2017**, *356*, 1026–1030. [CrossRef] [PubMed]
54. Kobayashi, K.; Kashima, K.; Higuchi, K.; Arakawa, T. [The mechanisms of gastrointestinal mucosal injury and repair]. *Nihon Rinsho.* **1998**, *56*, 2215–2222. [PubMed]
55. Kang, J.Y.; Teng, C.H.; Chen, F.C. Effect of capsaicin and cimetidine on the healing of acetic acid induced gastric ulceration in the rat. *Gut* **1996**, *38*, 832–836. [CrossRef]

molecules

MDPI

Article

Synergistic Effects of AgNPs and Biochar: A Potential Combination for Combating Lung Cancer and Pathogenic Bacteria

Maha N. Abu Hajleh [1], Muhamad Al-limoun [2], Amjad Al-Tarawneh [3], Tahani J. Hijazin [2], Moath Alqaraleh [4], Khaled Khleifat [5,*], Osama Y. Al-Madanat [6], Yaseen Al Qaisi [2], Ahmad AlSarayreh [2], Ali Al-Samydai [4], Haitham Qaralleh [5] and Emad A. S. Al-Dujaili [7,*]

1 Department of Cosmetic Science, Pharmacological and Diagnostic Research Centre, Faculty of Allied Medical Sciences, Al-Ahliyya Amman University, Amman 19328, Jordan; m.abuhajleh@ammanu.edu.jo

2 Department of Biological Sciences, Faculty of Science, Mutah University, P.O. Box 7, Mutah 61710, Jordan; moallimoun@mutah.edu.jo (M.A.-l.); thijazeen@yahoo.com (T.J.H.); yastq@yahoo.com (Y.A.Q.); ahmsar@mutah.edu.jo (A.A.)

3 Prince Faisal Center for Dead Sea, Environmental and Energy Research, Mutah University, Al-Karak 61710, Jordan; amjtar@hotmail.com

4 Pharmacological and Diagnostic Research Center (PDRC), Faculty of Pharmacy, Al-Ahliyya Amman University, Amman 19328, Jordan; alqaralehmoath@yahoo.com (M.A.); a.alsamydai@ammanu.edu.jo (A.A.-S.)

5 Department of Medical Analysis, Faculty of Science, Mutah University, Al-Karak 61710, Jordan; haitham@mutah.edu.jo

6 Department of Chemistry, Faculty of Science, Mutah University, Al-Karak 61710, Jordan; madanat@mutah.edu.jo

7 Centre for Cardiovascular Science, Queen's Medical Research Institute, University of Edinburgh, Edinburgh EH8 9YL, UK

* Correspondence: alkh_kha@hotmail.com (K.K.); ealduja1@exseed.ed.ac.uk (E.A.S.A.-D.); Tel.: +44-131-242-6777 (K.K.)

Abstract: The synthesis of reliable biological nanomaterials is a crucial area of study in nanotechnology. In this study, Emericella dentata was employed for the biosynthesis of AgNPs, which were then combined with synthesized biochar, a porous structure created through biomass pyrolysis. The synergistic effects of AgNPs and biochar were evaluated through the assessment of pro-inflammatory cytokines, anti-apoptotic gene expression, and antibacterial activity. Solid biosynthesized AgNPs were evaluated by XRD and STEM, with STEM images revealing that most of the AgNPs ranged from 10 to 80 nm, with over 70% being less than 40 nm. FTIR analysis indicated the presence of stabilizing and reducing functional groups in the AgNPs. The nanoemulsion's zeta potential, hydrodynamic diameter, and particle distribution index were found to be −19.6 mV, 37.62 nm, and 0.231, respectively. Biochar, on the other hand, did not have any antibacterial effects on the tested bacterial species. However, when combined with AgNPs, its antibacterial efficacy against all bacterial species was significantly enhanced. Furthermore, the combined material significantly reduced the expression of anti-apoptotic genes and pro-inflammatory cytokines compared to individual treatments. This study suggests that low-dose AgNPs coupled with biochar could be a more effective method to combat lung cancer epithelial cells and pathogenic bacteria compared to either substance alone.

Keywords: synergism; biochar; AgNPs; anticancer; anti-inflammatory; antibacterial

1. Introduction

Nanoscience, one of the most prominent areas of modern research, explores the composition, structure, and properties of nanoparticles. Since nanotechnologies are applied in several other disciplines, such as engineering [1], medicine, pharmacy, environmental remediation [2], and sustainable fuel production [3,4], they are recognized as one of the most current and active study areas [5,6]. The last ten years have seen a tremendous global expansion of the vast multidisciplinary field of nanotechnology [7,8]. Nanomaterials that have been created or modified using biotechnology are the focus of nanotechnology [9]. Fungal processes are used to create nanoparticles of metals, which have a wide range of uses such as materials, textiles, in food preservation, disease detection and control, and wound healing [10]. Other physical and chemical processes for creating nanoparticles (NPs) use hazardous substances and are expensive [11]. Due to their nanotoxicity, the biological method is currently used as a temporary option because it poses fewer environmental and health risks [12,13]. Therefore, environmentally friendly, straightforward, and efficient methods have been adopted for NP biosynthesis, which is crucial due to their lower toxicity and benign ecological impact. The behavior, biodistribution, effectiveness, and safety of nanoparticles are influenced by their physicochemical characteristics. To assess the functional qualities of the produced particles, the characterization of NPs is important. Various techniques can be used, including atomic force microscopy (AFM), scanning electron microscopy (SEM), transmission electron microscopy (TEM), and X-ray photoelectron spectroscopy (XPS) [14,15]. Silver nanoparticles (AgNPs) are primarily employed in medicine for their therapeutic and diagnostic applications in addition to their antimicrobial properties. Due to their unique physical, chemical, and optical properties, silver nanoparticles are attracting growing interest [16]. Antibacterial and anticancer activities are already present in silver nanoparticles [17,18]. It may be possible to treat cancers that stop responding to chemotherapy or radiotherapy by combining AgNPs' natural anticancer properties with anticancer pharmaceuticals, or by using these AgNPs as concurrent target-directed drug delivery platforms for anticancer drugs [19].

Biochar, a pyrolyzed material with a high carbon content can be made from a range of organic materials [20,21]. Biochar has a porous structure that enables it to hold and collect small molecules including nanoparticles [22]. Combining biochar with AgNPs may boost both compounds' potential antibacterial properties by lowering the doses of harmful bioactive molecules [23]. Recent findings have shown that biochar reduces the bioavailability of AgNPs through the complexion of surfaces, inhibiting their solubility capacity, and releasing damaging Ag+ ions into the growth media [24]. Previously, similar results were reported indicating that the presence of biochar caused tissue Ag levels to drop by at least a factor of two and efficiently prevent their bioaccumulation [25]. In addition, there have been few reports of the potential health risks associated with utilizing biochar. Further investigations are required to determine whether biochar can be used to boost the activity of silver nanoparticles against cancer cell lines and diverse microbial infections [26]. The aim of this study was to biosynthesize novel fungal-mediated AgNPs, describe their characteristics, and investigate AgNPs' antibacterial, anti-inflammatory, and anticancer properties using the A549 cell line, either alone or in combination with biochar.

2. Results

2.1. Silver Nanoparticles (AgNPs) and Biochar

Although there has been a lot of interest in AgNP biosynthesis, to our knowledge, this is the first report employing the fungus isolate *Emericella dentata* to produce AgNPs. The production of AgNPs was optimized at 10 g biomass and 1.0 mM $AgNO_3$ at 35 °C and pH 7.0 for 96 h. The test flask developed a brown hue because of the bioreduction of $AgNO_3$ salt via the prepared mycelia filtrate, which did not happen in the control experiment (Figure 1a). A silver nanoparticle SPR peak is visible in Figure 1b UV–vis spectrum at 438 nm.

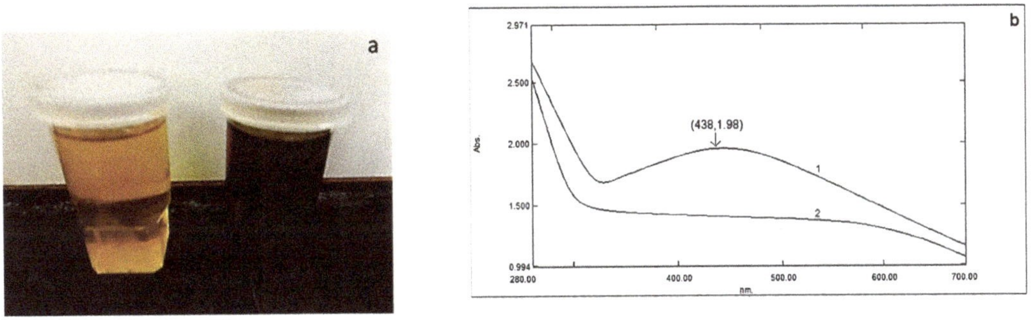

Figure 1. Bio-reduced 1.0 mM $AgNO_3$ by Emericella dentata at 35 °C: (**a**) color change and (**b**) UV–visible spectra. Line 1 represents the spectrum for the filtrate while line 2 shows the spectrum for the AgNP suspension.

The study of date seed (DS) biochar produced at a temperature of 550 °C for pyrolysis revealed a pH of 7.9, an organic matter of 98.56%, fixed carbon of 60.2%, a porosity of 73%, a biochar yield of 25%, and water holding capacity (WHC) of 59.7% (Table 1).

Table 1. Some physical and chemical properties of pyrolyzed DS biochar at 550 °C (n = 3); the results were reported as mean ± SD.

DS Biochar Parameters	Pyrolysis Temperature (550 °C)
pH	7.9 ± 0.15
Porosity (%)	73 ± 4.0
Organic matter (%)	98.56 ± 3.95
Biochar yield (%)	25.2 ± 3.2
Water holding capacity (% WHC)	59.7 ± 4.25

A STEM image (Figure 2a,b [27]) shows the porous surface of used biochar, and the nanoparticles' STEM image (Figure 2c) shows AgNPs as spherical objects with a size range from 10 to 80 nm. The STEM image of biochar combined with nanoparticles was distorted due to sample charge, the existence of nonconducting carbon stabilizer, and nanoparticle aggregates form bigger composites (Figure 2d); it was fuzzy at higher magnification, making it challenging to determine the structure of the observed AgNPs. STEM micrographs demonstrate that AgNPs decreased in size throughout the drying process, making them smaller than those detected by DLS analysis, where >90% of the AgNPs depicted were smaller than 80 nm, and >70% of the latter were about 40 nm or less (Figure 2e,f).

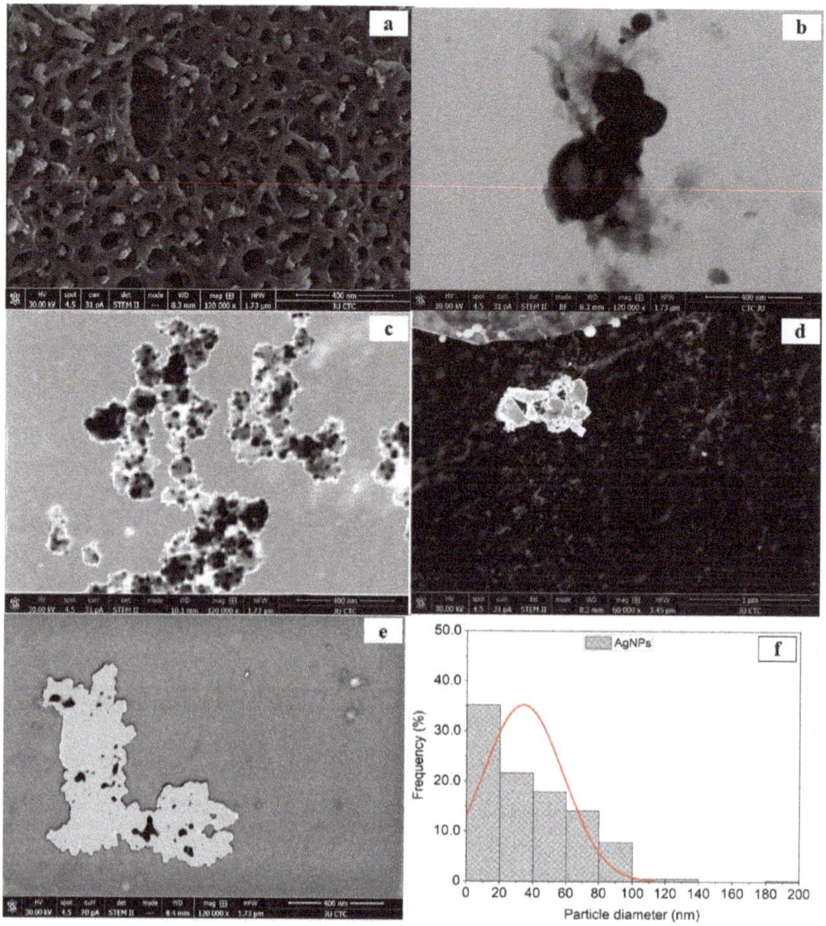

Figure 2. (**a**) STEM micrographs of 400 nm images of biochar, (**b**) STEM micrographs of 400 nm images of biochar [27], (**c**) 400 nm image of silver nanoparticles synthesized by the reaction of 1.0 mM silver nitrate with Emericella dentata filtrate, (**d**) 1000 nm image of combined biochar and AgNPs, (**e**) 400 nm combination of AgNPs and biochar, and (**f**) % frequency of AgNPs size distribution. (Figure 2b shows the identical detail as Figure 2a in [27] and is shown here for easier comparison).

2.2. Particle Size and Zeta Potential

AgNPs were found to have a particle distribution index of 0.231 and a zeta potential of −19.6 mV, both of which indicate that they are hydrodynamically stable. Their hydrodynamic size diameter averaged up to 45 nanometers. (Figure 3a). The zeta values used to describe the nanoparticle size distribution revealed that 97.3% of the AgNPs were 37.62 nm in size (Figure 3b).

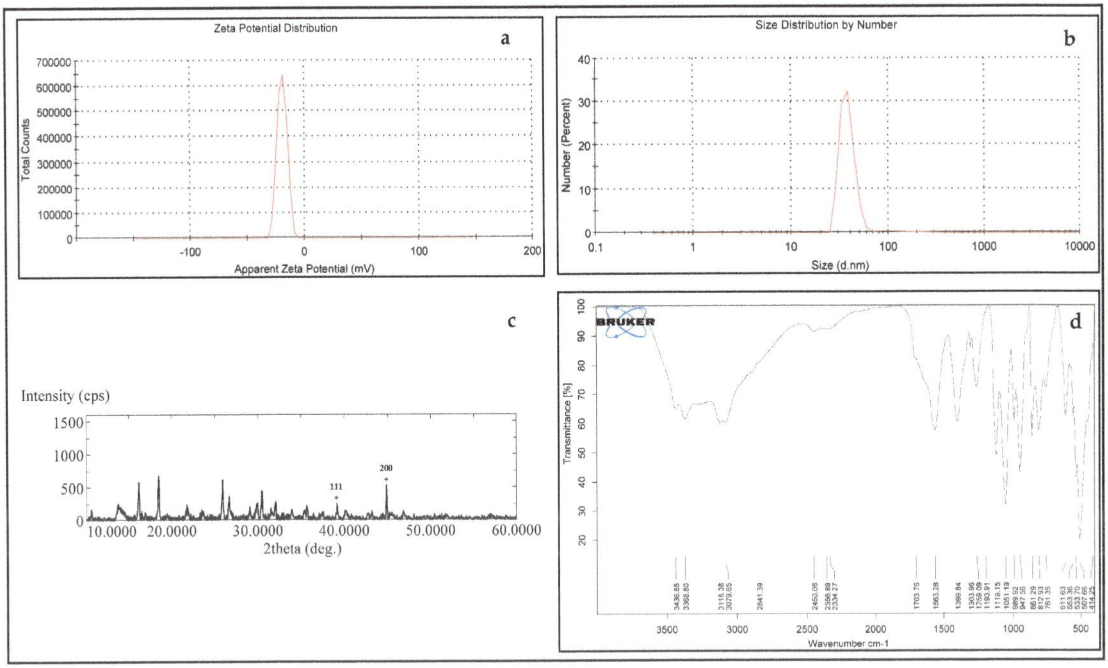

Figure 3. (**a**) Zeta potential distribution of silver nanoparticles [27]; (**b**) the size distribution by the intensity of AgNPs [27]; (**c**) XRD analysis of silver nanoparticles biologically prepared by Emericella dentata filtrate (* assign the reflection planes of the face-centered cubic structure of silver) [27]; and (**d**) ATR-IR of silver nanoparticles biologically prepared by Emericella dentata filtrate. (Figure 3a–c were taken from Figures 1A,B, and 3 in our previous published work [27] and are repeated here for easier comparison).

2.3. XRD Spectra Analysis

The crystalline nature of the biosynthesized Ag nanoparticles was confirmed by X-ray diffraction analysis (Figure 3c). Two distinct diffraction peaks at 2θ values of 38.1° and 44.1° (assigned with stars) can be assigned to the (1 1 1) and (2 0 0) planes, respectively. The appearance of these patterns indicates that the formation of silver nanoparticles are face-centered cubic structures (fcc) and crystalline in nature (JCPDS file no. 84-0713 and 04-0783) [28]. The appearance of several unassigned peaks observed in the XRD spectrum could be related to the crystallization of the bioorganic compounds from fungi during the preparation of the AgNPs, which further confirms the formation of ligand interaction between the silver nanoparticles and the bio-organic compounds from the fungi extract.

2.4. ATR-IR Spectra Analysis

The ATR-IR spectra of silver nanoparticles produced biologically (Figure 3d) show numerous distinct peaks at 633, 989, 1110, 1663, 1704, and 2450, which demonstrated the presence of several organic functional groups that act as reducing and stabilizing agents on the surfaces of silver nanoparticles. The analysis of this spectrum showed a broad band from 3080 to 3437 cm^{-1} assigned to the aromatic amines O–H stretching and the ~N–H stretching vibrations of amide. The presence of the main amine group of proteins is shown by the brevity of the broad peak at 2450 cm^{-1}. The appearance of several bands in the regions between 600 and 900 cm^{-1} corresponds to the C-H aromatic out of the plane. The band at 1259 cm^{-1} could be related to the formation of C-O-C stretching in aromatic rings. The strong wide peak between 1400 and 1450 cm^{-1} corresponds to C-H stretching, while the weak band at around 1520 cm^{-1} represents the formation of the C=C aromatic. Bands in the range of 2900–2990 cm^{-1} correspond to C-H stretching. The presence of the amide in the protein's C=O stretching vibration is indicated by the peaks at 1704, 1663, and 1110 cm^{-1}. The stretching frequencies of the amino and amino-methyl stretching groups of proteins have obvious peaks around 1340 cm^{-1}. These organizations may oversee the synthesis and conformation of the biological system that accompanies the silver nanoparticles.

2.5. Antimicrobial Activity of Silver Nanoparticles

It might be possible that antibiotic resistance could be slowed down by employing innovative approaches, such as the interaction between perfectly treated biochar and silver nanoparticles (AgNPs). The disc diffusion method and the microdilution procedures were used to assess the potential interactions between AgNPs and biochar (Table 2).

Table 2. Inhibition zones and MIC values of AgNPs, biochar, and AgNPs + biochar.

Micro-Organism	AgNPs		Biochar		AgNPs + Biochar	
	Inhibition Zone (mm)	MIC µg/mL	Inhibition Zone (mm)	MIC µg/mL	Inhibition Zone (mm)	MIC µg/mL
B. cereus (ATCC 11778)	20.5 ± 0.5	6.38	0.0	Nd	24.5 ± 0.5	2.13
L. monocytogene (ATCC 7644)	18.5 ± 0.5	6.38	0.0	Nd	20.5 ± 0.0	2.13
P. aeruginosa *	12.5 ± 0.5	19.15	0.0	Nd	14.5 ± 0.4	6.38
S. typhi (ATCC 14028)	15.5 ± 0.5	6.38	0.0	Nd	19.5 ± 0.6	2.13
S. aureus *	18.5 ± 0.5	6.38	0.0	Nd	21.5 ± 0.5	2.13
E. coli *	14.0 ± 0.0	19.15	0.0	Nd	16.5 ± 0.0	6.38
P. aeruginosa ATCC 10145 *	12.3 ± 0.0	19.15	0.0	Nd	16.5 ± 0.5	6.38
E. coli ATCC 25922 *	13.5 ± 0.6	19.15	0.0	Nd	15.0 ± 0.6	6.38
S. epidermidis *	17.5 ± 0.7	6.38	0.0	Nd	19.5 ± 0.0	2.13
E. coli 0157:H7 (ATCC 43888)	14.5 ± 0.6	19.15	0.0	Nd	17.0 ± 0.6	6.38

Nd: not detected. The bacterial strains marked with an asterisk are presented in the table for comparison and have been previously studied [27] as well.

The diameters of the inhibitory zones detected by AgNPs alone against *B. cereus*, *L. monocytogene*, *S. epidermidis*, *S. aureus*, *E. coli*, *P. aeruginosa* and *P. aeruginosa* ATCC 10145, *E. coli* 0157:H7, and *E. coli* ATCC 25922 are shown in Table 2. However, none of the bacteria tested were inhibited by the biochar when used alone. The combination of silver nanoparticles (AgNPs) and biochar resulted in a significant increase ($p < 0.05$) in the antibacterial activity of AgNPs against all types of bacteria. When biochar and AgNPs were combined in a ratio of 1:1, the resulting inhibitory zones had the following dimensions: 24.5, 20.5, 14.5, 19.5, 21.5, 16.5, 16.5, 15.0, 19.5, and 17.0 mm for all the microorganisms listed in Table 2. The results of the minimal inhibitory concentration (MIC) were matched by parallel results from the inhibition zone. All the bacteria employed had a MIC when using AgNPS alone ranging between 6.38 and 19.15 (µg/mL). However, the combined treatment of AgNPs and biochar reduced the MIC values to start from 2.13 µg/mL for *B. cereus*, *L. monocytogene*, *S. epidermidis*, and *S. aureus*, and to 6.38 µg/mL for the other investigated bacteria, with a definite reduction in MIC of up to 70% in each case.

2.6. Cytotoxicity Effect of AgNPs and Biochar on A549 Cells

The antiproliferative effects of biochar, AgNPs, and their interactions were investigated on fibroblast and A549 (ATCC CCL-185) cell lines. At dosages of 3 and 6 µg/mL, the antiproliferative effects of biochar on human periodontal ligament fibroblast cell lines (PDL) were negligible. However, at doses of 12 µg/mL or higher, there was a discernible inhibitory effect of up to 20% at a concentration of 200 µg/mL (Figure 4a). On the other hand, silver nanoparticles were able to suppress fibroblast cell lines' (PDL) viability at doses ranging from 12 to 200 µg/mL (Figure 4b). The manner of inhibition was concentration dependent. The cytotoxic effect of biochar on the A549 cell line is demonstrated in Figure 5a, which shows a maximum 40% inhibition of the A549 cell line by biochar at a concentration of 200 µg/mL. When AgNPs were tested against the A549 cell line (Figure 5b), a substantial level of cytotoxicity was seen at doses ranging from 6 to 200 µg/mL, which resulted an in inhibitory effect of up to 90% at the highest concentration tested. For comparison, untreated cells were used as a control. As a result, a constant concentration of 3 µg/mL AgNPs was chosen for future synergy testing against the A549 cell line. The 3 µg/mL dose of AgNPs and various amounts of biochar were applied to the A549 cell line, and the results revealed that the combination was more effective than utilizing each one of them separately (Figure 6). These findings demonstrate that lower AgNP concentrations produced a reasonable level of cytotoxicity and that biochar and AgNPs interact differently when used in combination compared to the use of either agent separately.

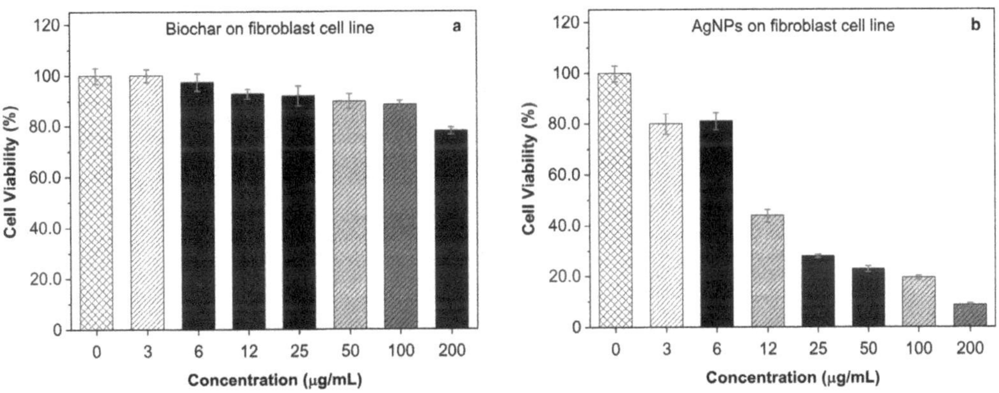

Figure 4. The antiproliferative activity of (**a**) increasing concentrations of biochar and (**b**) increasing concentrations of AgNPs on fibroblast cell line evaluated by MTT assay. The results represent the percentage of cell viability under different concentrations of biochar and AgNPs. All results are expressed as the mean of the three measurements ± SD (n = 3–4 independent replicates).

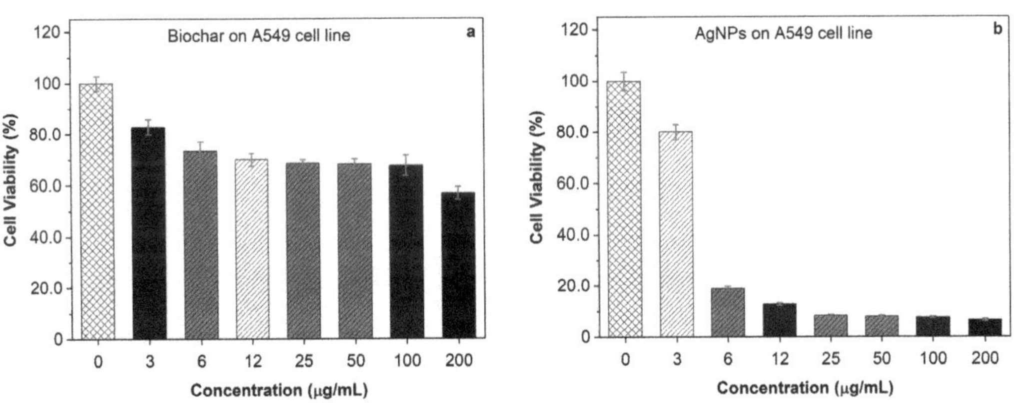

Figure 5. The antiproliferative activity of (**a**) increasing concentrations of biochar and (**b**) increasing concentrations of AgNPs on the A549 cell line evaluated by MTT assay. The results represent the percentage of cell viability under different concentrations of biochar and AgNPs. All results are expressed as the mean of the three measurements ± SD (n = 3–4 independent replicates).

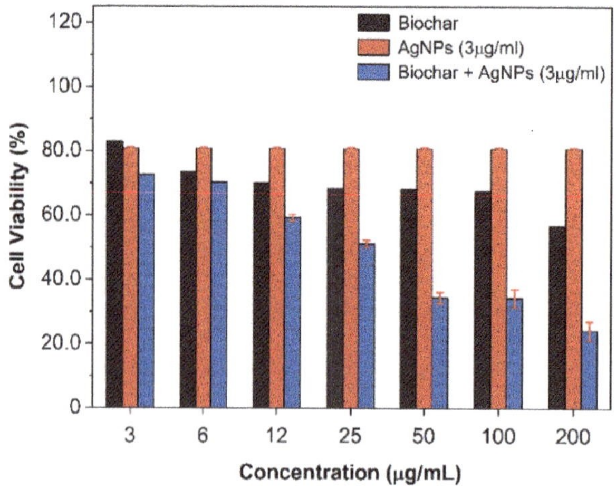

Figure 6. The antiproliferative activity of combined 3 μg/mL AgNPs and increasing concentrations of biochar on the A549 cell line evaluated by MTT assay. The results show cell viability at various biochar concentrations and 3 μg/mL AgNPs. All results are expressed as the mean of the three measurements ± SD (n = 3–4 independent replicates).

2.7. Effect of AgNPs and Biochar on the Expression of Gene Regulation

2.7.1. Pro- and Anti-Apoptotic Genes in A549 Cells

AgNPs, biochar, and their combinations were studied for their synergistic effects on the expression of pro- and anti-apoptotic genes in A549 cells (Figure 7b). AgNPs (3 μg/mL), biochar (50 μg/mL), or both combined (AgNPs (3 μg/mL) plus biochar (50 μg/mL)) were applied to A549 cells for 24 h. Whilst the IC50 value of biochar alone exerted no significant influence on the expression of caspase 3 and anti-apoptotic genes, including BCL-2 and cyclin D1, the effect of 3 μg/mL of AgNPs alone and biochar with AgNPs produced a statistically significant ($p < 0.05$) upregulation of caspase 3 (the pro-apoptotic genotype) in the A549 cell line compared to untreated cells. However, there was a downregulation of anti-apoptotic genes, including BCL-2 and cyclin D1. In comparison to a single treatment, the combination of AgNPs and biochar significantly reduced the expression of anti-apoptotic genes severalfold. AgNPs combined with biochar trigger apoptosis in A549 lung cancer cells, as demonstrated by our experiments using caspase 3.

2.7.2. The Expression of IL-1β, IL-6, and TNF-α in the A549 Cell Line

Combined treatment with AgNPs and biochar decreased IL-1β and IL-6 levels while raising TNF-α production (Figure 7a). Pro-inflammatory cytokines, IL-1β and IL-6, were negatively regulated in the A549 cell line when exposed to AgNPs (3 μg/mL), and a combination of biochar (50 μg/mL) and AgNPs (3 μg/mL) in comparison to untreated cells (Figure 7b). On the other hand, the IC50 value of biochar alone had an upregulating impact on IL-1β and IL-6 expression. Additionally, the combination of biochar with AgNPs at 3 μg/mL and AgNPs at 3 μg/mL alone significantly upregulated the anti-inflammatory cytokine TNF-α.

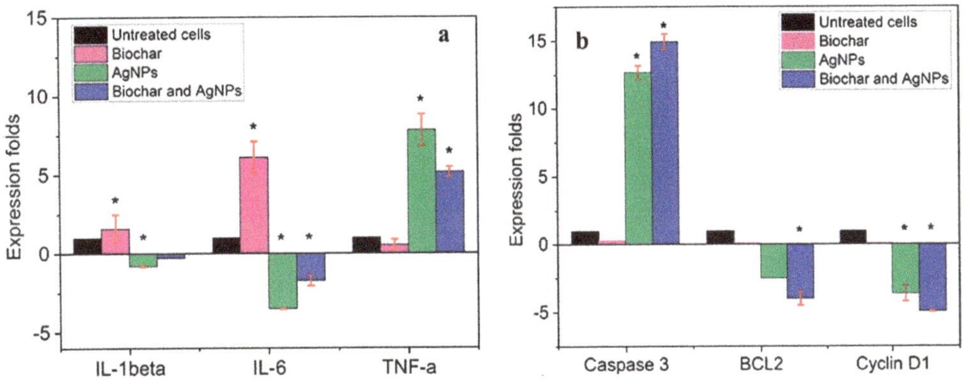

Figure 7. Effect of AgNPs and biochar on the (**a**) expression of caspase 3, BCL-2, and Cylin D1 in the A549 cell line (cells were treated with biochar using the IC50 value and 3 μg/mL of AgNPs) (**b**) the expression of IL-1beta, IL-6, and TNF alpha in the A549 cell line (cells were treated with biochar using the IC50 value and 3 μg/mL of AgNPs). All results are expressed as means of three dependent replicates ± SD. *: $p < 0.05$, compared to control untreated cells.

3. Discussion

An effective and green production of silver nanoparticles using natural reducing, capping, and stabilizing agents was proposed [29,30]. Recently, there has been a lot of interest in AgNP biosynthesis, and this is the first report employing the fungus isolate *Emericella dentata* to produce AgNPs. The process was optimized for 10 g biomass and 1.0 mM $AgNO_3$ at 35 °C and pH 7.0, which took 96 h. It is usually perceived that the size and form of the silver nanoparticles correspond to their absorption peak [31,32]. The reaction mixture's characteristic brown color was attributed to the Ag nanoparticles' surface plasmon resonance (SPR) [32]. Although the method of nanoparticle generation is not entirely understood, two putative pathways have been proposed: the quinine shuttle and NADH-dependent nitrate reductase [31,33,34]. It was found that AgNPs have a zeta potential of −19.6 mV, an average hydrodynamic size diameter of approximately 45 nm, and a particle distribution index of 0.231. These characteristics indicate that AgNPs seem to be very durable. Earlier, it was proposed [29,30] that a polydisperse distribution can be inferred if the PDI (DLS) is greater than 0.2. Particles with a high charge tend to have larger Z values because they are more resistant to self-assembly due to their electrostatic resilience. The density distribution in our collection revealed a broad spectrum of shapes. If the relationship between particle size and light scattering was considered, it could be possible that a tiny portion of a bigger component oversees the motion. The sample's optical properties and the size distribution data obtained from the density distribution were used to construct a relative number that was presented in the number distribution summary [31,32]. Measurements of nanoparticle size distribution zeta indicated that 97.3% of the AgNPs were 37.62 nm in size. Images obtained using scanning transmission electron microscopy (STEM) showed that the particles being investigated were composed of a very large number of extremely minute particles that are smaller than 0.5 μm in size. The analysis of the STEM measurement data was carried out with the assistance of ImageJ, a robust image-processing application that is available for free and under an open-source license [3].

The analysis of one hundred measurements of particle size suggested that biosynthesized AgNPs are round and have an average size of 30 ± 4.3 nm. It was observed that magnification caused the image to blur, making it difficult to determine the structure of the newly synthesized AgNPs. Nanoparticle aggregation into larger composites, the presence of nonconducting carbon stabilizers, and sample charging could also be potential explanations. The nanoparticles seen in the scanning electron microscopy images were spherical and ranged in size from about 10 to 80 nm. STEM images showed a smaller number of AgNPs after drying than were detected by DLS analysis. In fact, smaller than 45 nm is normal for AgNPs, according to several studies [31,33,34]. Porous surfaces were generated because of the volatilization of organic material in DS biochar. Between temperatures of 350 and 550 °C, the pores and deep pathways in biochar became increasingly visible. During the process of increasing the decomposition temperature from 350 to 550 °C, the porosity increased from 31% to 69% [35,36]. Thus, a synergistic potential between AgNPs and biochar was revealed, using 550 °C as the pyrolysis temperature for biochar production.

Silver nanoparticle production was confirmed by the XRD pattern and the presence of distinctive peaks. The detected diffraction peaks confirmed the crystalline nature of produced AgNPs [6,28]. Similar results were reported during the preparation of Ag nanoparticles using edible mushroom extract [35] and geranium leaves [37]. The exhibited peaks in ATR-IR spectra of recently prepared silver nanoparticles demonstrated the presence of several organic functional groups that act as reducing and stabilizing agents on the surfaces of silver nanoparticles [38,39]. The antibacterial potential interactions between AgNPs and biochar were evaluated using the disc diffusion method and MIC utilizing microdilution techniques. AgNPs and biochar together considerably improved the antibacterial activity of AgNPs against all bacterial species. However, none of the studied bacteria were inhibited by biochar alone, which was consistent with previous reports [40]. AgNPs may be helpful in food preservation and packaging due to their effectiveness against *L. monocytogenes* and other foodborne pathogens. AgNPs probably inhibited *B. cereus* and *L. monocytogenes* by interacting with the cell wall [41,42].

Increasing doses of AgNPs were tested on cancer cell lines generated from the A549 cell line as well as fibroblast cells. The A549 cell lines were treated with 3 μg/mL of AgNPs to evaluate the effects of the treatment on gene regulation. When administered to fibroblasts, silver nanoparticles displayed their cytotoxicity at concentrations of 12 μg/mL and above, but their antiproliferative effects on A549 cells were visible at concentrations of 6 μg/mL and higher. On the other hand, it was found that anti-apoptotic genes such as BCL-2 and cyclin D1 encountered severalfold downregulation when they were present in A549 cells that had been treated with 3 μg/mL AgNPs or a combination of 3 μg/mL AgNPs and 50 μg/mL biochar for a period of 24 h. When the A549 cell line was treated with varied concentrations of AgNPs, the effect of the lowest concentration utilized (3 μg/mL of AgNPs) showed that there was a statistically significant rise in caspase 3, the genotype that is associated with pro-apoptotic behavior. Other studies have shown that bioactive substances can influence several anti-apoptotic genes, thereby preventing these genes from performing their immediate protective function against apoptosis and leading to the death of apoptotic cells. This death of apoptotic cells can be attributed to the fact that these genes are unable to perform their immediate protective function against apoptosis [43–45].

The administration of AgNPs induced a reduction in the levels of both IL-1β and IL-6, while concurrently leading to an increase in TNF-α levels. It was found that TNF-α was the link between inflammation and cancer and appears to be a critical mediator in this association [46]. TNF-α is a key therapeutic target in several chronic inflammatory disorders [43,47,48]. Such outcomes might be connected, at least in part, to the capacity of biochar's porous structure to trap and manage the release of such tiny AgNP particles. This was examined when maize plants responded to biochar (2% w/v) and AgNPs (100–1000 mg/mL) in a hydroponic exposure media [49,50]. It has been observed that surface complexation by biochar might lower Ag+ ions in the growth media by reducing the bioavailability of AgNPs. Combining biochar with AgNPs mitigated their phytotoxicity by decreasing absorption and tissue accumulation of Ag+ ions by a factor of four to eight. Moreover, the reduced oxidative stress seen in plants treated with combined AgNPs and biochar was reflected in the increased activities of antioxidant enzymes [49,50]. Biochar can be used when antimicrobial agents are used to treat antibiotic-resistant bacteria or drugs for chemotherapies aimed at improving cancer treatment along with silver nanoparticles (AgNPs). Our findings provide substantial evidence for the claim that date seed biochar controls AgNP absorption and release. As a result, the biochar becomes more selective for lung cells, assisting in reducing the toxicity and release of AgNPs. The interaction of silver nanoparticles with biochar also leads to their immobilization, which lowers the degree of bioavailability in their surroundings [49]. In conclusion, biochar has the potential to prove useful as a nano-carrier in the fight against antibiotic-resistant pathogens and in the enhancement of treatment.

4. Material and Methods

4.1. Fungal Strain

The fungus strain W7B employed in this experiment was isolated from soil samples that were taken from the southern Jordanian region of Al-Karak. By using ITS sequencing, the fungus strain's species was determined (Macrogen, Seoul, Republic of Korea). A sequence similarity analysis using the NCBI database revealed that the ITS sequence of the fungus W7B was 100% identical to that of the *Emericella dentata*, whose accession number is MH032749 according to its identification sheet from Macrogen. The specific bioinformatics report that was supplied by Macrogen for our isolate revealed a 100% match with Emericella dentata, and the report displayed the closest match in comparison to other species as shown in the phylogenic tree.

4.2. Bacterial Strains and Reagents

Sigma-Aldrich (Milwaukee, WI 53209, USA) supplied all the chemicals and media used. The organisms used in the antibacterial assay were Gram-positive and Gram-negative. Some of these strains with ATCC numbers were taken as pure cultures purchased from Ben Hayyan Aqaba International Laboratories, Aqaba, Jordan, while others were isolated from UTI patients treated at Karak Government Hospital (KGH) and identified using a VITEK® 2 Compact instrument. This is a highly automated system used for identification and antimicrobial susceptibility testing (bioMerieux, Marcy-l'Étoile, France). The strains of bacteria were sustained by subculturing them on nutrient agar regularly and keeping them at 4 °C before use. All solutions were prepared with deionized water of the highest purity [51].

4.3. Raw Materials for Biochar and Processing Conditions

After harvesting the date fruit, date seeds (DSs) were acquired locally. Deionized water was used to clean the air-dried seeds. The seeds were then dried and placed in a desiccator for subsequent analysis and the generation of biochar [36].

4.4. Date Seeds' (DSs) Physicochemical Characteristics

Following 24 h incubation in an oven at 105 °C, the seeds were weighed to measure their wet weight. After drying in a muffle furnace set to 550 °C for two hours, the seeds were heat-treated. Equations (1)–(3) were used to calculate moisture and organic matter [52].

$$\text{Total organic matter} = \text{Dry}_{\text{wt}} - \text{Ash}_{\text{wt}} \tag{1}$$

where Dry_{wt} is the weight of the biochar after it has been dried at 105 °C for twenty-four hours and Wet_{wt} is the initial biochar weight prior to drying.

$$\text{Total organic matter (\%)} = \left(\frac{\text{organic matter}}{\text{Dry}_{\text{wt}}}\right) \times 100\% \tag{2}$$

$$\text{\% Moisture content} = \left(\frac{(\text{Wet}_{\text{wt}} - \text{Dry}_{\text{wt}})}{\text{Dry}_{\text{wt}}}\right) \times 100 \tag{3}$$

The pyrolysis of dehydrated date seeds under the lack of oxygen in a muffle furnace using a sealed porcelain crucible at a temperature of 550 °C for two hours was the method used to make DS biochar. In preparation for its usage in the subsequent trials, the DS biochar was reduced to a particle size of 2 mm by subsequent crushing and screening. Equation (4) was utilized to determine the amount of DS biochar that was produced [53].

$$\text{DS biochar yield } (\%) = \left(\frac{\text{weight of biochar}}{\text{weight of dry sample}}\right) \times 100 \tag{4}$$

Transmission electron microscopy (TEM) imaging was used to study the microstructure of DS biochar. The pH level of the DS biochar was studied according to Greenberg et al. [54]. The porosity and water absorption of DS biochar were determined using the Archimedes method in accordance with the accepted method (ASTM C20) as described by Sutcu et al. [55]. This was done to establish the DS biochar's porosity and water absorption. Equation (5) determined % porosity using the estimated parameters, which are as follows:

$$\text{Porosity percentage } (\%) = \left(\frac{\text{open pore volume}}{\text{total volume}}\right) \times 100 = \left(\frac{(\text{Sat}_{\text{wt}} - \text{Dry}_{\text{wt}})}{\text{Sat}_{\text{wt}} - \text{Sus}_{\text{wt}}}\right) \times 100 \tag{5}$$

where Sat_{wt} is the weight of the biochar when it has boiled in water for two hours, and Sus_{wt} is the weight of the biochar after it has been submerged in water for twelve hours.

4.5. AgNPs Biosynthesis

The technique previously mentioned by Gurunathan et al. was used to examine the fungal strain's capacity to produce AgNPs [56]. One mL of approximately 10^4 spore suspension of the fungal isolate *Emericella dentata* was first grown aerobically at 30 °C for 96 h in broth medium (pH 7.0) containing 1.0% (*w*/*v*) glucose, 1.0% (*w*/*v*) yeast extract, and 0.5% (*w*/*v*) NaCl. Filtration was used to collect the fungal biomass, which was completely washed with sterilized distilled water before being resuspended in 100 mL of buffered, sterilized, and deionized water (pH 7.0) and incubated for 72 h in an orbital shaker at 30 °C and 150 rpm. By adding another filtration step, the liquid component of the biomass–deionized water suspension was obtained. Silver nitrate was then added to the filtrate that had been collected. The produced mixture was incubated at a controlled temperature (30 °C) in a shaker incubator (150 rpm) in the dark until a change from a light yellow to a dark brown color was evident.

4.5.1. AgNPs Characterization

Using a UV-1800 spectrophotometer, we measured the absorbance of the resulting brown color, which indicated the synthesis of AgNPs. The reaction solution was centrifuged at 15,000 rpm for 20 min on several occasions to remove the bio-formed silver nanoparticles (MIKRO 200 R, Hettich, Westphalia, Germany). After being washed in deionized water, the nanoparticles were resuspended. Once the silver nanoparticle pellet was recovered, it was dried in a vacuum (VWR 1410 Vacuum Oven, Radnor, PA, USA). TEM images of the manufactured AgNPs' size distribution, shape, and form were captured using an FEI Versa 3D Dual Beam equipment (FEI, Malvern, PA, USA). MAXima-X XRD-7000 was used to determine the crystalline nature of the synthesized AgNPs. Proteins and other molecular structures were identified using a Bruker Alpha FTIR spectrometer as potential factors in AgNP stability [6,57–59].

4.5.2. The Size Distribution of the Particles and Their Zeta Potential

The Zeta-sizer Nano ZS90 was utilized so that both the particle size of the AgNPs as well as their zeta potential could be determined (Malvern Instruments, Malvern, UK). The investigation was conducted at 25 °C and a dispersion angle of 90 degrees utilizing samples of varying intensities that had been prepared with deionized water and distilled water, respectively.

4.6. The Antibacterial Activity of Silver Nanoparticles, Biochar, and Their Combination

The biosynthesized AgNPs, biochar, and their combination were tested against Gram-positive bacteria such as *S. epidermidis*, *S. aureus*, *Bacillus cereus* (ATCC 11778), *Listeria monocytogene* (ATCC 7644) as well as Gram-negative bacteria such as *Escherichia coli* 0157:H7 (ATCC 43888), *E. coli, P. aeruginosa, P. aeruginosa* (ATCC 10145), *Salmonella Typhi* (ATCC 14028), and *E. coli* (ATCC 25922). All the ATCC bacterial strains were supplied by Ben Hayyan–Aqaba International Laboratories, Jordan, and were maintained on MH agar until use. Using the Kirby–Bauer disk diffusion susceptibility test technique, the antibacterial activity of AgNPs, biochar, and their combination against the previously described pathogenic bacteria was assessed [60]. Using a sterile cotton swab, the bacterial strains were dispersed on Mueller–Hinton agar (MHA) (Merck, Darmstadt, Germany). The stock solution for AgNPs, biochar, and their combination were prepared as follows: 1 mg/mL AgNP solution (AgNPs-S), and 1 mg/mL biochar solution (BS) which was kept for 24 h at 25 °C while being shaken. The phosphate-buffered water used as the aqueous solution had a pH of 7.4 (Invitrogen, Waltham, MA, USA). AgNPs-S+BS mixture was made by combining 100 µL of AgNPs-S and 100 µL of BS solutions, and both were vortexed multiple times before use. To obtain 10 µg/disc of AgNPs and 10 µg/disc of biochar, as well as a combined 5 µg/disc of biochar and 5 µg/disc of AgNPs, 10 µL of AgNPs-S, BS, and AgNPs-S+BS were then poured onto each of the sterile 6 mm discs that had been placed on the plate. A center disc, without AgNPs, biochar, or their combination was maintained as control. The plates were then incubated for 24 h in a 37 °C incubator. The presence of growth-inhibitory zones was regularly checked after incubating the plates. The size of the zones of inhibition (ZOIs) was reported after being measured with a ruler. Each test was repeated three times [61–63].

4.6.1. MIC Determination

Using the broth micro-dilution method described by the Clinical and Laboratory Standards Institute (Wayne and Clinical and Laboratory Standards Institute 2012). The MIC of AgNPs, which is defined as the lowest concentration of AgNPs at which there is no detectable bacterial growth, was determined. The test was performed in triplicate using the nutrient broth for bacterial growth on 96-well microtiter plates. Each well of the microtitre plate was kept at a final bacterial concentration of 5×10^5 CFU mL^{-1}. Several concentrations of AgNPs, ranging from 0.016 to 1024 µg/mL, were examined for their effects on various bacteria. The growth of each of these different bacteria was not inhibited by biochar alone using multiple concentrations. In fact, for all the synergistic testing with varied AgNP concentrations, a fixed biochar concentration of 50 µg/mL was used. Two controls were utilized in the experiment: a positive control, which was a broth that had been combined with bacterial inoculum, and a negative control, which was a broth that was sterile and had not been inoculated. The bacterial microtitre plates were kept in an incubator for a duration of 24 h at a temperature of 37 °C. Then, an estimate of the MIC values was determined by a manual calculation [64].

4.6.2. Cancer Cell Lines' Culture

Human lung cancer cell line A549 (ATCC CCL-185) and human periodontal ligament fibroblast cell line (PDL) were employed. The human lung cancer cell line A549 (epithelial cell, lung; derived from the metastatic site; CCL-185™) was obtained from the University of Jordan, Amman, Jordan. Human periodontal ligament fibroblasts (PDL) were isolated from the ligament that fastens the molars to the jawbone. Both cell lines were propagated in DMEM with 10% FBS, 10 mM HEPES buffers, 100 µg/L L-glutamine, 50 µg/L gentamicin, 100 µg/L penicillin, and 100 mg/L streptomycin in a humidified 5% CO_2 incubator at 37 °C.

4.6.3. Cell Harvesting and Counting

First, all the cells were rinsed in flasks measuring 75 cm^2 with 3–5 mL of phosphate buffer saline (PBS). Next, 1–2 mL of trypsin was added to each flask, and the process was repeated until the cells were able to detach from one another. After the fresh medium was added to each cell line in an amount that was comparable, the mixture was pipetted thoroughly to dislodge any clumps and create a single-cell suspension that was consistent throughout. For each individual cell line, the frequency and ratio of cell propagation were uniquely characterized. After attaining the necessary number of cells, the cells were multiplied through propagation once every two to three days. After combining 25 μL of the collected cell suspension with 100 μL of a trypan blue dye solution containing 4% *w*/*v* of trypan blue, the cells were then counted by moving the cell suspension to the edges of a hemacytometer slide [65].

4.6.4. Cytotoxicity Assay

Both the biochar and the AgNPs were tested separately (3–200 μg/mL) as well as together for their potential to be cytotoxic to cancer cells. Untreated cells were used as control. The viability of the cells present in the culture was utilized as the basis for cytotoxicity studies. After the cells had been plated into 96-well plates with a density of 1×10^4 cells per well and cultured for 24 h at 37 °C in DMEM, the cells were treated for an additional 48 h in DMEM containing various doses of biochar and AgNPs. The MTT assay was then carried out in the following manner: the media were first discarded, and the cells in each well were then incubated at 37 °C for four hours with 20 μL of an MTT solution containing 5 mg/mL of the substance. The MTT solution was then discarded and 200 μL of dimethyl sulfoxide (DMSO) was added to dissolve the insoluble formazan crystals. Optical density readings were taken at 570 and 630 nm (data were collected from three independent wells). Primary cell cultures of human periodontal ligament fibroblasts (PDL) and human lung cancer (cell lines of A549 ATCC CCL-185) were utilized for the verification of selective cytotoxicity with the goal of obtaining the lowest antiproliferative IC50 values. All experiments were carried out in triplicates to ensure accuracy, and the IC50 antiproliferative activities were presented as the mean values with standard deviation (n = 3) [65,66].

4.6.5. Gene Expression Level Assay

Cancer cells were grown in 6-well plates with 1 μg/mL at a density of 1×10^6 cells per well [67]. The changes in fold expression of IL-6, IL-1β, TNF-α, Cyclin D1, BCL-2, and caspase-3 genes were measured after 24 h of incubation with the chosen concentrations of biochar and AgNPs [68].

4.6.6. Ribonucleic Acid (RNA) Extraction and Analysis

RNeasy Mini kit was employed to collect total RNA (QIAGEN, Germantown, MD, USA). Cell pellets were taken out of the −80 °C freezer, defrosted on ice, and then resuspended in 500 μL lysis solution containing 2-mercaptoethanol. To eliminate cellular debris, an equal volume of 500 μL of 70% ethanol solution was added to the filtering lysate and carefully vortexed. The cell lysates were then passed to the RNeasy Mini spin columns and spun at 10,000 revolutions per minute for 15 s. A binding column contained the whole RNA that had been trapped. The collection tubes were brought back to a binder column after the flow-through liquids were discarded. The tubes were subjected to 3 wash phases. A fresh collecting tube was then used to hold the binding columns. To extract the RNA, 50 μL of RNase-free water was added straight away to the spin columns' membranes and centrifuged at 10,000 rpm for one minute. Refined RNA was promptly collected and stored at −80 °C. Using Nanodrop ND-1000 spectrophotometers, the recovered total RNA's concentration and purity were assessed (Thermo Scientific, Wilmington, DE, USA). The optical densities at 260 nm and 280 nm were calculated. For most of the RNA-isolated specimens, the proportion (A260/A280) was between 1.8 and 2.1.

4.6.7. Complementary Deoxyribonucleic Acid (cDNA) Synthesis

cDNA was created utilizing a reverse transcription technique (Applied Biosystem, Waltham, MA, USA). An amount of 2 μg of total RNA and 1 μL of oligo-deoxythymidine primers were added to a microcentrifuge tube and heated on a thermocycler C1000 for five minutes at 65 °C (Bio-Rad, Hercules, CA, USA). The tubes were immediately centrifuged, after which they were placed in ice. The accompanying chemicals were used to create the 20 μL reaction solution: 1.4 μL of 25 mM $MgCl_2$ and 4 μL of a combination of 10 mM dNTPs, avian myeloblastosis virus reverse transcriptase (1 μL), recombinant RNasin® ribonuclease inhibitor (1 μL), Shirley, NY 11967, USA, and reverse-transcribed 10× buffers (2 μL) (AMV-RT). The following were the temperature requirements of cDNA synthesis: The microcentrifuge tubes were incubated for 30 min at 37 °C. The specimens were heated for five minutes at 95 °C as part of the denatured protein phase. Following a 5 min incubation period at 4 °C, microcentrifuge tubes were stored at −80 °C for later examination. Nanodrop ND-1000 spectrophotometers were used to measure the amount and quality of cDNA (Thermo Scientific, Wilmington, DE, USA). The optical densities at 260 nm and 280 nm were calculated, and for most of the cDNA retrieved specimens, the proportion (A260/A280) was between 1.6 and 1.8.

4.6.8. Relative Quantitative RT-PCR Analysis

Fast SYBR green kappa master mixes were used for relative quantitative assessments of the mRNA expression rates of the investigated enzyme (Biosystem, Foster City, CA, USA). In each PCR reaction, 200 nM of the forward primers and 200 nM of the reverse primers were mixed with a mixture of 1× concentration KAPA SYBR greens fast master solution, 1–2 μL of cDNA templates, and adjusted to a final volume of 20 μL. Table 3 contains a list of the primer combination sequences that were employed. The IQ5 multicolor real-time PCR detection system (Bio-Rad, USA) was used to carry out the PCR amplifications. Every process ended with melting curves that ranged from 70 to 95 °C. To normalize the expressions of the examined genes, glyceraldehyde-3-phosphate dehydrogenase (GAPDH) was employed as an internal reference gene. The efficiency of the PCR reaction was evaluated using the calibrating curves method for comparable quantitative measurements. The Pffafl technique (Equation (6)) was used to calculate the mRNA expression statistics [69].

$$RQ = \frac{(E_{target})^{\Delta Ct(target)}}{(E_{reference})^{\Delta Ct(reference)}} \quad (6)$$

where,

ΔCt(target) = Ct (target gene in calibration) − Ct (target gene in test);

ΔCt(reference) = Ct (reference gene in calibration) − Ct (reference gene in test).

The amplification efficiency was calculated using Equation (7):

$$E = 10^{-1/slope} \quad (7)$$

In one instance, the effectiveness was 2 (the effectiveness of both the targets and references genes is equal to 2), and the slopes were −3.32 if the number of references and targeted DNA areas are doubling each cycle, which is calculable assuming (Equation (8)):

$$\begin{aligned} RQ &= \frac{2^{\Delta Ct(target)}}{2^{\Delta Ct(reference)}} \\ &= 2^{[\Delta Ct(target)) - \Delta Ct(reference)]} \\ &= 2^{[(Ct(target,calibrator) - Ct(target,test)] - [(Ct(reference,calibrator) - Ct(reference,test)]} \\ &= 2^{-[(Ct(target,test)) - Ct(target,calibrator)] - [(Ct(reference,test) - Ct(reference,calibrator)]} \\ &= 2^{-\Delta\Delta Ct} \end{aligned} \quad (8)$$

Our results were obtained from three independently performed experiments.

Table 3. List of primer sequences used for the selected genes.

Gene Name or Symbol	Primer Sequence
Cyclin D1	Forward: 5′-ACC TGA GGA GCC CCA ACA A-3′ Reverse: 5′-TCT GCT CCT GGC AGG CC-3′
IL-6	Forward: 5′-GGTACATCCTCGACGGCATCT-3′; Reverse: 5′-GT GCCTCTTTGCTGCTTTCAC-3′
IL-1β	Forward: 5′-ATGGCAACTGTTCCTGAACTCAAC-3′ Reverse: 5′-CAGGACAGGTATAGATTCTTTCCTTT-3′
TNF-α	Forward: 5′-ATGAGCACAGAAAGCATGATCC-3′ Reverse: 5′-TCACAGAGCAATGACTCCAAAGTAG-3′
BCL-2	Forward: 5′-AAG CCG GCG ACG ACT TCT-3′ Reverse: 5′-GGT GCC GGT TCA GGT ACT-3′
caspase 3	Forward: 5′-AGCAAACCTCAGGGAAACATT-3′, Reverse: 5′-CTCAGAAGCACACAAACAAAACT-3′

4.7. Statistical Analysis

A non-parametric Mann–Whitney test was employed to investigate any significant group differences. Additionally, Dunnett's post hoc test was employed after a one-way analysis of variance (ANOVA) for data that were regularly distributed. SPSS version 22 was used to analyze the data (SPSS, Inc., Chicago, IL, USA). The remaining findings are displayed as the means and standard deviations (SD) of 3–4 separate studies. Dunnett's post hoc test was used to examine the statistical differences between the control and various treatment groups after performing an ANOVA on GraphPad Prism. A p-value of less than 0.05 was regarded as statistically significant for all statistical analyses. A statistical difference was deemed to be very significant if the p-value was <0.001.

5. Conclusions

In conclusion, this is the first investigation that uses AgNPs and biochar in combination against pathogenic bacteria and lung cancer cells. Although biochar by itself exhibited no antibacterial action, the combination of the two possessed synergistic antibacterial activity (14.5–21.5 mm inhibitory zones). The A549 (ATCC CCL-185) and fibroblast cell lines used in this work were susceptible to AgNPs alone, and the effect was more potent when combined with biochar. The present study found that silver nanoparticles produced by fungi and biochar possess cytotoxic properties that can be used in biomedical applications. Our findings showed that biosynthesized AgNPs with biochar in minute quantities could potentially be employed to treat drug-resistant bacteria and lung cancer epithelial cells.

Author Contributions: Conceptualization, E.A.S.A.-D., K.K. and M.A.; methodology, M.A.-l., A.A.-T., and M.A.; software, O.Y.A.-M. and Y.A.Q.; validation, K.K., A.A.-S. and H.Q.; formal analysis, K.K., M.A.-l., T.J.H., O.Y.A.-M. and A.A.-S.; investigation, M.N.A.H. and E.A.S.A.-D.; resources, K.K. and A.A.; data curation, M.A.; writing—original draft preparation, K.K., M.A.-l. and M.N.A.H.; writing—review and editing, K.K., M.N.A.H., E.A.S.A.-D., A.A.-S., H.Q., Y.A.Q. and T.J.H.; visualization, M.N.A.H. and H.Q.; supervision, K.K.; project administration, M.A.-l. All authors have read and agreed to the published version of the manuscript.

Funding: This research received no external funding.

Institutional Review Board Statement: Not applicable.

Informed Consent Statement: Not applicable.

Data Availability Statement: Not applicable.

Acknowledgments: The authors would like to express their appreciation to the Deanship of Scientific Research at Mutah University, Al-Karak, Jordan for their assistance in completing this work (420/2021).

Conflicts of Interest: The authors declare no conflict of interest.

Sample Availability: Not applicable.

Abbreviations

NPs: nanoparticles; AFM: atomic force microscopy; SEM: scanning electron microscopy; TEM: transmission electron microscopy; XPS: X-ray photoelectron spectroscopy; AgNPs: silver nanoparticles; DS: date seed; Fcc: face-centered cells; MIC: minimal inhibitory concentration; SPR: surface plasmon resonance; STEM: scanning transmission electron microscopy; XRD: X-ray diffraction; BS: biochar solution; ZOIs: zones of inhibition; PBS: phosphate buffer saline; DMSO: dimethyl sulfoxide; GAPDH: glyceraldehyde-3-phosphates dehydrogenases; ANOVA: one-way analysis of variance; SD: standard deviation.

References

1. Ombaka, L.M.; McGettrick, J.D.; Oseghe, E.O.; Al-Madanat, O.; Rieck genannt Best, F.; Msagati, T.A.M.; Davies, M.L.; Bredow, T.; Bahnemann, D.W. Photocatalytic H_2 production and degradation of aqueous 2-chlorophenol over B/N-graphene-coated Cu^0/TiO_2: A DFT, experimental and mechanistic investigation. *J. Environ. Manag.* **2022**, *311*, 114822. [CrossRef]
2. Alsalka, Y.; Al-Madanat, O.; Hakki, A.; Bahnemann, D.W. Boosting the H_2 production efficiency via photocatalytic organic reforming: The role of additional hole scavenging system. *Catalysts* **2021**, *11*, 1423. [CrossRef]
3. Al-Madanat, O.; Curti, M.; Günnemann, C.; AlSalka, Y.; Dillert, R.; Bahnemann, D.W. TiO_2 photocatalysis: Impact of the platinum loading method on reductive and oxidative half-reactions. *Catal. Today* **2021**, *380*, 3–15. [CrossRef]
4. Al-Madanat, O.; Alsalka, Y.; Dillert, R.; Bahnemann, D.W. Photocatalytic H_2 production from naphthalene by various TiO_2 photocatalysts: Impact of pt loading and formation of intermediates. *Catalysts* **2021**, *11*, 107. [CrossRef]
5. Satalkar, P.; Elger, B.S.; Shaw, D.M. Defining Nano, Nanotechnology and Nanomedicine: Why Should It Matter? *Sci. Eng. Ethics* **2016**, *22*, 1255–1276. [CrossRef] [PubMed]
6. Khleifat, K.; Alqaraleh, M.; Allimoun, M.; Alfarrayeh, I.; Khatib, R.; Qaralleh, H.; Alsarayreh, A.; Al Qaisi, Y.; Hajleh, M.A. The Ability of *Rhizopus stolonifer* MR11 to Biosynthesize Silver Nanoparticles in Response to Various Culture Media Components and Optimization of Process Parameters Required at Each Stage of Biosynthesis. *J. Ecol. Eng.* **2022**, *23*, 8. [CrossRef]
7. Gomes, H.I.O.; Martins, C.S.M.; Prior, J.A.V. Silver Nanoparticles as Carriers of Anticancer Drugs for Efficient Target Treatment of Cancer Cells. *Nanomaterials* **2021**, *11*, 964. [CrossRef]
8. Bayda, S.; Adeel, M.; Tuccinardi, T.; Cordani, M.; Rizzolio, F. The History of Nanoscience and Nanotechnology: From Chemical-Physical Applications to Nanomedicine. *Molecules* **2019**, *25*, 112. [CrossRef]
9. Abu Hajleh, M.N.; Abu-Huwaij, R.; AL-Samydai, A.; Al-Halaseh, L.K.; Al-Dujaili, E.A. The revolution of cosmeceuticals delivery by using nanotechnology: A narrative review of advantages and side effects. *J. Cosm. Dermatol.* **2021**, *20*, 3818–3828. [CrossRef]
10. Khan, I.; Saeed, K.; Khan, I. Nanoparticles: Properties, applications and toxicities. *Arab. J. Chem.* **2019**, *12*, 908–931. [CrossRef]
11. Abu Hajleh, M.N.; AL-Samydai, A.; Al-Dujaili, E.A. Nano, micro particulate and cosmetic delivery systems of polylactic acid: A mini review. *J. Cosm. Dermatol.* **2020**, *19*, 2805–2811. [CrossRef] [PubMed]
12. Khleifat, K.M.; Abboud, M.M.; Al-Mustafa, A.H. Effect of *Vitreoscilla* hemoglobin gene (vgb) and metabolic inhibitors on cadmium uptake by the heterologous host *Enterobacter aerogenes*. *Process Biochem.* **2006**, *41*, 930–934. [CrossRef]
13. Mathur, P.; Jha, S.; Ramteke, S.; Jain, N.K. Pharmaceutical aspects of silver nanoparticles. *Artif. Cells Nanomed. Biotechnol.* **2018**, *46*, 115–126. [CrossRef]
14. Zhang, X.F.; Gurunathan, S. Combination of salinomycin and silver nanoparticles enhances apoptosis and autophagy in human ovarian cancer cells: An effective anticancer therapy. *Int. J. Nanomed.* **2016**, *11*, 3655–3675. [CrossRef]
15. Zhang, X.F.; Liu, Z.G.; Shen, W.; Gurunathan, S. Silver Nanoparticles: Synthesis, Characterization, Properties, Applications, and Therapeutic Approaches. *Int. J. Mol. Sci.* **2016**, *17*, 1534. [CrossRef] [PubMed]
16. Krishnan, P.D.; Banas, D.; Durai, R.D.; Kabanov, D.; Hosnedlova, B.; Kepinska, M.; Fernandez, C.; Ruttkay-Nedecky, B.; Nguyen, H.V.; Farid, A.; et al. Silver Nanomaterials for Wound Dressing Applications. *Pharmaceutics* **2020**, *12*, 821. [CrossRef]
17. Talapko, J.; Matijević, T.; Juzbašić, M.; Antolović-Požgain, A.; Škrlec, I. Antibacterial Activity of Silver and Its Application in Dentistry, Cardiology and Dermatology. *Microorganisms* **2020**, *8*, 1400. [CrossRef]
18. Alahmad, A.; Al-Zereini, W.A.; Hijazin, T.J.; Al-Madanat, O.Y.; Alghoraibi, I.; Al-Qaralleh, O.; Al-Qaraleh, S.; Feldhoff, A.; Walter, J.G.; Scheper, T. Green Synthesis of Silver Nanoparticles Using *Hypericum perforatum* L. Aqueous Extract with the Evaluation of Its Antibacterial Activity against Clinical and Food Pathogens. *Pharmaceutics* **2022**, *14*, 1104. [CrossRef]
19. Lara, H.H. Bactericidal effect of silver nanoparticles against multidrug-resistant bacteria. *World J. Microbiol. Biotechnol.* **2010**, *26*, 615–621. [CrossRef]
20. El Hanandeh, A.; Mahdi, Z.; Imtiaz, M.S. Modelling of the adsorption of Pb, Cu and Ni ions from single and multi-component aqueous solutions by date seed derived biochar: Comparison of six machine learning approaches. *Environ. Res.* **2021**, *192*, 110338. [CrossRef]

21. Osman, A.I.; Fawzy, S.; Farghali, M.; El-Azazy, M.; Elgarahy, A.M.; Fahim, R.A.; Maksoud, M.A.; Ajlan, A.A.; Yousry, M.; Saleem, Y.; et al. Biochar for agronomy, animal farming, anaerobic digestion, composting, water treatment, soil remediation, construction, energy storage, and carbon sequestration: A review. *Environ. Chem. Lett.* **2022**, *20*, 2385–2485. [CrossRef] [PubMed]
22. Ghramh, H.A.; Ibrahim, E.H.; Kilnay, M. Majra Honey Abrogated the Normal and Cancer Cells Proliferation Inhibition by *Juniperus procera* Extract and Extract/Honey Generated AgNPs. *Anticancer Agents Med. Chem.* **2020**, *20*, 970–981. [CrossRef]
23. Palem, R.R.; Shimoga, G.; Kang, T.J.; Lee, S.H. Fabrication of multifunctional Guar gum-silver nanocomposite hydrogels for biomedical and environmental applications. *Int. J. Biol. Macromol.* **2020**, *159*, 474–486. [CrossRef]
24. Kumar, N.; Chamoli, P.; Misra, M.; Manoj, M.K.; Sharma, A. Advanced metal and carbon nanostructures for medical, drug delivery and bio-imaging applications. *Nanoscale* **2022**, *14*, 3987–4017. [CrossRef] [PubMed]
25. Kvolik, S.; Dobrosevic, B.; Marczi, S.; Prlic, L.; Glavas-obrovac, L. Different apoptosis ratios and gene expressions in two human cell lines after sevoflurane anaesthesia. *Acta Anaesthesiol. Scand.* **2009**, *53*, 1192–1199. [CrossRef]
26. Hosny, M.; Fawzy, M.; Eltaweil, A.S. Green synthesis of bimetallic Ag/ZnO@Biohar nanocomposite for photocatalytic degradation of tetracycline, antibacterial and antioxidant activities. *Sci. Rep.* **2022**, *12*, 7316. [CrossRef] [PubMed]
27. Alqaraleh, M.; Khleifat, K.M.; Abu Hajleh, M.N.; Farah, H.S.; Ahmed, K.A.A. Fungal-mediated silver nanoparticle and biochar synergy against colorectal cancer cells and pathogenic bacteria. *Antibiotics* **2023**, *12*, 597. [CrossRef] [PubMed]
28. Vanaja, M.; Annadurai, G. *Coleus aromaticus* leaf extract mediated synthesis of silver nanoparticles and its bactericidal activity. *Appl. Nanosci.* **2013**, *3*, 217–223. [CrossRef]
29. Ahmad, A.; Mukherjee, P.; Senapati, S.; Mandal, D.; Khan, M.I.; Kumar, R.; Sastry, M. Extracellular biosynthesis of silver nanoparticles using the fungus Fusarium oxysporum. *Colloids Surf. B Biointerfaces* **2003**, *28*, 313–318. [CrossRef]
30. Ankamwar, B.; Damle, C.; Ahmad, A.; Sastry, M. Biosynthesis of gold and silver nanoparticles using *Emblica officinalis* fruit extract, their phase transfer and transmetallation in an organic solution. *J. Nanosci. Nanotechnol.* **2005**, *5*, 1665–1671. [CrossRef]
31. Jaidev, L.R.; Narasimha, G. Fungal mediated biosynthesis of silver nanoparticles, characterization and antimicrobial activity. *Colloids Surf. B Biointerfaces* **2010**, *81*, 430–433. [CrossRef]
32. Al-limoun, M.; Qaralleh, N.H.; Khleifat, M.K.; Al-Anber, M.; Al-Tarawneh, A.; Al-sharafa, K.; Kailani, M.H.; Zaitoun, M.A.; Matar, S.A.; Al-soub, T. Culture Media Composition and Reduction Potential Optimization of Mycelia-free Filtrate for the Biosynthesis of Silver Nanoparticles Using the Fungus *Tritirachium oryzae* W5H. *Curr. Nanosci.* **2020**, *16*, 757–769. [CrossRef]
33. Padalia, H.; Moteriya, P.; Chanda, S. Green synthesis of silver nanoparticles from marigold flower and its synergistic antimicrobial potential. *Arab. J. Chem.* **2015**, *8*, 732–741. [CrossRef]
34. Chau, Y.F.; Yeh, H.H.; Tsai, D.P. Surface Plasmon Resonances Effects on Different Patterns of Solid-silver and Silver-shell Nanocylindrical Pairs. *J. Electromagn. Waves Appl.* **2010**, *24*, 1005–1014. [CrossRef]
35. Philip, D. Biosynthesis of Au, Ag and Au–Ag nanoparticles using edible mushroom extract. *Spectrochim. Acta A Mol. Biomol. Spectrosc.* **2009**, *73*, 374–381. [CrossRef]
36. Demirbas, A. Effects of temperature and particle size on bio-char yield from pyrolysis of agricultural residues. *J. Anal. Appl. Pyrolysis* **2004**, *72*, 243–248. [CrossRef]
37. Shankar, S.S.; Ahmad, A.; Sastry, M. Geranium leaf assisted biosynthesis of silver nanoparticles. *Biotechnol. Prog.* **2003**, *19*, 1627–1631. [CrossRef] [PubMed]
38. Lehto, J.; Louhelainen, J.K.; Kłosińska, T.; Drożdżek, M.; Alén, R. Characterization of alkali-extracted wood by FTIR-ATR spectroscopy. *Biomass Convers. Biorefin.* **2018**, *8*, 847–855. [CrossRef]
39. Osorio-Echavarría, J.; Osorio-Echavarría, J.; Ossa-Orozco, C.P.; Gómez-Vanegas, N.A. Synthesis of silver nanoparticles using white-rot fungus *Anamorphous Bjerkandera* sp. R1: Influence of silver nitrate concentration and fungus growth time. *Sci. Rep.* **2021**, *11*, 3842. [CrossRef]
40. Yıldızlı, G.; Coral, G.; Ayaz, F. Biochar as a Biocompatible Mild Anti-Inflammatory Supplement for Animal Feed and Agricultural Fields. *Chem. Biodivers.* **2021**, *18*, e2001002. [CrossRef]
41. Rai, M.; Yadav, A.; Gade, A. Silver nanoparticles as a new generation of antimicrobials. *Biotechnol. Adv.* **2009**, *27*, 76–83. [CrossRef]
42. Patra, J.K.; Baek, K.H. Antibacterial Activity and Synergistic Antibacterial Potential of Biosynthesized Silver Nanoparticles against Foodborne Pathogenic Bacteria along with its Anticandidal and Antioxidant Effects. *Front. Microbiol.* **2017**, *8*, 167. [CrossRef] [PubMed]
43. Cao, X.X.; Mohuiddin, I.; Ece, F.; McConkey, D.J.; Smythe, W.R. Histone deacetylase inhibitor downregulation of bcl-xl gene expression leads to apoptotic cell death in mesothelioma. *Am. J. Respir. Cell Mol. Biol.* **2001**, *25*, 562–568. [CrossRef]
44. Xu, H.W.; Huang, Y.J.; Xie, Z.Y.; Lin, L.; Guo, Y.C.; Zhuang, Z.R.; Lin, X.P.; Zhou, W.; Li, M.; Huang, H.H.; et al. The expression of cytoglobin as a prognostic factor in gliomas: A retrospective analysis of 88 patients. *BMC Cancer* **2013**, *13*, 247. [CrossRef] [PubMed]
45. Gurunathan, S.; Kang, M.H.; Kim, J.H. Combination Effect of Silver Nanoparticles and Histone Deacetylases Inhibitor in Human Alveolar Basal Epithelial Cells. *Molecules* **2018**, *23*, 2046. [CrossRef] [PubMed]
46. Karin, M.; Lawrence, T.; Nizet, V. Innate immunity gone awry: Linking microbial infections to chronic inflammation and cancer. *Cell* **2006**, *124*, 823–835. [CrossRef]
47. Ahmed, S.T.; Ivashkiv, L.B. Inhibition of IL-6 and IL-10 Signaling and Stat Activation by Inflammatory and Stress Pathways. *J. Immunol.* **2000**, *165*, 5227–5237. [CrossRef]

48. Yang, L.; Guo, P.; Wang, P.; Wang, W.; Liu, J. IL-6/ERK signaling pathway participates in type I IFN-programmed, unconventional M2-like macrophage polarization. *Sci. Rep.* **2023**, *13*, 1827. [CrossRef]
49. Abbas, Q.; Liu, G.; Yousaf, B.; Ali, M.U.; Ullah, H.; Ahmed, R. Effects of biochar on uptake, acquisition and translocation of silver nanoparticles in rice (*Oryza sativa* L.) in relation to growth, photosynthetic traits and nutrients displacement. *Environ. Pollut.* **2019**, *250*, 728–736. [CrossRef]
50. Abbas, Q.; Yousaf, B.; Ullah, H.; Ali, M.U.; Zia-ur-Rehman, M.; Rizwan, M.; Rinklebe, J. Biochar-induced immobilization and transformation of silver-nanoparticles affect growth, intracellular-radicles generation and nutrients assimilation by reducing oxidative stress in maize. *J. Hazard. Mater.* **2020**, *390*, 121976. [CrossRef]
51. Khleifat, K.M.; Sharaf, E.F.; Al-limoun, M.O. Biodegradation of 2-Chlorobenzoic Acid by *Enterobacter cloacae*: Growth Kinetics and Effect of Growth Conditions. *Bioremediation J.* **2015**, *19*, 207–217. [CrossRef]
52. Manariotis, I.D.; Fotopoulou, K.N.; Karapanagioti, H.K. Preparation and Characterization of Biochar Sorbents Produced from Malt Spent Rootlets. *Ind. Eng. Chem. Res.* **2015**, *54*, 9577–9584. [CrossRef]
53. Mohawesh, O.; Coolong, T.; Aliedeh, M.; Alqaraleh, S. Greenhouse evaluation of biochar to enhance soil properties and plant growth performance under arid environment. *Bulg. J. Agric. Sci.* **2018**, *24*, 1012–1019. [CrossRef]
54. Greenberg, I.; Kaiser, M.; Polifka, S.; Wiedner, K.; Glaser, B.; Ludwig, B. The effect of biochar with biogas digestate or mineral fertilizer on fertility, aggregation and organic carbon content of a sandy soil: Results of a temperate field experiment. *J. Plant Nutr. Soil Sci.* **2019**, *182*, 824–835. [CrossRef]
55. Sutcu, M.; Erdogmus, E.; Gencel, O.; Gholampour, A.; Atan, E.; Ozbakkaloglu, T. Recycling of bottom ash and fly ash wastes in eco-friendly clay brick production. *J. Clean. Prod.* **2019**, *233*, 753–764. [CrossRef]
56. Gurunathan, S.; Lee, K.J.; Kalishwaralal, K.; Sheikpranbabu, S.; Vaidyanathan, R.; Eom, S.H. Antiangiogenic properties of silver nanoparticles. *Biomaterials* **2009**, *30*, 6341–6350. [CrossRef] [PubMed]
57. AlSalka, Y.; Al-Madanat, O.; Curti, M.; Hakki, A.; Bahnemann, D.W. Photocatalytic H2 evolution from oxalic acid: Effect of cocatalysts and carbon dioxide radical anion on the surface charge transfer mechanisms. *ACS Appl. Energy Mater.* **2020**, *3*, 6678–6691. [CrossRef]
58. Al-Madanat, O.; Alsalka, Y.; Curti, M.; Dillert, R.; Bahnemann, D.W. Mechanistic insights into hydrogen evolution by photocatalytic reforming of naphthalene. *ACS Catal.* **2020**, *10*, 7398–7412. [CrossRef]
59. AlSalka, Y.; Al-Madanat, O.; Hakki, A. TiO_2-based photocatalytic hydrogen production: How to transfer it to an applicable approach? *Appl. Catal. A Gen.* **2023**, *662*, 119287. [CrossRef]
60. Loo, Y.Y.; Rukayadi, Y.; Nor-Khaizura, M.A.R.; Kuan, C.H.; Chieng, B.W.; Nishibuchi, M.; Radu, S. In Vitro Antimicrobial Activity of Green Synthesized Silver Nanoparticles Against Selected Gram-negative Foodborne Pathogens. *Front. Microbiol.* **2018**, *9*, 1555. [CrossRef]
61. Khleifat, K.M.; Tarawneh, K.A.; Ali Wedyan, M.; Al-Tarawneh, A.A.; Al Sharafa, K. Growth kinetics and toxicity of *Enterobacter cloacae* grown on linear alkylbenzene sulfonate as sole carbon source. *Curr. Microbiol.* **2008**, *57*, 364–370. [CrossRef]
62. Khleifat, K.M.; Matar, S.A.; Jaafreh, M.; Qaralleh, H.; Al-limoun, M.O.; Alsharafa, K.Y. Essential Oil of *Centaurea damascena* Aerial Parts, Antibacterial and Synergistic Effect. *J. Essent. Oil-Bear. Plants* **2019**, *22*, 356–367. [CrossRef]
63. Qaralleh, H.; Khleifat, K.M.; Al-Limoun, M.O.; Alzedaneen, F.Y.; Al-Tawarah, N. Antibacterial and synergistic effect of biosynthesized silver nanoparticles using the fungi *Tritirachium oryzae* W5H with essential oil of *Centaurea damascena* to enhance conventional antibiotics activity. *Adv. Nat. Sci. Nanosci. Nanotechnol.* **2019**, *10*, 025016. [CrossRef]
64. Wypij, M.; Jędrzejewski, T.; Trzcińska-Wencel, J.; Ostrowski, M.; Rai, M.; Golińska, P. Green Synthesized Silver Nanoparticles: Antibacterial and Anticancer Activities, Biocompatibility, and Analyses of Surface-Attached Proteins. *Front. Microbiol.* **2021**, *12*, 632505. [CrossRef] [PubMed]
65. Al-Tawarah, N.M.; Qaralleh, H.; Khlaifat, A.M.; Nofal, M.N.; Alqaraleh, M.; Khleifat, K.M.; Al-limoun, M.O.; Al Shhab, M.A. Anticancer and Antibacterial Properties of *Verthemia Iphionides* Essential Oil /Silver Nanoparticles. *Biomed. Pharmacol. J.* **2020**, *13*, 1175–1184. [CrossRef]
66. Alqaraleh, M.; Kasabri, V. The Antiglycation Effect of Monomethyl Branched Chained Fatty Acid and Phytochemical Compounds and their Synergistic Effect on Obesity Related Colorectal Cancer Cell Panel. *Romanian J. Diabetes Nutr. Metab. Dis.* **2019**, *26*, 361–369. [CrossRef]
67. Karna, S.K.L.; Ahmad, F.; Lone, B.A.; Pokharel, Y.R. Knockdown of PTOV1 and PIN1 exhibit common phenotypic anti-cancer effects in MDA-MB-231 cells. *PLoS ONE* **2019**, *14*, e0211658. [CrossRef]
68. Jabir, M.S.; Saleh, Y.M.; Sulaiman, G.M.; Yaseen, N.Y.; Sahib, U.I.; Dewir, Y.H.; Alwahibi, M.S.; Soliman, D.A. Green Synthesis of Silver Nanoparticles Using *Annona muricata* Extract as an Inducer of Apoptosis in Cancer Cells and Inhibitor for NLRP3 Inflammasome via Enhanced Autophagy. *Nanomaterials* **2021**, *11*, 384. [CrossRef]
69. Pfaffl, M.W.; Hageleit, M. Validities of mRNA quantification using recombinant RNA and recombinant DNA external calibration curves in real-time RT-PCR. *Biotechnol. Lett.* **2001**, *23*, 275–282. [CrossRef]

molecules

MDPI

Review

Nanoparticle Tracking Analysis: An Effective Tool to Characterize Extracellular Vesicles

Gabrielle Kowkabany and Yuping Bao *

Chemical and Biological Engineering, The University of Alabama, Tuscaloosa, AL 35487, USA; gakowkabany@crimson.ua.edu
* Correspondence: ybao@eng.ua.edu; Tel.: +1-205-348-9869

Abstract: Extracellular vesicles (EVs) are membrane-enclosed particles that have attracted much attention for their potential in disease diagnosis and therapy. However, the clinical translation is limited by the dosing consistency due to their heterogeneity. Among various characterization techniques, nanoparticle tracking analysis (NTA) offers distinct benefits for EV characterization. In this review, we will discuss the NTA technique with a focus on factors affecting the results; then, we will review the two modes of the NTA techniques along with suitable applications in specific areas of EV studies. EVs are typically characterized by their size, size distribution, concentration, protein markers, and RNA cargos. The light-scattering mode of NTA offers accurate size, size distribution, and concentration information in solution, which is useful for comparing EV isolation methods, storage conditions, and EV secretion conditions. In contrast, fluorescent mode of NTA allows differentiating EV subgroups based on specific markers. The success of fluorescence NTA heavily relies on fluorescent tags (e.g., types of dyes and labeling methods). When EVs are labeled with disease-specific markers, fluorescence NTA offers an effective tool for disease detection in biological fluids, such as saliva, blood, and serum. Finally, we will discuss the limitations and future directions of the NTA technique in EV characterization.

Keywords: extracellular vesicles; exosomes; nanoparticle-tracking analysis; fluorescent labeling

1. Introduction

Extracellular vesicles (EVs) are membrane-enclosed particles naturally secreted by various cells [1]. EVs play significant roles in regulating cell–cell communication [2,3], directing cell behaviors [4–6], and are able to cross biological barriers [7]. Recently, numerous studies have shown that EVs are effective tools for disease diagnosis, such as neurological disorders [8–10], cardiac diseases [11], cancer progression [12–14], and metastasis [15,16]. However, the clinical translation of EVs is hindered by the lack of standardization in EV quantification [17]. The challenges of EV quantification result from their intrinsic heterogeneity. First, EVs have large heterogeneity in size (e.g., exosomes of 30–130 nm, microvesicles up to 1000 nm, and micro-sized apoptotic body) and EV cargos (e.g., miRNA and protein biomarkers) [18]. Second, EVs can be secreted from diverse sources, production conditions can vary greatly, and the secretion process is highly dynamic [19]. Many isolation and purification methods are available, such as ultracentrifugation, microfluidic separation, immunoaffinity capture, filtration, etc. [20–24]. All of these factors consequently lead to large variations and inconsistency in EV dosing during preclinical and clinical studies (e.g., 10^9–10^{14} EVs/dose or 5 μg–6 mg proteins/dose). The inconsistency in dosing makes it impractical to cross-compare the therapeutic potentials of EVs. The large dose disparity further highlights the limitation in quantification methods during manufacturing and the crucial need to establish a consistent EV dosing strategy [25–27]. Therefore, there is an urgent need to establish consistency in EV quantification [28].

Many strategies have been developed to characterize EVs, and complementary techniques are typically used to obtain desirable information, such as transmission electron microscopy (TEM) for size and morphology, especially cryo-electron microscopy [29], enzyme-linked immunosorbent assay (ELISA), or flow cytometry and immunostaining for surface marker confirmation, and protein profiling by mass spectrometry [30,31]. Furthermore, emerging techniques continue to be developed, such as Raman tweezers microspectroscopy for chemical composition without labeling [29]. Regardless of potential applications, proper choices of characterization techniques for EV analysis are critical [32]. Among various characterization techniques, nanoparticle-tracking analysis (NTA) has proven to be one of the most useful methods for EV characterization, as it provides information about EV size, size distribution, and concentration in solution. In conjunction with fluorescent labeling of EV-specific biomarkers or disease markers, NTA in fluorescent mode allows for distinguishing different subpopulations and for disease detection in biological fluids.

In this review, we will discuss the NTA technique in both light scattering and fluorescent mode. In particular, we will highlight the factors affecting the specific information for NTA analysis. For example, practical considerations in the size and concentration measurement of EVs for light-scattering mode will be covered along with their practical applications. Beyond the size, size distribution, and EV concentration, it is critical to characterize protein and RNA markers to confirm EV phenotypes. With specific fluorescent labeling of EV protein markers, the fluorescent mode of NTA allows for the characterization of EVs in much specificity. The fluoresce-based NTA greatly depends on the fluorescent tags for EV labeling. The types of fluorescent tags not only influence the quality of NTA results but also define suitable applications. Here, special attention will be given to EV detection in biological fluids for potential disease diagnosis. Finally, we will discuss NTA's limitations and future direction to address the need for standardization.

2. NTA Technique

NTA is a widely used technique to visualize and characterize EVs, providing various information from a single technique, such as size, size distribution, concentration, surface biomarkers, etc. [33]. NTA tracks the Brownian motion of nanoparticles in a solution using a laser beam, which uses a high-sensitivity camera to capture the scattered light from nanoparticles in real-time. By analyzing trajectories of nanoparticles frame by frame within a certain period, the diffusion coefficient of each particle is calculated from its motion, and the hydrodynamic diameter is subsequently calculated using the Stokes–Einstein equation. Currently, there are two modes of NTA based on detecting signals either from the scattered lights from EVs or fluorescent emission of fluorescence-labeled EVs, as illustrated in Figure 1. NTA instruments currently have four choices of lasers (e.g., 405, 488, 532, or 642 nm).

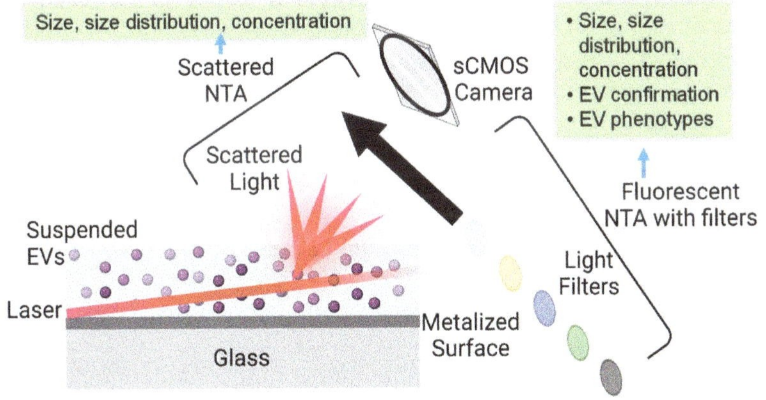

Figure 1. Illustration of NTA measurement principle in scattering and fluorescent modes along with obtained EV information, where the various colored circles indicated that different wavelength of emission lights can be collected by the selection of appropriate filter.

Along with the appropriate filters, a wide range of fluorescent tags can be used to facilitate fluorescence measurements of EVs. The light-scattering mode NTA has the same working principle as dynamic light scattering (DLS), both of which track the Brownian motion of the objects by detecting the scattered lights [34]. DLS is another commonly used technique to characterize EVs in solution [32]. DLS only provides information on EV size and size distribution by analyzing the scattered light intensities. However, NTA generates a number-based size and size distribution by visualization. Compared to NTA, DLS does not offer information related to concentration or numbers because it analyzes all particles in solution simultaneously [35]. In addition, DLS has challenges in analyzing polydisperse samples, where scattered lights from larger objects dominant over the smaller ones. One benefit of DLS over NTA is the upper detection threshold of around 6 μm versus 1 μm for NTA [36]. In general, the size obtained from DLS is slightly larger than that from NTA because of the intrinsic heterogeneity of EVs and the domination of scattered light by larger-sized objects [37].

Typically, the light-scattering mode of NTA provides accurate size and concentration information in solution. The measured EV sizes typically agree well with other techniques, such as TEM [38]. However, sample conditions greatly affect NTA measurements, such as sample dilution, EV purity, measurement temperature, etc. In addition, the instrument settings, video acquisition, and data analysis settings all require calibration and optimization for consistent results [39]. It has been shown that the types of standards to calibrate the instrument were also important for EV measurement [39]. A comparison of measured EV size and concentration by the same operator using two NanoSight NS500 instruments at different laboratories suggested a large variation between EV size and concentration depending on applied instrument settings and technical conditions [40]. In the study, both intra-assay (within a day, n = 6) and inter-assay (day-to-day, n = 6) variations of EVs from different isolated methods were studied. It was suggested that the intra-assay variation, day-to-day variation, and operator variation were not significant on the same instrument. However, significant variation was observed between two instruments using identical software settings, which was attributed to instrument-optimized settings. This study emphasized the importance of consistent instrumental settings, standard operating procedures, and data analysis protocols. Therefore, proper sample preparation with standardized protocols is critical for NTA analysis of EVs to ensure accurate size and concentration. These conditions (e.g., sample dilution, choice of buffers, and removal of aggregates or contaminants) can significantly influence the NTA results. In addition, regular calibration of NTA instruments is essential to ensure accurate size and concentration measurements, such as camera settings, laser alignment, and temperature control. Finally, data acquisition and analysis parameters, such as frame rate, camera shutter speed, and tracking setting, also need attention. It is desirable that these parameters are optimized according to the sample to be measured to improve the reliability of the measurements. Therefore, it is critical to include instrumental settings and operating conditions when reporting experimental data of EVs from NTA.

When operated properly, NTA measurement provides fast and accurate information on EV size, size distribution, and concentration. For example, NTA-measured sizes of EVs isolated from conditioned media of human placenta-derived mesenchymal cells by differential centrifugation agreed well with the sizes obtained from TEM [38]. The size distribution obtained from NTA measurement provides insights into the heterogeneity of the EV populations because different types of EVs (exosomes, microvesicles, and apoptotic bodies) have distinct size ranges. However, the light-scattering mode of NTA cannot differentiate EVs from other nanosized objects, such as protein aggregates, contaminations, and salt precipitates. Consequently, the fluorescent mode of NTA was developed, which detects fluorescently labeled EVs. Switching from scattering to fluorescence mode, a long-pass filter is normally used to block the excitation wavelength. The fluorescent mode of NTA not only provides more accurate size and concentration information but also allows for the confirmation of EV types. When EV samples are analyzed in both light scattering and fluorescent modes, the percentage of EVs with labeled specific protein markers can be obtained in the solution. With the capability of multiple labeling, biomarker-positive or negative EVs allow the establishment of EV profiling as a supporting method for EV quantification.

In summary, NTA provides real-time EV analysis in solution, yielding accurate information regarding EV size, size distribution, and phenotypes. If EV samples are properly prepared and NTA instrument parameters are well calibrated, NTA quantification is highly valuable for a number of EV studies, such as the evaluation of isolation methods, dynamic studies of EV production and release, and EV detection based on surface markers. The selection of light-scattering mode vs. fluorescent mode will depend on the study needs and the information to be obtained.

3. EV Characterization with Light Scattering Mode of NTA

In the scattering mode of NTA, the solution sample is illuminated by a laser and the scattered light from the particles in solution is captured by a camera. The software algorithms analyze the particle trajectories to determine their hydrodynamic diameter and concentration. However, the light-scattering mode of NTA does not provide EV-specific information. Compared to other techniques, such as TEM and immunostaining, NTA is noninvasive with quick data acquisition, offering an effective tool for quickly comparing EV isolation methods, storage and EV release conditions. Numerous EV studies have utilized NTA as the primary characterization tool for EV size and concentration measurement. First, the scattering mode of NTA provides a high-resolution size distribution profile, enabling the characterization of the heterogeneity of EV populations based on the size distribution (e.g., exosomes, microvesicles, and apoptotic bodies). For example, NTA has a typical measurement size range of 50 nm~1 μm [36] with improved upper bound size around 2 μm for carefully prepared samples [41]. Compared to exosomes and microvesicles, apoptotic bodies are much larger (up to 5 μm) [42,43], which directly affects the measurement accuracy because of the lower particle number per analyzing volume and possible particle overlaps [36,37].

On the other hand, exosomes smaller than 50 nm are challenging for NTA to analyze. For uniform EVs less than 50 nm, DLS can provide a more reliable analysis of size and size distribution. Comfort et al. reported a detailed NTA protocol for quantifying the size and concentration of EVs isolated from mouse perigonadal adipose tissue and human plasma [33]. By analyzing EVs of different subpopulations from the human placenta and plasma using NTA, Soo et al. recommended several considerations for sample preparation [44]. First, the light-scattering mode of NTA has a low size detection limit of ~50 nm, smaller than which may not be quantified accurately. Second, NTA has an effective EV concentration of 10^8–10^9, but the accuracy of size measurement decreases for polydisperse samples. Tian et al. [45] recently presented a study to search critical parameters for the standardization of size and concentration determination of nanomaterials by NTA using polystyrene and SiO_2 standard nanoparticles. The search result suggested an optimal concentration of 10^8–10^9 particles/mL. Therefore, a proper sample concentration is critical for NTA camera detection with all EVs that are detectable but without overlaying.

Because NTA provides accurate size and concentration information, the NTA technique has been the most useful tool to quantify EV yields from different conditions and monitor EV storage conditions. For example, the size and concentration of EVs isolated from human induced pluripotent stem cells and mesenchymal stem cells were accurately quantified by NTA [46]. NTA is also highly valuable for evaluating isolation efficiency and cross-comparison of EV isolation methods of various samples [47]. The NTA size measurement of EVs isolated from conditioned media of placenta-derived mesenchymal cells had a good agreement with TEM results of negative stained EVs [36]. Another study by Ekström et al. [48] isolated EVs from lymphatic drain fluids of seven patients with breast cancer the day after axillary lymph node dissection and subsequently quantified EV concentration by NTA, along with other techniques. NTA EV concentration coupled with protein quantification was used to evaluate the efficiency of the EV isolation process, and the ratio of EV number and protein amount served as an indicator of EV purity. NTA concentration quantification of urinary EVs isolated from the urine of 32 patients with varying levels of albuminuria showed the need for cautious interpretation of NTA concentration of EVs in biological fluids containing high proteins [49].

The accurate size and concentration measurement of NTA offers an effective tool for studying the stability of EVs. EV membrane disruption will not only change EV size but also decrease EV concentration. For example, the storage conditions (e.g., −80, −20, and 4 °C) of EVs isolated from HEK293T cells were studied by NTA in scattering mode as a function of time [50]. With increasing storage time, the disruption of EV membranes led to a reduction of EV concentrations. Therefore, NTA-based concentration quantification was more accurate and effective in monitoring the integrity of EVs compared to bulk RNA or protein quantification. Accurate determination of EV concentration is also critical for dose-response studies in therapeutic applications. EV number per unit volume has been one of the most commonly used EV dosing strategies in preclinical and clinical studies, where NTA has been the primary technique used to quantify the dose of EVs [25].

Given that NTA provides EV size and concentration information in real-time in solution, it allows for monitoring of EV release, aiding in optimizing culture conditions and treatment times to enhance EV yield. Monitoring the dynamic production of EVs from cultured cells over time can provide insights into cellular processes and the effects of treatments. For example, the exosome and microvesicle release from human lymphoblastoid T-cell lines Jurkat and CEM were stimulated with known potentiators (ionophores monensin and A23187) and quantified by NTA [44]. NTA quantification suggested that the release of microvesicles and exosomes was dependent on the time and concentration of potentiators. In the same study, NTA was applied to effectively monitor microvesicle release from peripheral blood monocyte-derived dendritic cells treated with bacterial lipopolysaccharide.

Furthermore, NTA has served as a great tool to study EVs isolated from body fluids, such as saliva, whole blood, urine, etc. For example, NTA was shown to effectively detect neuronal EVs in saliva for early detection of neurodegenerative diseases [51]. Despite the demonstrated effectiveness of NTA in studying EV concentration in biofluids, the quality of the results is highly dependent on sample preparation and instrumentation settings. Because NTA in light-scattering mode cannot differentiate EVs from other nanoparticles, the quantification of EV size and concentration in biological fluids with high protein contents will further increase the difficulty. A study using NTA to analyze EVs from neat biofluids (human serum and pericardial fluid) of patients undergoing cardiac surgery and from healthy controls suggested that several factors affected the NTA results, such as contamination from lipoproteins, sample freeze–thaw cycles without filtration, video frame, and EV numbers per frame [52]. To ensure cross-comparison among various studies, it is important to establish standard operating procedures for sample preparation, purity, and reference methods and materials. Sometimes, the types of NTA instruments also contribute to the consistency variation among EV characterization. For example, Bachurski et al. have compared the accuracy and repeatability of EV analysis from two NTA instruments (Malvern's NanoSight NS300 and Particle Metrix's ZetaView) [53]. In this study, the size and concentration of EVs from human serum and cell culture supernatants were compared as a function of serial dilutions for sample preparation and freeze–thaw cycles. The results suggested that ZetaView provided a more accurate and repeatable depiction of EV concentration, whereas NanoSight NS300 supplied size measurements of higher resolution.

NTA has been demonstrated to be an effective tool to quantify the size and concentration of EVs in cell culture and human body fluids, which has been explored as a diagnostic tool for disease detection. A study by Roni et al. compared EV concentration in patients' saliva based on NTA quantification, which could be directly correlated to the progression of cognitive impairment in Alzheimer's disease [54]. This study suggested that NTA-based EV quantification could be potentially used for early detection and cost-effective screening of diseases. Similarly, it was also shown that NTA could be used to detect EVs in other biological fluids, such as urine [55]. However, NTA is typically not very effective in analyzing small-sized EVs. Parsons et al. [56] developed a protocol to improve the precision and reproducibility of NTA to study EVs in the range of 50–120 nm in plasma [56]. It was suggested that increasing video replicates led to a reduction in overall variance and increased reproducibility.

In summary, the light-scattering mode of NTA is a non-destructive technique, allowing for further analysis of the same sample. The fast and accurate size and concentration measurement of NTA has demonstrated effectiveness in comparing EV isolation methods, studying EV purity and storage conditions, and monitoring EV production and release. In addition, NTA measurement highly depends on the EV isolation methods and sources. To ensure consistent results, many factors need to be considered, such as standard sample preparation protocols, consistent instruments, data acquisition and analysis settings. Despite the indisputable benefits in characterizing EV size, size distribution, and concentration, NTA in the light-scattering mode cannot differentiate the EVs from other nanoobjects, such as protein aggregates and other contaminants, which indicates the need for fluorescent NTA.

4. EV Characterization with Fluorescent Mode of NTA

The fluorescent mode of NTA is an advanced version of the NTA technique, which combines both scattered light and fluorescence detection. This approach is particularly powerful for confirming EVs through labeling EV-specific protein markers. In the fluorescent mode of NTA, EVs can be labeled with fluorescent molecules that specifically bind either to typical EV markers, such as tetraspanin (e.g., CD9, CD63, and CD81) or cytosolic protein (e.g., TSG101, ALIX, and syntenin) or target a specific disease protein marker. Switching from scattering to fluorescence mode, a long-pass filter is used to block the excitation wavelength and fluorescent emission from the labeled EVs are detected. Beyond the size and concentration, the fluorescent emission from the labeled EVs allows for the differentiation of labeled EVs from non-labeled ones in a mixed population. The most determent factor for fluorescent NTA is EV labeling (e.g., types of tags and labeling methods). In this section, we will first discuss EV labeling and then review the practical applications of fluorescent NTA in EV analysis.

4.1. EV Labeling

Fluorescent labeling of EVs refers to the incorporation of fluorescent molecules into EVs. The fluorescent labeling enables direct visualization of EVs with high specificity and sensitivity using the fluorescent mode of NTA. Numerous methods have been developed to label EVs, which will be discussed in detail in terms of choices of fluorescent tags, labeling strategies, and suitable applications. Depending on the labeling biomarkers, fluorescence NTA can be applied to study EVs for diverse bio-applications in vitro and in vivo [57].

The fluorescent labeling of EVs can take place at the EV membrane, surface proteins, or internal cargos [58], as illustrated in Figure 2. First, the most common EV labeling is to use lipophilic dyes (e.g., PKH67, DiI, and DiO), which have a fluorescent head group and a long hydrophobic tail capable of inserting into EVs [59]. Membrane dye labeling has high labeling efficiency with strong fluorescent signals and minimal interference of internal cargo. In addition, the labeling process is relatively straightforward and quick [57] with developed labeling protocols [60]. Because membrane-labeling dyes stain all EVs, the quantification of EVs labeled with membrane dyes by fluorescence NTA provides the total counts of EVs regardless of phenotypes. On the other hand, the membrane dyes are non-specific and label any lipid-containing particles; therefore, the purity of the isolated EVs is critical to using membrane dyes as EV labels. For example, Chen et al. [61] systematically investigated the correlation of labeling efficiency with EV purity, suggesting that a 60–80% labeling efficiency for EVs isolated from conditioned cell culture media with EV purity of ~88% and ~40–70% labeling efficiency for EVs isolated from platelet-free plasma with

EV purity of ~73%. In addition, the insertion of dyes into the lipid bilayer of EVs may affect their structure and function. The higher the labeling efficiency, the brighter the fluorescent signal, but a significant amount of lipophilic dye insertion could alter the size and structure of EVs. It was shown that excessive labeling with PKH26 could alter the membrane integrity of EVs [61]. Compared to PKH26, di-8-ANEPPS and DiI showed higher and more uniform EV labeling, with nearly 100% labeling efficiency for di-8-ANEPPS and 70–100% for DiI [61]. Unfortunately, dye aggregates and micelle structures were observed for all tested membrane dyes in this study [61], indicating a general issue of the membrane dyes for EV labeling.

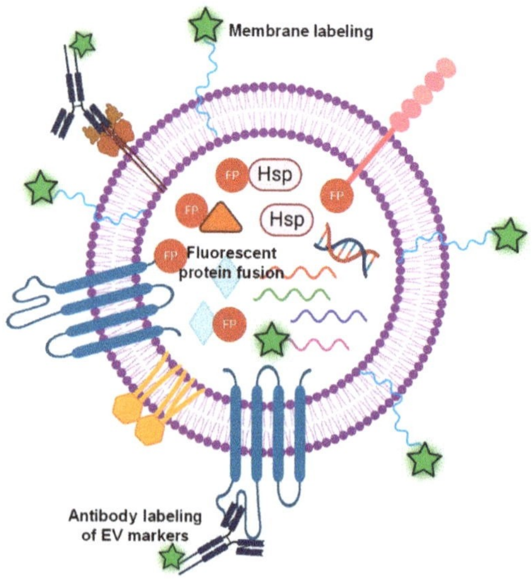

Figure 2. Illustration of various labeling strategies of EVs, such as lipophilic dyes for non-specific EV labeling, a fluorescent antibody targeting EV surface markers, or fluorescent protein (FP) fused to either surface proteins or internal cytosolic proteins, and mRNA labeling.

Similarly, Midekessa et al. [62] investigated the effects of labeling conditions of lipophilic CellMask™ Green dyes on EVs isolated from human choriocarcinoma cells and different biological fluids using fluorescence NTA. By comparing EVs purified with different methods and EVs from biological fluids, it was found that the increased dye concentration significantly decreased the observed EV size. This observed size shift indicated the need to emphasize the optimization of dye concentrations to preserve the size of EVs after labeling. However, another comparison study [63] by fluorescent NTA showed that EVs labeled with lipophilic fluorescent dye molecules increased EV sizes at all labeling conditions. In contrast, a membrane-permeable dye that localized inside EVs did not affect the EV size, such as CFSE (5-(and-6)-carboxyfluorescein diacetate succinimidyl ester).

In addition to the alteration of EV structure, the labeling conditions must be carefully evaluated in salt-containing buffers or media, where most of these lipid dyes generally have low water solubility, readily forming micelles or aggregates. A study by Cha et al. [64] described a facile method with efficient EV labeling using lipophilic fluorescent dyes by adjusting the ionic strength of buffers with NaCl. Using cell-derived EVs labeled with DiI as a model system, it was found that a low-salt condition (20 mM) improved EV-labeling efficiency by a factor of 290 compared to high-salt concentration (150 mM). Another concern about using lipophilic dyes for EV labeling is the complete removal of unincorporated dyes that could cause background fluorescence [65]. A systematic study of EV purification efficiency after the labeling with various purification methods was performed using fluorescent mode NTA. It was found that the purification step must be carefully performed to ensure the accurate characterization of labeled EVs [66]. Therefore, the proper selection of purification methods and labeling conditions are important to membrane dye labeling. It was shown that increasing NaCl concentration in purification buffers after labeling induced aggregate formation of free dye molecules, which could be effectively removed through filtration [64]. Therefore, using a high salt concentration to reduce off-target labeling could be developed into a general method [64]. Besides the advancement of labeling and purification methods, new lipophilic fluorescent dyes have also been explored. Shimomura et al. [67] recently reported the development of a new type of dye consisting of a fluorescent cyanine group with an attached amphiphilic moiety that showed excellent EV labeling with no aggregation and less EV alteration based on the characterization by fluorescent NTA [67]. Alternatively, the fluorescent probes can be encapsulated into the lumen of EVs by incubating dye molecules permeable to bilayer membranes or nanoparticles by physical diffusion or active uptake, electroporation or sonication [68]. It was found that luminal labeling of EVs has less effect on the EV sizes [59].

One of the main drawbacks of membrane dye labeling is that it is non-specific, which means it cannot provide EV-specific information. Therefore, to obtain EV-specific information, the surface protein markers of EVs are commonly labeled with fluorescent antibodies specific for biomarkers of interest. By far, many different fluorescent antibodies have been developed against EV-specific surface markers (e.g., CD63, CD81, and CD9) that are characteristic of the EVs of interest. When EV-specific antibodies are conjugated to fluorescent dyes (e.g., FITC or Alexa Fluor—AF), EVs can be labeled directly and visualized by fluorescent NTA. For example, Cho reported the multifluorescence of single EVs and direct characterization by a modified form of fluorescent NTA [69]. Specifically, EVs were labeled with a blue fluoresce dye (AF405) conjugated antibody against CD81, a green fluorescent dye (AF488), a conjugated CD9 antibody, and a red fluorescent dye (AF647) CD63 antibody. The labeled EVs were subsequently characterized with fluorescent NTA with three excitation wavelengths (405, 488, and 638 nm). This study not only demonstrated the effectiveness of specific EV labeling via EV marker antibodies but also showed the feasibility of characterization of individual EVs using the fluorescent mode of NTA. The fluorescent antibody labeling provides high specificity, enabling specific detection and analysis of labeled EVs within a heterogeneous population. It also provides quantitative data on the concentration and size distribution of specific EV subpopulations. Therefore, this labeling strategy is best suited for EV confirmation and detection. For therapeutic applications or cell–cell communication studies, labeling surface protein markers may hinder the biological functions of EVs. In addition, the effectiveness of labeling with fluorescent antibodies depends on the antibody specificity, number of protein surface markers, and fluorescent stability.

Alternatively, EV-specific surface proteins or structural proteins within EVs can be tagged through genetic modification of EV-producing cells, yielding fluorescent protein-fused EV proteins. Fluorescent protein can be fused to EV protein markers either as recombinant proteins on the EV membrane or as internal cargo proteins in the EV lumen. Once established, fluorescent labeling is consistent and reliable. This labeling strategy enables facile functional analysis of EV components. For example, green fluorescent protein (GFP) has been fused to typical EV markers, CD63 [70] and CD81 [71], allowing for quantification and subpopulation determination of EVs by fluorescent mode NTA. However, this EV-labeling process requires genetic modification of the parent cells, which can be time-consuming and not applicable to all EVs. For example, the CD81 genes of humans (Hus) or Chinese hamsters (CHOs) were fused with GFP via a flexible peptide linker and then were expressed in CHO cells as recombinant proteins. Subsequently, GFP-labeled EVs were isolated from those transfected CHO cells, and EV concentration and yield across the EV purification process were quantified using the fluorescent mode of NTA. NTA concentration of EVs isolated from the CD81-GFP (CHO) and CD81-GFP

(Hu) cell lines showed that the CD81-GFP (CHO) cell line did not secrete non-fused GFP while the expression of non-fused GFP from the CD81-GFP (Hu) cells was observed. EV concentrations were higher in the CD81-GFP (CHO) cells compared to the CD81-GFP (Hu) cells. For fused fluorescent protein fusion EV labeling, a systematic study of EVs with GFP fused CD63 showed the highest fluorescent protein per EV no more than 40–60% [72]. Some of the GFP-tagged EV showed quenched fluorescence either due to non-EV particles or the presence of truncated GFP. In addition, GFPs typically suffer from background interference, while RFPs are less bright. Most recently, a study by Mao et al. demonstrated effective EV labeling with a super-bright far-red fluorescence protein, mKate2 [73]. This dye is considered the next-generation fluorescent label with super brightness and far-red emission, high pH stability and photostability, low cytotoxicity, and low background interference. The fluorescent mode of NTA showed effective incorporation of mKate2-tagged protein into EV membranes with 90% labeling efficiency and without altering the EV size [73]. Additionally, the EV surface proteins can be labeled directly via click chemistry [74,75] to covalently attach fluorescent probes to the EV surface. This strategy can utilize a wide range of fluorescent probes with numerous linkers being developed [68]. However, chemical modification may affect the functionality and integrity of EVs.

Labeling EV protein markers is somehow limited by the number of surface proteins for enough fluorescent signals. Although fluorescent labeling with membrane dyes (e.g., PKH27, PKH67, etc.) provides an adequate signal for EV detection, this approach is non-specific and a higher amount of dye labeling was shown to alter the EV size and structural integrity. Recently, a study by Baldwin et al. [76] demonstrated the feasibility of determining the miRNA content of EVs isolated from A549 lung cancer cells using the fluorescent mode of NTA. In this study, miR-21 was fluorescently labeled by the hybridization of miRNA with fluorescently labeled, miRNA-specific molecular beacons encapsulated in cationic lipoplex nanoparticles that fuse non-specifically with negatively charged EVs. A stoichiometric analysis of miR-21 in EVs released from A549 lung cancer cells was analyzed in relation to the total EV population from the light-scattering mode of NTA. The result reported a threshold number of 33 miR-21 copies per EV required for fluorescence tracking. This study demonstrated the feasibility of fluorescent NTA analysis of fluorescent-labeled miRNA, which could potentially be used for EV sizing, concentration quantification, phenotyping, and identifying specific EV subpopulations in patient samples for diagnostic applications.

As discussed above, numerous fluorescent tags and labeling methods have been developed with their own pros and cons [77], as summarized in Table 1. By far, the photostability of most dyes remains a major concern for long-time tracking [78]. A study by Thane et al. [79] demonstrated reproducible NTA size and concentration quantification of fluorescently labeled EVs with quantum dots (QDs). In conjunction with the light-scattering mode, this study suggested that NTA offered an effective tool to estimate EV fraction with a specific biomarker. QDs are nanocrystals with bright and stable fluorescent emission, ideally suited for NTA applications. However, conjugation of larger inorganic nanoparticles could affect antibody activities.

Table 1. A summary of various EV-labeling strategies.

Dye Types	Binding Location	Advantages	Disadvantages	Example
Lipophilic dye	EV membrane	High labeling efficiency, easy operation	Non-specific, aggregation, alteration of EV size and structure	Refs. [52–55]
Membrane permeable probes	EV lumen	Easy operation, minimal alteration of EV membrane	Non-specific, labeling efficiency-dependent labeling methods, possible EV structural disruption	Refs. [52,56,61]

Table 1. *Cont.*

Dye Types	Binding Location	Advantages	Disadvantages	Example
Fluorescent protein fusion	EV surface or cytosolic proteins	High specificity and high efficiency, minimal alteration of EV protein function	Not applicable to all EVs, genetic modification of cells, and non-fused proteins.	Refs. [62–66]
Fluorescent antibody labeling	EV surface protein markers	Highly specificity	Limited number of surface proteins, alteration of protein function	Refs. [62,69]
Dye conjugation	EV surface proteins	High efficiency, versatile	Protein function alteration, precise chemical modification	Refs. [67,68]

In summary, choosing an appropriate fluorescent labeling method for EVs depends on the specific requirements of the study, such as the need for specificity, sensitivity, and functional integrity. It is important to balance these factors to achieve reliable and meaningful results.

4.2. Application of Fluorescent Mode of NTA in EV Characterization

The fluorescent mode of NTA is a powerful technique for EV characterization, offering insights into EV phenotypes, precise EV size profiles, etc. Therefore, fluorescent NTA has significant potential in the study of EVs for various in vitro and in vivo applications, such as accurate size and concentration quantification in a mixed solution and EV phenotype confirmation for disease detection. In this section, we will review the emerging applications of fluorescent NTA in EV characterization.

Quantification of EV size and concentration: Compared to the light-scattering mode, the fluorescent mode of NTA provides more accurate size, size distribution, and concentration of EVs, especially for EVs with low purity. For example, NTA number quantification of EVs from plasma via CD 63 antibody labeling showed a significantly higher concentration of EVs in plasma melanoma patients than in healthy donors [80]. This study suggested the potential of the fluorescent mode of NTA in disease detection. In another study, EVs isolated from the serum of hepatocellular carcinoma patients were labeled with lipophilic membrane dye and quantified by fluorescent mode of NTA for total EVs [81]. In the same study, isolated EVs were labeled with fluorescent antibodies against alpha-fetoprotein (AFP) and glypican (3GPC3) markers. NTA concentration quantification of GPC3- and AFP-positive EVs in hepatocellular carcinoma patient serum were compared to that from healthy controls, indicating a positive correlation of serum concentration of GPC3-positive EVs with tumor size. Therefore, this study demonstrated a proof-of-principle to use patient serum-derived EVs as a diagnostic tool. Furthermore, by comparing the fluorescently labeled EVs with the EV concentration of light-scattering mode, the fluorescent mode of NTA could effectively study contaminants and subpopulations [77].

Confirmation of EV subpopulation: In addition to accurate determination of size and concentration, NTA in fluorescent mode allows for the identification of EV phenotypes based on specific biomarker labeling [76]. EVs are intrinsically heterogeneous, where EV subgroups reflect various information related to biogenesis and characteristics of the secreting cells. Fluorescence-mode NTA was used to study purified and non-purified EVs from different cell sources, where the EVs were fluorescently labeled with both specific dyes and antibodies for EV identification. It was shown that the fluorescent mode of NTA effectively confirmed the presence of two EV subpopulations (85 nm and 135 nm) by tagging the typical EV marker, CD63, fused with GFP and expressed in Hela cell line [70]. In addition to the size and concentration of EVs, the fluorescent mode of NTA was shown to effectively detect EVs from human placental and plasma as small as ~50 nm and EV phenotypes were confirmed through labeling with QDs conjugated with NDOG2 antibody specifically against placental alkaline phosphatase [82].

EVs can be fluorescently labeled with non-specific membrane markers for total EV counts or labeled with antibodies specifically targeting surface markers of certain EV types, where the comparison of these two EV concentrations yields the accurate percentage of a specific EV type. For example, by proper labeling with fluorescent probes, fluorescent NTA provides a way to identify the size and concentration of an EV subpopulation in biological samples [83]. Another protocol development study [84] directly compared EV quantification by fluorescence NTA when EVs were labeled with either general membrane dye for total EV counts or with QD-conjugated antibody against disease-positive markers on EVs for quantification of certain EV groups [84].

A study by Desgeorges et al. [85] reported the NTA quantification of EVs isolated from umbilical cord mesenchymal stromal cells using fluorescent mode. The comparison of EV concentrations from light-scattering mode versus fluorescence mode allowed for the determination of the percentage of protein marker-positive EVs within a mixed particulate solution. When EVs are labeled with multiple fluorescence tags, fluorescent NTA can detect multifluorescence from single EVs by a modified form of fluorescent NTA [69]. Using EVs derived from HEK293 cells as a model system, multifluorescence labeling was demonstrated by tagging CD81 with blue dye-conjugated antibody, CD9 with green fluorescent dye-conjugated antibody, and CD63 with red fluorescent dye antibody. EVs with multilabeling were analyzed effectively on a single EV level by a modified form of fluorescent NTA, where four lasers of different wavelengths are modulated in a time-sequential manner with on-off pattern (e.g., scattering with 520 nm laser → 405 nm laser excitation → scattering with 520 nm laser → 488 nm laser excitation → scattering with 520 nm laser → 638 nm laser excitation), as illustrated in Figure 3a. The scattering NTA mode provides total counts of EVs while florescent NTA mode generates EV counts of a specific group, such as 405 nm excitation for CD81-positive EV number, 488 nm excitation for CD 9-positive EV counts, and 638 excitation for CD63 EV counts. By analyzing the fluorescence detected by NTA, it suggested that only 20% of EVs had one or more EV-associated tetraspanin markers (CD9, CD69, and CD81), and the majority of EVs are not fluorescent (either EVs lacking those markers or contaminants) (Figure 3b). This NTA design enabled not only single EV characterization but also the determination of localization of EV-associated tetraspanin markers (CD9, CD69, and CD81) in a single EV.

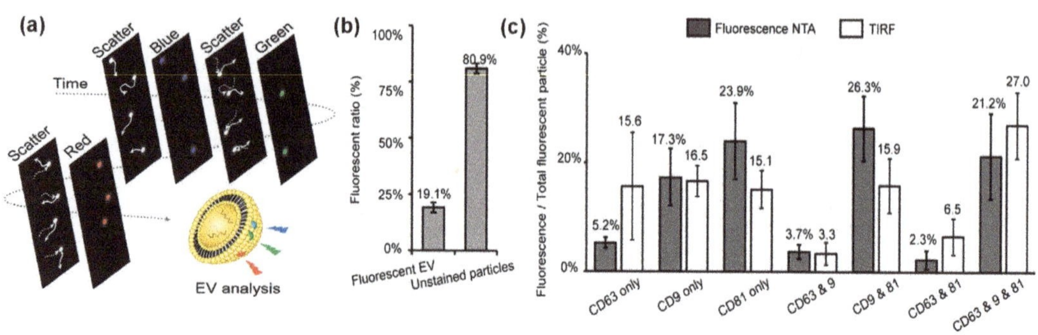

Figure 3. Single EV analysis by a multifluorescence NTA with time-sequential illumination where CD81, CD9, and CD63 markers were labeled by blue, green and red fluorescence, respectively: (**a**) illustration of the detection process, (**b**) relative percentage of EVs with and without fluorescent labels, and (**c**) comparison of detection of EVs with three CD markers by NTA and TIRF. (Copyright © 2021 American Chemical Society).

The quantifications of EVs labeled with multiple CD markers were compared with results from total internal reflection fluorescence (TIRF) microscopy, resulting in results and trends for EVs labeled with single markers, dual markers, and triple markers (Figure 3c). TIRF microscopy is a highly effective optical tool that offers high resolution and instinctive results without additional processing [86]. Therefore, the comparison of these two techniques also inferred that the NTA is a reliable method for EV analysis with multiple labels.

Monitoring EV release: The accurate EV count allows fluorescent NTA to monitor the dynamic process of EV release and uptake in real-time, providing valuable information about their biological functions. For example, the fluorescent mode of NTA was applied to study the effects of cell culturing conditions on the release of large-sized EVs (e.g., microvesicles and apoptotic bodies) from human umbilical vein endothelial cells [87]. The NTA quantification suggested that cell density and conditioning time greatly affected the concentration and size distribution of EVs. In another study [88], the fluorescent mode of NTA was applied to study EV secretion from colorectal and glioblastoma cancer cells. shRNAs targeting RAB27A, a trafficking-associated protein, were known to facilitate EV secretion towards the plasma membrane. Therefore, shRNAs were used to alter EV release in colorectal and glioblastoma cancer cells. NTA quantification of EV concentration showed increased EV section under rotenone treatment or hypoxia conditions.

EV detection in biological fluids: The fluorescent mode of NTA is increasingly used in disease detection and diagnosis by studying fluorescently labeled EVs with specific disease markers. By leveraging the specificity and sensitivity of fluorescent labeling, disease-specific EVs provide valuable insights for early diagnosis. For example, EVs in urine carry specific markers of kidney damage, such as podocyte-specific proteins, e.g., podocin. By labeling both typical EV marker CD63 and disease-specific marker podocin with ant-CD63 and anti-podocin antibodies, fluorescent NTA effectively detected and quantified podocin-positive EVs in urine [55]. A study by Dlugolecka et al. [89] presented a comprehensive EV phenotyping using the fluorescent mode of NTA for EVs isolated from bronchopulmonary lavage fluid of patients with non-small cell lung cancer. The NTA quantification of EVs from bronchopulmonary lavage fluid was compared with patient plasma-derived EVs, where EVs were labeled with lipophilic membrane dye CMDR and fluorescent antibodies against CD63 and CD9. The NTA-based phenotyping of EVs in plasma and bronchoalveolar lavage fluid highlighted the importance of sample composition and EV purity to EV analysis by fluorescent NTA.

Furthermore, it was demonstrated that fluorescent NTA can be used to characterize EVs from human blood at a single particle level [90]. In this study, EVs were isolated from human whole blood and labeled with PKH67, a common lipophilic green fluorescent dye for membrane labeling. The NTA results were further validated by several typical EV surface markers, such as CD63, CD9, vimentin, and lysosomal-associated membrane protein 1. Similarly, small-sized EVs in saliva were effectively quantified by fluorescent NTA. The NTA quantification of EV concentration showed a much higher EV concentration in Parkinson's disease patients than in the healthy control, serving as a diagnostic tool for PD [91]. This study further suggested that fluorescent NTA could be used as a potential tool to monitor disease progression with clinically acceptable sensitivity. However, a detailed analysis of small-sized EVs isolated from urine by several complementary methods suggested that the NTA evaluation of EVs is best supported by other methods [92]. In addition, the MISEV2018 guideline recommended that at least one tetraspanin (e.g., CD9, CD63, and CD81) and one cytosolic protein (e.g., TSG101, ALIX, and syntenin) should be detected for the positive identification of EVs. Moreover, the presence of non-EV-specific membrane markers (e.g., GM130) is an indication of potential contamination.

In summary, fluorescent mode NTA is a powerful tool for EV characterization, offering enhanced specificity and sensitivity compared to light-scattering mode NTA. It is particularly valuable for identifying and quantifying specific EV subpopulations, studying EV-cell interactions, and investigating the functional properties of EVs. It is important to optimize the experimental conditions to minimize operational effects from dye selection, labeling methods, and the needs of specific applications. The choice of fluorescent markers and the sensitivity of the NTA instrument are also critical for accurate detection and analysis.

5. Conclusions and Perspective

In summary, it is indisputable that NTA is a valuable tool for EV characterization, providing insights into EV size, size distribution, concentration, and heterogeneity. Many factors are important for NTA results in characterizing EVs, such as proper sample preparation in terms of EV concentration, presence of contaminants, instrumentation calibration (e.g., types, size, and concentration of calibration standards), and data acquisition and analysis parameters. Therefore, it is always a good practice to include an instrumentation setting when presenting NTA data in a publication. For the two modes of NTA, the light-scattering mode of NTA only provides size and concentration information but cannot differentiate EVs from other nanoparticles, such as protein aggregates. In contrast, the fluorescent mode of NTA offers a more accurate determination of the size and concentration of EVs because it only measures the labeled EVs. In addition, the fluorescent mode of NTA allows for the confirmation of specific types of EVs based on EV protein markers. However, the fluorescent NTA is highly dependent on the fluorescent labeling of EVs, which is affected by the labeling of fluorescent probes and labeling methods.

Despite some limitations, NTA continues to play a crucial role in advancing our understanding of EV biology and its implications in health and disease, such as the identification of EVs as disease markers, monitoring EV release and cell–cell communication. In particular, the fluorescent mode of NTA is highly valuable for disease detection by using EVs in body fluids. While NTA provides valuable EV information, it is often used in conjunction with other techniques, such as TEM, immunostaining, and flow cytometry, for comprehensive EV characterization. Continuous advancements in NTA technology will further enhance the importance of NTA in EV characterization for reproducible and comparable data across studies. First, it is important to improve the standardization and reproducibility of this technique in characterizing EVs through further advancement. These improvements can include (1) developing standardized protocols for sample preparation, data acquisition and analysis to ensure reproducibility across different laboratories, (2) establishing reference materials and calibration standards to improve the accuracy of NTA measurements, and (3) developing automated NTA systems to reduce user-dependent variability and increase throughput for large-scale studies. In addition, the sensitivity and resolution of this technique may be further improved, such as increasing the sensitivity of NTA to detect smaller EVs (<30 nm) and applying computational methods to enhance the resolution and accuracy of size distribution profiles.

Furthermore, integrating NTA with other techniques may offer additional possibilities, such as Raman spectroscopy, surface plasmon resonance, and mass spectrometry, to provide comprehensive characterization of EVs, including their molecular composition and surface markers. Finally, exploring the possibilities of integrating NTA with artificial intelligence by implementing machine-learning algorithms to enhance data analysis and automating particle tracking will provide deeper insights into EV populations and their heterogeneity.

Author Contributions: G.K.: illustration, Y.B.; writing—original draft preparation and supervision. All authors have read and agreed to the published version of the manuscript.

Funding: Bao acknowledges the University of Alabama Center for Convergent Bioscience and Medicine (CCBM) Pilot Innovation Fund (SP14596) and the Breast Cancer Research Foundation of Alabama (A23-0129).

Conflicts of Interest: The authors declare no conflicts of interest.

References

1. van Niel, G.; D'Angelo, G.; Raposo, G. Shedding light on the cell biology of extracellular vesicles. *Nat. Rev. Mol. Cell Biol.* **2018**, *19*, 213–228. [CrossRef] [PubMed]
2. Gurung, S.; Perocheau, D.; Touramanidou, L.; Baruteau, J. The exosome journey: From biogenesis to uptake and intracellular signalling. *Cell Commun. Signal.* **2021**, *19*, 47. [CrossRef] [PubMed]
3. Hessvik, N.P.; Llorente, A. Current knowledge on exosome biogenesis and release. *Cell. Mol. Life Sci.* **2018**, *75*, 193–208. [CrossRef]

4. He, C.J.; Zheng, S.; Luo, Y.; Wang, B. Exosome Theranostics: Biology and Translational Medicine. *Theranostics* **2018**, *8*, 237–255. [CrossRef]
5. Lobb, R.J.; Lima, L.G.; Moller, A. Exosomes: Key mediators of metastasis and pre-metastatic niche formation. *Semin. Cell Dev. Biol.* **2017**, *67*, 3–10. [CrossRef]
6. Steinbichler, T.B.; Dudas, J.; Riechelmann, H.; Skvortsova, I.I. The role of exosomes in cancer metastasis. *Semin. Cancer Biol.* **2017**, *44*, 170–181. [CrossRef] [PubMed]
7. Elliott, R.O.; He, M. Unlocking the Power of Exosomes for Crossing Biological Barriers in Drug Delivery. *Pharmaceutics* **2021**, *13*, 122. [CrossRef]
8. Andjus, P.; Kosanović, M.; Milićević, K.; Gautam, M.; Vainio, S.J.; Jagečić, D.; Kozlova, E.N.; Pivoriūnas, A.; Chachques, J.C.; Sakaj, M.; et al. Extracellular Vesicles as Innovative Tool for Diagnosis, Regeneration and Protection against Neurological Damage. *Int. J. Mol. Sci.* **2020**, *21*, 6859. [CrossRef]
9. Wang, X.; Yang, H.; Liu, C.; Liu, K. A new diagnostic tool for brain disorders: Extracellular vesicles derived from neuron, astrocyte, and oligodendrocyte. *Front. Mol. Neurosci.* **2023**, *16*, 1194210. [CrossRef]
10. Ashish, K.; Michael, A.N.; Gagan, D. Emergence of extracellular vesicles as 'liquid biopsy' for neurological disorders: Boom or Bust. *Pharmacol. Rev.* **2024**, *76*, 199–227. [CrossRef]
11. Davidson, S.M.; Boulanger, C.M.; Aikawa, E.; Badimon, L.; Barile, L.; Binder, C.J.; Brisson, A.; Buzas, E.; Emanueli, C.; Jansen, F.; et al. Methods for the identification and characterization of extracellular vesicles in cardiovascular studies: From exosomes to microvesicles. *Cardiovasc. Res.* **2023**, *119*, 45–63. [CrossRef] [PubMed]
12. Lee, Y.; Ni, J.; Beretov, J.; Wasinger, V.C.; Graham, P.; Li, Y. Recent advances of small extracellular vesicle biomarkers in breast cancer diagnosis and prognosis. *Mol. Cancer* **2023**, *22*, 33. [CrossRef] [PubMed]
13. Morimoto, M.; Maishi, N.; Hida, K. Acquisition of drug resistance in endothelial cells by tumor-derived extracellular vesicles and cancer progression. *Cancer Drug Resist.* **2024**, *7*, 1. [CrossRef]
14. Zhang, C.; Qin, C.; Dewanjee, S.; Bhattacharya, H.; Chakraborty, P.; Jha, N.K.; Gangopadhyay, M.; Jha, S.K.; Liu, Q. Tumor-derived small extracellular vesicles in cancer invasion and metastasis: Molecular mechanisms, and clinical significance. *Mol. Cancer* **2024**, *23*, 18. [CrossRef]
15. Urabe, F.; Patil, K.; Ramm, G.A.; Ochiya, T.; Soekmadji, C. Extracellular vesicles in the development of organ-specific metastasis. *J. Extracell. Vesicles* **2021**, *10*, e12125. [CrossRef]
16. Dong, Q.; Liu, X.; Cheng, K.; Sheng, J.; Kong, J.; Liu, T. Pre-metastatic Niche Formation in Different Organs Induced by Tumor Extracellular Vesicles. *Front. Cell Dev. Biol.* **2021**, *9*, 733627. [CrossRef]
17. Nelson, B.C.; Maragh, S.; Ghiran, I.C.; Jones, J.C.; DeRose, P.C.; Elsheikh, E.; Vreeland, W.N.; Wang, L. Measurement and standardization challenges for extracellular vesicle therapeutic delivery vectors. *Nanomedicine* **2020**, *15*, 2149–2170. [CrossRef] [PubMed]
18. Doyle, L.M.; Wang, M.Z. Overview of Extracellular Vesicles, Their Origin, Composition, Purpose, and Methods for Exosome Isolation and Analysis. *Cells* **2019**, *8*, 727. [CrossRef]
19. Almeria, C.; Kreß, S.; Weber, V.; Egger, D.; Kasper, C. Heterogeneity of mesenchymal stem cell-derived extracellular vesicles is highly impacted by the tissue/cell source and culture conditions. *Cell Biosci.* **2022**, *12*, 51. [CrossRef]
20. Gao, J.; Li, A.; Hu, J.; Feng, L.; Liu, L.; Shen, Z. Recent developments in isolating methods for exosomes. *Front. Bioeng. Biotechnol.* **2023**, *10*, 1100892. [CrossRef]
21. Liangsupree, T.; Multia, E.; Riekkola, M.L. Modern isolation and separation techniques for extracellular vesicles. *J. Chromatogr. A* **2021**, *1636*, 461773. [CrossRef] [PubMed]
22. Liu, W.Z.; Ma, Z.J.; Kang, X.W. Current status and outlook of advances in exosome isolation. *Anal. Bioanal. Chem.* **2022**, *414*, 7123–7141. [CrossRef] [PubMed]
23. Whitford, W.; Guterstam, P. Exosome manufacturing status. *Future Med. Chem.* **2019**, *11*, 1225–1236. [CrossRef]
24. Ahn, S.H.; Ryu, S.W.; Choi, H.; You, S.; Park, J.; Choi, C. Manufacturing Therapeutic Exosomes: From Bench to Industry. *Mol. Cells* **2022**, *45*, 284–290. [CrossRef]
25. Gupta, D.; Zickler, A.M.; El Andaloussi, S. Dosing extracellular vesicles. *Adv. Drug Deliv. Rev.* **2021**, *178*, 113961. [CrossRef]
26. Salmond, N.; Williams, K.C. Isolation and characterization of extracellular vesicles for clinical applications in cancer—Time for standardization? *Nanoscale Adv.* **2021**, *3*, 1830–1852. [CrossRef] [PubMed]
27. Lenzini, S. Establishing a working range for effective MSC-EV dose. *RoosterBio Blog*, 16 December 2021.
28. Claridge, B.; Lozano, J.; Poh, Q.H.; Greening, D.W. Development of Extracellular Vesicle Therapeutics: Challenges, Considerations, and Opportunities. *Front. Cell Dev. Biol.* **2021**, *9*, 734720. [CrossRef] [PubMed]
29. Tatischeff, I.; Larquet, E.; Falcón-Pérez, J.M.; Turpin, P.Y.; Kruglik, S.G. Fast characterisation of cell-derived extracellular vesicles by nanoparticles tracking analysis, cryo-electron microscopy, and Raman tweezers microspectroscopy. *J. Extracell. Vesicles* **2012**, *1*, 19179. [CrossRef]
30. Askeland, A.; Borup, A.; Østergaard, O.; Olsen, J.V.; Lund, S.M.; Christiansen, G.; Kristensen, S.R.; Heegaard, N.H.H.; Pedersen, S. Mass-Spectrometry Based Proteome Comparison of Extracellular Vesicle Isolation Methods: Comparison of ME-kit, Size-Exclusion Chromatography, and High-Speed Centrifugation. *Biomedicines* **2020**, *8*, 246. [CrossRef]

31. Manouchehri Doulabi, E.; Fredolini, C.; Gallini, R.; Löf, L.; Shen, Q.; Ikebuchi, R.; Dubois, L.; Azimi, A.; Loudig, O.; Gabrielsson, S.; et al. Surface protein profiling of prostate-derived extracellular vesicles by mass spectrometry and proximity assays. *Commun. Biol.* **2022**, *5*, 1402. [CrossRef]
32. Szatanek, R.; Baj-Krzyworzeka, M.; Zimoch, J.; Lekka, M.; Siedlar, M.; Baran, J. The Methods of Choice for Extracellular Vesicles (EVs) Characterization. *Int. J. Mol. Sci.* **2017**, *18*, 1153. [CrossRef] [PubMed]
33. Comfort, N.; Cai, K.; Bloomquist, T.R.; Strait, M.D.; Ferrante, A.W., Jr.; Baccarelli, A.A. Nanoparticle Tracking Analysis for the Quantification and Size Determination of Extracellular Vesicles. *J. Vis. Exp.* **2021**, *169*, e62447. [CrossRef]
34. Wu, S.; Zhao, Y.; Zhang, Z.; Zuo, C.; Wu, H.; Liu, Y. The Advances and Applications of Characterization Technique for Exosomes: From Dynamic Light Scattering to Super-Resolution Imaging Technology. *Photonics* **2024**, *11*, 101. [CrossRef]
35. Kesimer, M.; Gupta, R. Physical characterization and profiling of airway epithelial derived exosomes using light scattering. *Methods* **2015**, *87*, 59–63. [CrossRef]
36. Filipe, V.; Hawe, A.; Jiskoot, W. Critical evaluation of Nanoparticle Tracking Analysis (NTA) by NanoSight for the measurement of nanoparticles and protein aggregates. *Pharm. Res.* **2010**, *27*, 796–810. [CrossRef]
37. Geng, T.; Paek, S.Y.; Leung, E.; Chamley, L.W.; Wu, Z. Comparing extracellular vesicles from four different cell origins for intracellular drug delivery to pancreatic cancer cells: Small or large vesicles? *J. Drug Deliv. Sci. Technol.* **2024**, *93*, 105416. [CrossRef]
38. Bagrov, D.V.; Senkovenko, A.M.; Nikishin, I.I.; Skryabin, G.O.; Kopnin, P.B.; Tchevkina, E.M. Application of AFM, TEM, and NTA for characterization of exosomes produced by placenta-derived mesenchymal cells. *J. Phys. Conf. Ser.* **2021**, *1942*, 012013. [CrossRef]
39. Gardiner, C.; Ferreira, Y.J.; Dragovic, R.A.; Redman, C.W.; Sargent, I.L. Extracellular vesicle sizing and enumeration by nanoparticle tracking analysis. *J. Extracell. Vesicles* **2013**, *2*, 19671. [CrossRef]
40. Vestad, B.; Llorente, A.; Neurauter, A.; Phuyal, S.; Kierulf, B.; Kierulf, P.; Skotland, T.; Sandvig, K.; Haug, K.B.F.; Øvstebø, R. Size and concentration analyses of extracellular vesicles by nanoparticle tracking analysis: A variation study. *J. Extracell. Vesicles* **2017**, *6*, 1344087. [CrossRef]
41. Hubert, M.; Yang, D.T.; Kwok, S.C.; Rios, A.; Das, T.K.; Patel, A.; Wuchner, K.; Antochshuk, V.; Junge, F.; Bou-Assaf, G.M.; et al. A Multicompany Assessment of Submicron Particle Levels by NTA and RMM in a Wide Range of Late-Phase Clinical and Commercial Biotechnology-Derived Protein Products. *J. Pharm. Sci.* **2020**, *109*, 830–844. [CrossRef]
42. Zhang, X.; Yang, J.; Ma, S.; Gao, X.; Wang, G.; Sun, Y.; Yu, Y.; Wang, Z.; Tian, W.; Liao, L. Functional diversity of apoptotic vesicle subpopulations from bone marrow mesenchymal stem cells in tissue regeneration. *J. Extracell. Vesicles* **2024**, *13*, e12434. [CrossRef] [PubMed]
43. Gregory, C.D.; Rimmer, M.P. Extracellular vesicles arising from apoptosis: Forms, functions, and applications. *J. Pathol.* **2023**, *260*, 592–608. [CrossRef]
44. Soo, C.Y.; Song, Y.; Zheng, Y.; Campbell, E.C.; Riches, A.C.; Gunn-Moore, F.; Powis, S.J. Nanoparticle tracking analysis monitors microvesicle and exosome secretion from immune cells. *Immunology* **2012**, *136*, 192–197. [CrossRef] [PubMed]
45. Tian, Y.; Tian, D.; Peng, X.; Qiu, H. Critical parameters to standardize the size and concentration determination of nanomaterials by nanoparticle tracking analysis. *Int. J. Pharm.* **2024**, *656*, 124097. [CrossRef] [PubMed]
46. Liu, S.; Mahairaki, V.; Bai, H.; Ding, Z.; Li, J.; Witwer, K.W.; Cheng, L. Highly Purified Human Extracellular Vesicles Produced by Stem Cells Alleviate Aging Cellular Phenotypes of Senescent Human Cells. *Stem Cells* **2019**, *37*, 779–790. [CrossRef] [PubMed]
47. Lee, Y.; Ni, J.; Wasinger, V.C.; Graham, P.; Li, Y. Comparison Study of Small Extracellular Vesicle Isolation Methods for Profiling Protein Biomarkers in Breast Cancer Liquid Biopsies. *Int. J. Mol. Sci.* **2023**, *24*, 15462. [CrossRef]
48. Ekström, K.; Crescitelli, R.; Pétursson, H.I.; Johansson, J.; Lässer, C.; Olofsson Bagge, R. Characterization of surface markers on extracellular vesicles isolated from lymphatic exudate from patients with breast cancer. *BMC Cancer* **2022**, *22*, 50. [CrossRef]
49. McNicholas, K.; Li, J.Y.; Michael, M.Z.; Gleadle, J.M. Albuminuria is not associated with elevated urinary vesicle concentration but can confound nanoparticle tracking analysis. *Nephrology* **2017**, *22*, 854–863. [CrossRef]
50. Görgens, A.; Corso, G.; Hagey, D.W.; Jawad Wiklander, R.; Gustafsson, M.O.; Felldin, U.; Lee, Y.; Bostancioglu, R.B.; Sork, H.; Liang, X.; et al. Identification of storage conditions stabilizing extracellular vesicles preparations. *J. Extracell. Vesicles* **2022**, *11*, e12238. [CrossRef]
51. Sharma, V.; Nikolajeff, F.; Kumar, S. Employing nanoparticle tracking analysis of salivary neuronal exosomes for early detection of neurodegenerative diseases. *Transl. Neurodegener.* **2023**, *12*, 7. [CrossRef]
52. Shearn, A.I.U.; Aday, S.; Ben-Aicha, S.; Carnell-Morris, P.; Siupa, A.; Angelini, G.D.; Clayton, A.; Boulanger, C.; Punjabi, P.; Emanueli, C.; et al. Analysis of Neat Biofluids Obtained During Cardiac Surgery Using Nanoparticle Tracking Analysis: Methodological Considerations. *Front. Cell Dev. Biol.* **2020**, *8*, 367. [CrossRef] [PubMed]
53. Bachurski, D.; Schuldner, M.; Nguyen, P.H.; Malz, A.; Reiners, K.S.; Grenzi, P.C.; Babatz, F.; Schauss, A.C.; Hansen, H.P.; Hallek, M.; et al. Extracellular vesicle measurements with nanoparticle tracking analysis—An accuracy and repeatability comparison between NanoSight NS300 and ZetaView. *J. Extracell. Vesicles* **2019**, *8*, 1596016. [CrossRef] [PubMed]
54. Rani, K.; Rastogi, S.; Vishwakarma, P.; Bharti, P.S.; Sharma, V.; Renu, K.; Modi, G.P.; Vishnu, V.Y.; Chatterjee, P.; Dey, A.B.; et al. A novel approach to correlate the salivary exosomes and their protein cargo in the progression of cognitive impairment into Alzheimer's disease. *J. Neurosci. Methods* **2021**, *347*, 108980. [CrossRef]

55. Sałaga-Zaleska, K.; Kuchta, A.; Bzoma, B.; Chyła-Danił, G.; Safianowska, A.; Płoska, A.; Kalinowski, L.; Dębska-Ślizień, A.; Jankowski, M. Nanoparticle Tracking Analysis of Urinary Extracellular Vesicle Proteins as a New Challenge in Laboratory Medicine. *Int. J. Mol. Sci.* **2023**, *24*, 12228. [CrossRef]
56. Parsons, M.E.M.; McParland, D.; Szklanna, P.B.; Guang, M.H.Z.; O'Connell, K.; O'Connor, H.D.; McGuigan, C.; Ní Áinle, F.; McCann, A.; Maguire, P.B. A Protocol for Improved Precision and Increased Confidence in Nanoparticle Tracking Analysis Concentration Measurements between 50 and 120 nm in Biological Fluids. *Front. Cardiovasc. Med.* **2017**, *4*, 68. [CrossRef] [PubMed]
57. He, Y.; Xing, Y.; Jiang, T.; Wang, J.; Sang, S.; Rong, H.; Yu, F. Fluorescence labeling of extracellular vesicles for diverse bio-applications in vitro and in vivo. *Chem. Commun.* **2023**, *59*, 6609–6626. [CrossRef]
58. Liu, Q.; Huang, J.; Xia, J.; Liang, Y.; Li, G. Tracking tools of extracellular vesicles for biomedical research. *Front. Bioeng. Biotechnol.* **2022**, *10*, 943712. [CrossRef]
59. Dehghani, M.; Gaborski, T.R. Chapter Two—Fluorescent labeling of extracellular vesicles. In *Methods in Enzymology*; Spada, S., Galluzzi, L., Eds.; Academic Press: Cambridge, MA, USA, 2020; Volume 645, pp. 15–42. [CrossRef]
60. Santelices, J.; Ou, M.; Hui, W.W.; Maegawa, G.H.B.; Edelmann, M.J. Fluorescent Labeling of Small Extracellular Vesicles (EVs) Isolated from Conditioned Media. *Bio-Protocol* **2022**, *12*, e4447. [CrossRef]
61. Chen, C.; Cai, N.; Niu, Q.; Tian, Y.; Hu, Y.; Yan, X. Quantitative assessment of lipophilic membrane dye-based labelling of extracellular vesicles by nano-flow cytometry. *J. Extracell. Vesicles* **2023**, *12*, 12351. [CrossRef]
62. Midekessa, G.; Godakumara, K.; Dissanayake, K.; Hasan, M.M.; Reshi, Q.U.; Rinken, T.; Fazeli, A. Characterization of Extracellular Vesicles Labelled with a Lipophilic Dye Using Fluorescence Nanoparticle Tracking Analysis. *Membranes* **2021**, *11*, 779. [CrossRef]
63. Dehghani, M.; Gulvin, S.M.; Flax, J.; Gaborski, T.R. Systematic Evaluation of PKH Labelling on Extracellular Vesicle Size by Nanoparticle Tracking Analysis. *Sci. Rep.* **2020**, *10*, 9533. [CrossRef] [PubMed]
64. Cha, M.; Jeong, S.H.; Bae, S.; Park, J.H.; Baeg, Y.; Han, D.W.; Kim, S.S.; Shin, J.; Park, J.E.; Oh, S.W.; et al. Efficient Labeling of Vesicles with Lipophilic Fluorescent Dyes via the Salt-Change Method. *Anal. Chem.* **2023**, *95*, 5843–5849. [CrossRef] [PubMed]
65. Hartjes, T.A.; Mytnyk, S.; Jenster, G.W.; van Steijn, V.; van Royen, M.E. Extracellular Vesicle Quantification and Characterization: Common Methods and Emerging Approaches. *Bioengineering* **2019**, *6*, 7. [CrossRef]
66. Rautaniemi, K.; Zini, J.; Löfman, E.; Saari, H.; Haapalehto, I.; Laukka, J.; Vesamäki, S.; Efimov, A.; Yliperttula, M.; Laaksonen, T.; et al. Addressing challenges in the removal of unbound dye from passively labelled extracellular vesicles. *Nanoscale Adv.* **2022**, *4*, 226–240. [CrossRef] [PubMed]
67. Shimomura, T.; Seino, R.; Umezaki, K.; Shimoda, A.; Ezoe, T.; Ishiyama, M.; Akiyoshi, K. New Lipophilic Fluorescent Dyes for Labeling Extracellular Vesicles: Characterization and Monitoring of Cellular Uptake. *Bioconjug. Chem.* **2021**, *32*, 680–684. [CrossRef]
68. Barjesteh, T.; Mansur, S.; Bao, Y. Inorganic Nanoparticle-Loaded Exosomes for Biomedical Applications. *Molecules* **2021**, *26*, 1135. [CrossRef]
69. Cho, S.; Yi, J.; Kwon, Y.; Kang, H.; Han, C.; Park, J. Multifluorescence Single Extracellular Vesicle Analysis by Time-Sequential Illumination and Tracking. *ACS Nano* **2021**, *15*, 11753–11761. [CrossRef]
70. Selenina, A.V.; Kulichkova, V.A.; Tomilin, A.N.; Tsimokha, A.S. Nanoparticle tracking analysis of extracellular vesicles reveals two populations of exosomes. *J. Phys. Conf. Seri.* **2018**, *1124*, 031006. [CrossRef]
71. Carrillo Sanchez, B.; Hinchliffe, M.; Bracewell, D.G. GFP-tagging of extracellular vesicles for rapid process development. *Biotechnol. J.* **2022**, *17*, 2100583. [CrossRef]
72. Corso, G.; Heusermann, W.; Trojer, D.; Görgens, A.; Steib, E.; Voshol, J.; Graff, A.; Genoud, C.; Lee, Y.; Hean, J.; et al. Systematic characterization of extracellular vesicle sorting domains and quantification at the single molecule—Single vesicle level by fluorescence correlation spectroscopy and single particle imaging. *J. Extracell. Vesicles* **2019**, *8*, 1663043. [CrossRef]
73. Mao, K.; Lv, Y.; Huo, F.; Hu, E.; Zhang, R.; Fu, Y. The fluorescence mKate2 labeling as a visualizing system for monitoring small extracellular vesicles. *Biotechnol. J.* **2024**, *19*, 2400128. [CrossRef] [PubMed]
74. Smyth, T.; Petrova, K.; Payton, N.M.; Persaud, I.; Redzic, J.S.; Graner, M.W.; Smith-Jones, P.; Anchordoquy, T.J. Surface Functionalization of Exosomes Using Click Chemistry. *Bioconjug. Chem.* **2014**, *25*, 1777–1784. [CrossRef] [PubMed]
75. Salunkhe, S.; Dheeraj; Basak, M.; Chitkara, D.; Mittal, A. Surface functionalization of exosomes for target-specific delivery and in vivo imaging & tracking: Strategies and significance. *J. Controll. Release* **2020**, *326*, 599–614. [CrossRef]
76. Baldwin, S.; Deighan, C.; Bandeira, E.; Kwak, K.J.; Rahman, M.; Nana-Sinkam, P.; Lee, L.J.; Paulaitis, M.E. Analyzing the miRNA content of extracellular vesicles by fluorescence nanoparticle tracking. *Nanomed. Nanotechnol. Biol. Med.* **2017**, *13*, 765–770. [CrossRef]
77. Fortunato, D.; Mladenović, D.; Criscuoli, M.; Loria, F.; Veiman, K.L.; Zocco, D.; Koort, K.; Zarovni, N. Opportunities and Pitfalls of Fluorescent Labeling Methodologies for Extracellular Vesicle Profiling on High-Resolution Single-Particle Platforms. *Int. J. Mol. Sci.* **2021**, *22*, 10510. [CrossRef]
78. Simonsen, J.B. Pitfalls associated with lipophilic fluorophore staining of extracellular vesicles for uptake studies. *J. Extracell. Vesicles* **2019**, *8*, 1582237. [CrossRef]
79. Thane, K.E.; Davis, A.M.; Hoffman, A.M. Improved methods for fluorescent labeling and detection of single extracellular vesicles using nanoparticle tracking analysis. *Sci. Rep.* **2019**, *9*, 12295. [CrossRef] [PubMed]

80. Logozzi, M.; De Milito, A.; Lugini, L.; Borghi, M.; Calabrò, L.; Spada, M.; Perdicchio, M.; Marino, M.L.; Federici, C.; Iessi, E.; et al. High levels of exosomes expressing CD63 and caveolin-1 in plasma of melanoma patients. *PLoS ONE* **2009**, *4*, e5219. [CrossRef]
81. Koksal, A.R.; Ekmen, N.; Aydin, Y.; Nunez, K.; Sandow, T.; Delk, M.; Moehlen, M.; Thevenot, P.; Cohen, A.; Dash, S. A Single-Step Immunocapture Assay to Quantify HCC Exosomes Using the Highly Sensitive Fluorescence Nanoparticle-Tracking Analysis. *J. Hepatocell. Carcinoma* **2023**, *10*, 1935–1954. [CrossRef]
82. Dragovic, R.A.; Gardiner, C.; Brooks, A.S.; Tannetta, D.S.; Ferguson, D.J.P.; Hole, P.; Carr, B.; Redman, C.W.G.; Harris, A.L.; Dobson, P.J.; et al. Sizing and phenotyping of cellular vesicles using Nanoparticle Tracking Analysis. *Nanomed. Nanotechnol. Biol. Med.* **2011**, *7*, 780–788. [CrossRef]
83. McNicholas, K.; Michael, M.Z. Immuno-characterization of Exosomes Using Nanoparticle Tracking Analysis. *Methods Mol. Biol.* **2017**, *1545*, 35–42. [CrossRef] [PubMed]
84. Carnell-Morris, P.; Tannetta, D.; Siupa, A.; Hole, P.; Dragovic, R. Analysis of Extracellular Vesicles Using Fluorescence Nanoparticle Tracking Analysis. *Methods Mol. Biol.* **2017**, *1660*, 153–173. [CrossRef] [PubMed]
85. Desgeorges, A.; Hollerweger, J.; Lassacher, T.; Rohde, E.; Helmbrecht, C.; Gimona, M. Differential fluorescence nanoparticle tracking analysis for enumeration of the extracellular vesicle content in mixed particulate solutions. *Methods* **2020**, *177*, 67–73. [CrossRef] [PubMed]
86. Kwon, Y.; Park, J. Methods to analyze extracellular vesicles at single particle level. *Micro Nano Syst. Lett.* **2022**, *10*, 14. [CrossRef]
87. Oesterreicher, J.; Pultar, M.; Schneider, J.; Mühleder, S.; Zipperle, J.; Grillari, J.; Holnthoner, W. Fluorescence-Based Nanoparticle Tracking Analysis and Flow Cytometry for Characterization of Endothelial Extracellular Vesicle Release. *Int. J. Mol. Sci.* **2020**, *21*, 9278. [CrossRef]
88. Auger, C.; Brunel, A.; Darbas, T.; Akil, H.; Perraud, A.; Bégaud, G.; Bessette, B.; Christou, N.; Verdier, M. Extracellular Vesicle Measurements with Nanoparticle Tracking Analysis: A Different Appreciation of Up and Down Secretion. *Int. J. Mol. Sci.* **2022**, *23*, 2310. [CrossRef]
89. Dlugolecka, M.; Szymanski, J.; Zareba, L.; Homoncik, Z.; Domagala-Kulawik, J.; Polubiec-Kownacka, M.; Czystowska-Kuzmicz, M. Characterization of Extracellular Vesicles from Bronchoalveolar Lavage Fluid and Plasma of Patients with Lung Lesions Using Fluorescence Nanoparticle Tracking Analysis. *Cells* **2021**, *10*, 3473. [CrossRef] [PubMed]
90. Akhyari, P.; Lichtenberg, A.; Weber, A.; Wehmeyer, J.C.; Schmidt, V. Rapid Fluorescence-based Characterization of Single Extracellular Vesicles in Human Blood with Nanoparticle-tracking Analysis. *JoVE* **2019**, *143*, e58731. [CrossRef]
91. Rastogi, S.; Rani, K.; Rai, S.; Singh, R.; Bharti, P.S.; Sharma, V.; Sahu, J.; Kapoor, V.; Vishwakarma, P.; Garg, S.; et al. Fluorescence-tagged salivary small extracellular vesicles as a nanotool in early diagnosis of Parkinson's disease. *BMC Med.* **2023**, *21*, 335. [CrossRef]
92. Droste, M.; Tertel, T.; Jeruschke, S.; Dittrich, R.; Kontopoulou, E.; Walkenfort, B.; Börger, V.; Hoyer, P.F.; Büscher, A.K.; Thakur, B.K.; et al. Single Extracellular Vesicle Analysis Performed by Imaging Flow Cytometry and Nanoparticle Tracking Analysis Evaluate the Accuracy of Urinary Extracellular Vesicle Preparation Techniques Differently. *Int. J. Mol. Sci.* **2021**, *22*, 12436. [CrossRef]

molecules

MDPI

Review

Advancements in the Synthesis and Functionalization of Zinc Oxide-Based Nanomaterials for Enhanced Oral Cancer Therapy

Jinjin Pei [1], Prabhu Manickam Natarajan [2,*], Vidhya Rekha Umapathy [3], Bhuminathan Swamikannu [4], Nandini Manickam Sivaraman [5], Lakshmi Krishnasamy [5] and Chella Perumal Palanisamy [6,*]

1 Qinba State Key Laboratory of Biological Resources and Ecological Environment, 2011 QinLing-Bashan Mountains Bioresources Comprehensive Development C. I. C., Shaanxi Province Key Laboratory of Bio-Resources, College of Bioscience and Bioengineering, Shaanxi University of Technology, Hanzhong 723001, China; xnjinjinpei@163.com
2 Department of Clinical Sciences, d Centre of Medical and Bio-Allied Health Sciences and Research, College of Dentistry, Ajman University, Ajman P.O. Box 346, United Arab Emirates
3 Department of Public Health Dentistry, Thai Moogambigai Dental College and Hospital, Chennai 600 107, Tamil Nadu, India; drvidhyarekha@gmail.com
4 Department of Prosthodontics, Sree Balaji Dental College and Hospital, Pallikaranai, Chennai 600 100, Tamil Nadu, India; bhumi.sbdch@gmail.com
5 Department of Microbiology, Sree Balaji Medical College and Hospital, Bharath University, Chennai 600 100, Tamil Nadu, India; drnandini@bharathuniv.ac.in (N.M.S.); laksh45@gmail.com (L.K.)
6 Department of Chemical Technology, Faculty of Science, Chulalongkorn University, Bangkok 10330, Thailand
* Correspondence: prabhuperio@gmail.com (P.M.N.); chella.p@chula.ac.th (C.P.P.)

Abstract: The fabrication of zinc oxide-based nanomaterials (including natural and synthetic polymers like sulfated polysaccharide, chitosan, and polymethyl methacrylate) has potential to improve oral cancer treatment strategies. This comprehensive review explores the diverse synthesis methods employed to fabricate zinc oxide nanomaterials tailored for oral cancer applications. Several synthesis processes, particularly sol–gel, hydrothermal, and chemical vapor deposition approaches, are thoroughly studied, highlighting their advantages and limitations. The review also examines how synthesis parameters, such as precursor selection, the reaction temperature, and growth conditions, influence both the physicochemical attributes and biological efficacy of the resulting nanomaterials. Furthermore, recent advancements in surface functionalization and modification strategies targeted at improving the targeting specificity and pharmaceutical effectiveness of zinc oxide-based nanomaterials in oral cancer therapy are elucidated. Additionally, the review provides insights into the existing issues and prospective views in the field, emphasizing the need for further research to optimize synthesis methodologies and elucidate the mechanisms underlying the efficacy of zinc oxide-based nanoparticles in oral cancer therapy.

Keywords: ZnO nanomaterials; synthesis methods; surface functionalization; oral cancer

1. Introduction

Oral cancer remains a significant public health concern globally, with its incidence steadily rising in recent years [1]. Despite breakthroughs in treatment modalities such as surgery, chemotherapy, and radiotherapy, the long-term outlook for individuals with oral cancer remains poor, owing mostly to late-stage detection and the limited efficacy of available therapies against aggressive tumor morphologies [2]. As a result, there is a critical requirement to develop unique therapeutic techniques that can selectively target oral cancer cells while limiting systemic toxicity [3]. In this context, nanotechnology has become known as an exciting approach for enhancing cancer diagnosis and treatment [4]. Nanomaterials, with their unique physicochemical properties and tunable surface characteristics, offer versatile platforms for drug delivery, imaging, and targeted therapy [5,6]. Zinc oxide (ZnO)-based nanomaterials have gained popularity in recent years due to their biocompatibility, low toxicity, and photocatalytic characteristics. Furthermore, ZnO nanoparticles have inherent anticancer activities due to their production of reactive oxygen species (ROS) when exposed to light or UV radiation, making them promising candidates for cancer therapy [7].

The manufacturing of ZnO-based nanomaterials is crucial for their use in oral cancer therapy. Several synthesis methods have been established to produce ZnO nanoparticles with exact sizes, shapes, and surface characteristics [8]. Sol–gel, hydrothermal synthesis, chemical vapor deposition, and other novel procedures are among the options, each with its own set of benefits and drawbacks. Understanding the impact of synthesis factors such as precursor selection, reaction temperature, and growth conditions is critical for adapting the properties of ZnO nanoparticles to the specific needs of oral cancer applications [9]. Furthermore, surface functionalization and modification strategies play an essential role in enhancing the targeting specificity and therapeutic efficacy of ZnO-based nanomaterials. By conjugating targeting ligands or enclosing therapeutic agents within the structure of ZnO nanoparticles, researchers can achieve selective accumulations within tumor tissues and improve drug delivery efficiency while minimizing off-target effects. Moreover, surface modifications can also enhance the stability and biocompatibility of ZnO nanomaterials, facilitating their translation into clinical practice [10].

Despite the significant progress made in the field of ZnO-based nanomaterials for oral cancer applications, several challenges still need to be addressed. These include optimizing synthesis methodologies to improve reproducibility and scalability, elucidating the mechanisms underlying the anticancer activity of ZnO nanoparticles, and addressing concerns regarding their long-term biocompatibility and safety [11]. Additionally, the development of robust preclinical models that accurately recapitulate the complex tumor microenvironment of oral cancer is essential for evaluating the efficacy and safety of ZnO nanomaterials in vivo [12]. This comprehensive analysis aims to provide a thorough understanding of the synthesis of ZnO-based nanomaterials for oral cancer applications.. Various synthesis methods are used, the impact of synthesis parameters on nanomaterial properties, and the importance of surface functionalization in improving their therapeutic efficacy are analyzed. Furthermore, this review discussed current achievements in the field, as well as the challenges and future prospects for developing ZnO-based nanomaterials as effective oral cancer therapies. This review aims to enhance nanotechnology-based approaches for precise cancer therapy by integrating existing knowledge and recommending topics for future research.

2. Synthesis Methods for Zinc Oxide-Based Nanomaterials

Nanotechnology has revolutionized the field of materials science, offering precise control over the synthesis of nanomaterials with tailored properties for various applications, including cancer therapy [13]. In the context of oral cancer treatment, ZnO-based nanomaterials have garnered significant interest due to their inherent anticancer properties and biocompatibility. Numerous synthesis approaches have been established to produce ZnO nanoparticles with exact sizes, shapes, and surface properties [14]. This section delves into some of the most generally used synthesis methods for ZnO-based nanomaterials (Figure 1).

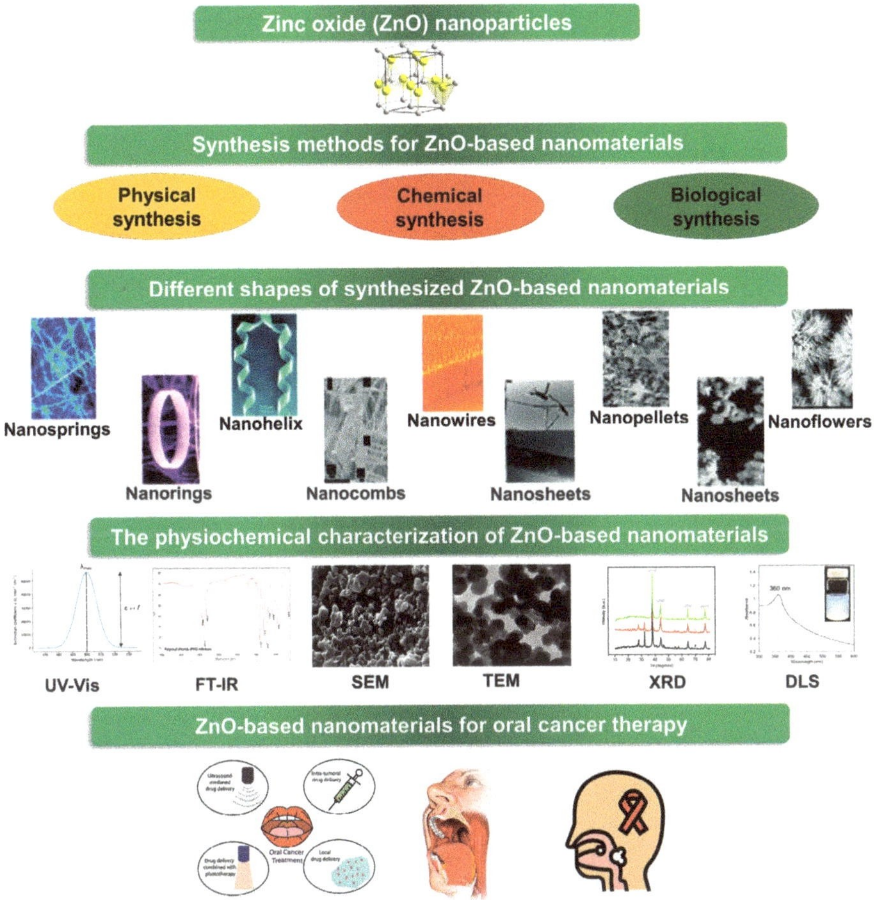

Figure 1. The fabrication of ZnO-based nanomaterials for oral cancer therapy.

2.1. Physical Synthesis Methods

Physical methods for the synthesis of zinc oxide-based nanomaterials rely on physical processes such as vapor deposition, laser ablation, and mechanical milling to fabricate nanostructures [15]. A list of some common physical synthesis methods includes: Chemical Vapor Deposition (CVD): In CVD, ZnO nanostructures are grown through the reaction of precursor vapors on a substrate at elevated temperatures. This method offers precise control over film thickness, morphology, and crystallinity [16]. Physical Vapor Deposition (PVD): PVD methods, such as sputtering and evaporation, are employed to physically deposit ZnO thin films or nanostructures onto substrates without involving chemical reactions [17]. Pulsed Laser Deposition (PLD): PLD involves the ablation of a ZnO target made by a pulsed laser in a vacuum or controlled atmosphere, resulting in the deposition of ZnO thin films or nanostructures on a substrate [18]. Electrodeposition: Electrodeposition is a physical method in which ZnO nanostructures are grown via electrodeposition from an aqueous solution containing zinc ions onto a conductive substrate under the influence of an electric field [19]. Molecular Beam Epitaxy (MBE): MBE is a highly controlled physical vapor deposition technique used to grow epitaxial ZnO thin films layer by layer on a substrate under ultra-high vacuum conditions [20]. Sputtering: Sputtering represents a physical vapor deposition method where energetic ions bombard a ZnO target, resulting in the ejection and deposition of atoms onto a substrate, thereby forming thin films or nanostructures [21]. Evaporation: Evaporation involves the heating of a ZnO source material in a vacuum chamber, causing it to evaporate and condense onto a substrate to form thin films or nanostructures [22]. Magnetron Sputtering: Magnetron sputtering is a variation of sputtering in which a magnetic field is applied to increase the efficiency of the ionization and deposition of ZnO thin films or nanostructures [21]. Physical Mixing and Milling: Physical mixing and milling methods entail mechanically grinding or milling bulk ZnO materials to diminish their size to a nanoscale. This approach proves fitting for generating ZnO nanoparticles or nanocomposites [23]. Gas Phase Synthesis: Gas phase synthesis methods such as aerosol techniques and gas-phase condensation involve the nucleation and growth of ZnO nanoparticles from vapor-phase precursors in a controlled gas environment [24]. These physical synthesis methods offer precise control over the size, morphology, and crystallinity of the resulting ZnO nanostructures, making them suitable for various applications in electronics, optoelectronics, catalysis, and sensing.

2.2. Chemical Synthesis Methods

Chemical methods for the synthesis of zinc oxide-based nanomaterials involve chemical reactions between precursor compounds to form ZnO nanostructures [15]. A list of some common chemical synthesis methods are briefly described in this section. The Sol–Gel Method: This process entails the hydrolysis and condensation of metal alkoxides or salts within a solution, leading to the formation of a sol, which subsequently undergoes gelation and drying processes to obtain ZnO nanoparticles [25]. Hydrothermal/Solvothermal Synthesis: ZnO nanostructures are created within high-temperature and high-pressure environments using aqueous or organic solvents. This method facilitates precise control over the synthesis, yielding diverse nanostructures like nanorods, nanowires, and nanosheets [26]. Precipitation Method: Zinc salts (e.g., zinc acetate, zinc nitrate) are precipitated in the presence of a base (e.g., sodium hydroxide, ammonium hydroxide) or a complexing agent, leading to the formation of ZnO nanoparticles [27]. Microemulsion Method: This involves the formation of nanoscale droplets (microemulsions) containing precursor compounds, followed by the reaction and nucleation of ZnO nanoparticles within these droplets [28]. Combustion Synthesis: ZnO nanoparticles are synthesized by the combustion of suitable precursors such as zinc nitrate mixed with a fuel source (e.g., urea, glycine), resulting in highly crystalline ZnO nanoparticles [29]. Template-Assisted Methods: Templates such as porous membranes, polymers, or self-assembled monolayers are used to control the size and shape of ZnO nanostructures during synthesis, including electrodeposition, electrospinning, and layer-by-layer assembly [30]. Microwave-Assisted Synthesis: Microwave irradiation promotes rapid heating and uniform nucleation, leading to reduced reaction times and improved crystallinity during the synthesis of ZnO nanostructures [31]. Complex Precursor Decomposition: Complex precursors containing Zn and organic ligands are decomposed thermally or hydrothermally to yield ZnO nanoparticles with controlled sizes and morphologies [32]. Spray Pyrolysis: ZnO nanoparticles are synthesized by the thermal decomposition of precursor solutions sprayed onto a heated substrate, allowing for the large-scale production of ZnO thin films or nanostructures [33]. These chemical synthesis methods offer versatility in controlling the size, shape, morphology, and properties of ZnO nanomaterials, making them suitable for various applications in electronics, optoelectronics, catalysis, sensors, and biomedical devices [34].

2.3. Biological Synthesis Methods

Biological approaches to synthesizing zinc oxide-based nanomaterials utilize biological agents, including plant extracts, microorganisms, or enzymes, serving as both reducing and stabilizing agents [35]. The list of some common biological synthesis methods includes: Plant-Mediated Synthesis: Plant extracts harboring phytochemicals like flavonoids, phenols, and terpenoids serve as both reducing and capping agents in the synthesis of ZnO nanoparticles. Various plant species including Aloe vera, Azadirachta indica (neem), and green tea have been utilized for this purpose [36]. Microbial Synthesis: Microorganisms such as bacteria, fungi, and yeast are employed to biosynthesize ZnO nanoparticles through the reduction of zinc salts in culture media. Microbial enzymes and metabolites play a crucial role in the reduction and stabilization of ZnO nanoparticles [37]. Algal-Mediated Synthesis: Algae are utilized for the green synthesis of ZnO nanoparticles due to their ability to secrete bioactive compounds and enzymes. Algal extracts or biomasses are used as reducing agents to convert zinc salts into ZnO nanoparticles [38]. Enzyme-Assisted Synthesis: Enzymes such as urease, alkaline phosphatase, and lysozyme are used to facilitate the biogenic synthesis of ZnO nanoparticles by catalyzing the reduction of zinc ions into ZnO in aqueous solutions [39]. Cell-Free Extracts: Cell-free extracts obtained from plants, microorganisms, or algae are used as bioreducing agents for the synthesis of ZnO nanoparticles. These extracts contain a rich mixture of biomolecules such as proteins, carbohydrates, and secondary metabolites that aid in nanoparticle formation [40]. Biogenic Precipitation: Biogenic precipitation involves the formation of ZnO nanoparticles through the biomineralization process mediated by biological entities. This method mimics the natural mineralization processes observed in organisms such as diatoms and mollusks [41]. Extracellular Synthesis: ZnO nanoparticles are synthesized extracellularly by microorganisms or plant cells, where the reduction and nucleation of zinc ions occurs outside the cell in the presence of biomolecules released by biological entities [42]. Intracellular Synthesis: ZnO nanoparticles are synthesized intracellularly within microbial or plant cells, where zinc ions are transported into the cell and reduced into ZnO nanoparticles in specialized organelles or compartments [43]. Biocomposite Formation: Biocomposite materials containing ZnO nanoparticles embedded within a biopolymeric matrix are synthesized using biological entities as reducing and stabilizing agents. These biocomposites exhibit enhanced properties for various applications [44]. Green Synthesis Approaches: Biological methods for ZnO nanoparticle synthesis are considered to be green and eco-friendly alternatives to conventional chemical methods, offering low toxicity, biocompatibility, and sustainability [45]. These biological synthesis methods offer advantages such as environmentally friendly synthesis routes, mild reaction conditions, and the potential for the large-scale production of ZnO nanoparticles for various applications including uses in biomedical, agricultural, and environmental sectors [46].

A wide range of synthesis methods are available for the fabrication of ZnO-based nanomaterials with tailored properties for various applications. Each method offers unique advantages and limitations (Table 1), and the choice of technique depends on factors such as the desired nanostructure morphology, scalability, and targeted applications (Table 2) [47]. Advances in synthesis techniques continue to drive the development of ZnO nanomaterials with enhanced performances and functionalities, paving the way for their widespread adoption in diverse technological fields [34].

Table 1. Unique insights into and a comparison of different synthesis methods of ZnO NPs.

S. No	Synthesis Methods		Advantages	Limitations
1.	Physical Synthesis Methods	Chemical Vapor Deposition	High control over film thickness, morphology, and crystallinity; suitable for large-scale production.	Requires high temperatures and sophisticated equipment; relatively high cost.
		Physical Vapor Deposition	Can deposit thin films without chemical reactions; versatile and precise.	Often requires vacuum conditions; may involve high-energy processes.
		Pulsed Laser Deposition	High purity and control over film composition; suitable for complex structures.	Expensive equipment; may have low deposition rates.
		Electrodeposition	Low-cost and scalable; allows fine control over nanostructure growth.	Limited to conductive substrates; may produce uneven films.
		Molecular Beam Epitaxy	Atomic-level control over layer composition; produces high-quality epitaxial films.	Extremely expensive and complex; low throughput.

Table 1. *Cont.*

S. No	Synthesis Methods		Advantages	Limitations
1.	Physical Synthesis Methods	Sputtering	High deposition rates; good for uniform thin films.	Requires vacuum and high-energy ions; potential for target contamination.
		Evaporation	Simple and straightforward; effective for thin films.	Limited to materials that can be evaporated; control over thickness can be challenging.
		Magnetron Sputtering	Enhanced ionization efficiency; better control over film properties.	More complex setup than regular sputtering; still requires a vacuum.
		Physical Mixing and Milling	Simple and cost-effective; good for producing nanoparticles.	Limited control over particle size and shape; potential contamination.
		Gas Phase Synthesis	Precise control over nanoparticle size; scalable for large production.	Requires specialized equipment; can be energy-intensive.
2.	Chemical Synthesis Methods	Sol–Gel Method	Versatile; allows fine control over nanoparticle size and distribution.	Requires careful control of reaction conditions; potential for organic solvent use.
		Hydrothermal/ Solvothermal Synthesis	High-quality nanostructures; precise control over shape and size.	High pressure and temperature conditions; longer reaction times.
		Precipitation Method	Simple and cost-effective; scalable.	Limited control over particle size and morphology; potential for agglomeration.
		Microemulsion Method	Good control over particle size and uniformity; mild reaction conditions.	Use of surfactants and organic solvents; may require complex purification.
		Combustion Synthesis	Fast and energy-efficient; high-purity products.	Exothermic reactions can be difficult to control; potential safety hazards.
		Template-Assisted Methods	Allows precise control over nanostructure shape and size.	Removal of templates can be challenging; potential for template contamination.
		Microwave-Assisted Synthesis	Rapid heating; reduced reaction times and energy consumption.	Requires microwave-specific equipment; uneven heating can occur.
		Complex Precursor Decomposition	Controlled release of ZnO; precise control over particle properties.	Complex synthesis and purification steps; potential for by-product formation.
		Spray Pyrolysis	Suitable for large-scale production; uniform thin films.	Requires high-temperature substrates; control over particle size can be difficult.
3.	Biological Synthesis Methods	Plant-Mediated Synthesis	Eco-friendly and sustainable; uses natural reducing agents.	Variability in plant extract composition; scalability can be challenging.
		Microbial Synthesis	Green synthesis route; utilizes natural biological processes.	Requires careful control of microbial culture conditions; slower reaction times.
		Algal-Mediated Synthesis	Utilizes bioactive compounds from algae; environmentally friendly.	Limited control over particle size and shape; scalability issues.
		Enzyme-Assisted Synthesis	High specificity and mild reaction conditions; eco-friendly.	High cost of enzymes; potential for enzyme denaturation.
		Cell-Free Extracts	Uses a rich mixture of biomolecules; green synthesis.	Variability in extract composition; reproducibility can be challenging.
		Biogenic Precipitation	Mimics natural mineralization processes; sustainable.	Slow process; limited control over particle properties.
		Extracellular Synthesis	Simple and eco-friendly; avoids cell lysis.	Lower yields; potential for extracellular contamination.

Table 1. *Cont.*

S. No	Synthesis Methods		Advantages	Limitations
3.	Biological Synthesis Methods	Intracellular Synthesis	Protects nanoparticles from aggregation; precise control within cells.	Requires cell lysis for extraction; complex purification needed.
		Biocomposite Formation	Enhanced properties for specific applications; eco-friendly.	Complex synthesis; limited scalability.
		Green Synthesis Approaches	Low toxicity and biocompatibility; environmentally sustainable.	Often slower and less efficient; may have lower yields.

Table 2. Other properties and a comparison and analysis of different synthesis methods of ZnO NPs.

S. No	Comparison and Analysis	Physical Methods	Chemical Methods	Biological Methods
1.	Control Over Nanostructure Properties	Physical methods generally offer precise control over size, morphology, and crystallinity but require sophisticated equipment and conditions.	Chemical methods provide versatility and scalability but often involve hazardous chemicals.	Biological methods are environmentally friendly and sustainable but can be less controllable and slower.
2.	Scalability	They are more easily scalable for industrial production.	They are more easily scalable for industrial production.	Biological methods face challenges in scaling up due to their variability in biological materials.
3.	Environmental Impact	Physical methods can be energy-intensive.	Chemical methods often involve toxic reagents and solvents.	Biological methods are the most environmentally friendly, using natural agents and mild conditions.
4.	Cost	Chemical methods vary widely in cost depending on the specific process and reagents used.	Physical methods often involve high initial capital investments in equipment.	Biological methods are typically less expensive due to the use of natural and renewable resources, but the complexity of control can increase costs.
5.	Application Suitability	Physical methods are suitable for high-tech applications requiring precise control, such as electronics and optoelectronics.	Chemical methods are versatile and suitable for a wide range of applications, including catalysis and sensing.	Biological methods are particularly suitable for biomedical and environmental applications due to their biocompatibility and eco-friendliness.

3. Influence of Synthesis Parameters on Nanomaterial Properties

The properties of ZnO-based nanomaterials crucially depend on various synthesis parameters, including precursor selection, reaction temperature, and growth conditions. By finely adjusting these parameters, it becomes possible to exert precise control over the nanoparticle size, shape, crystallinity, surface morphology, and surface chemistry. These factors subsequently impact the physicochemical properties and the biological behavior of the nanomaterials [48]. In this section, how these synthesis parameters influence the properties of ZnO-based nanomaterials specifically tailored for oral cancer applications is discussed.

3.1. Precursor Selection

The selection of a precursor is pivotal in shaping the chemical composition, purity, and crystallinity of ZnO-based nanomaterials. Typical precursors utilized for ZnO synthesis encompass zinc salts like zinc acetate, zinc nitrate, zinc chloride, and zinc sulfate, alongside ZnO nanoparticles or complexes [49]. The chemical composition and solubility of the precursor in the reaction medium significantly influences the nucleation and growth kinetics of ZnO nanoparticles. Zinc acetate, for example, is a commonly used precursor due to its high solubility in polar solvents and its ability to form homogeneous precursor solutions. On the other hand, zinc chloride is preferred for nonaqueous synthesis routes due to its high volatility and low solubility in water [50]. Additionally, the concentration of the precursor affects the rate of nucleation, the distribution of particle sizes, and the morphology of the ZnO nanoparticles. Higher precursor concentrations typically result in higher nucleation rates and smaller particle sizes due to the increased availability of zinc ions for nucleation and growth. However, excessively high precursor concentrations can lead to particle aggregation and Ostwald ripening, resulting in broad size distributions and irregular morphologies [51]. In addition to the choice of precursor, the presence of dopant ions or additives in the precursor solution can modify the properties of ZnO nanoparticles. Dopant ions, such as aluminum, indium, or gallium, can alter the bandgap, optical properties, and photocatalytic activity of the ZnO nanomaterials, making them suitable for specific applications, such as photodynamic therapy or imaging [52].

In physical synthesis methods such as Chemical Vapor Deposition (CVD) and Physical Vapor Deposition (PVD), a low precursor concentration can result in slower deposition rates, leading to thinner films and incomplete coverage, which negatively impacts the uniformity and crystallinity of ZnO films. Similarly, in electrodeposition, an insufficient precursor concentration can lead to lower nucleation rates, resulting in sparse and uneven nanostructure growth that compromises the film's density and uniformity. In Pulsed Laser Deposition (PLD), a reduced precursor concentration can decrease the ablation efficiency, leading to thinner films with potential defects and lower crystallinity [53].

In chemical synthesis methods, the effects of low precursor concentration are equally significant. In the sol–gel process, this can lead to incomplete hydrolysis and condensation, resulting in smaller and less-uniform nanoparticles, and a lower viscosity sol that affects the gelation process. In hydrothermal or solvothermal synthesis, lower precursor concentration slows nucleation and growth rates, producing smaller, less crystalline particles and potentially irregular shapes. The precipitation method can suffer from lower yields and a broader size distribution due to incomplete reactions. Microwave-assisted synthesis may experience reduced heating efficiency and slower reaction rates, affecting the size and uniformity of the nanoparticles produced [54].

Biological synthesis methods are also impacted by the precursor concentration. In plant-mediated synthesis, a low precursor concentration can lead to insufficient interactions between plant extracts and zinc ions, resulting in lower yields and smaller, less-uniform nanoparticles. Microbial synthesis can be limited by the availability of zinc ions for microbial reduction, leading to slower synthesis rates and lower yields. In enzyme-assisted synthesis, a low precursor concentration can result in an incomplete reduction of zinc ions, yielding smaller and less-crystalline nanoparticles, with enzymes potentially becoming less efficient [55].

Other factors such as temperature, pH, reaction time, surfactants, and solvents also significantly impact ZnO synthesis. Higher temperatures generally enhance reaction rates and crystallinity but can lead to larger particle sizes and potential agglomeration, while lower temperatures yield smaller particles with better size distribution control [48]. The pH of the reaction medium affects the solubility of the zinc precursors and the stability of the ZnO nanoparticles, with alkaline conditions favoring ZnO formation. Extended reaction times can improve crystallinity but may cause agglomeration and the loss of nanoscale properties. Surfactants and stabilizers help control particle size and shape by preventing agglomeration and guiding growth, though they must be optimized to avoid introducing impurities [51]. The choice of solvent influences the solubility of precursors, reaction kinetics, and the morphology of the ZnO nanostructures, with aqueous solvents being more environmentally friendly and organic solvents offering better control over particle size and shape [56].

The concentration of precursors is a crucial parameter in ZnO synthesis, influencing the physical and chemical properties of the nanomaterials [57]. Low precursor concentrations can lead to incomplete reactions, lower yields, and suboptimal nanostructure characteristics. Addressing the precursor concentration alongside factors like temperature, pH, reaction time, surfactants, and solvents provides the comprehensive understanding necessary for optimizing ZnO synthesis for various applications. By systematically studying these parameters, researchers can tailor the synthesis process to produce ZnO nanomaterials with the desired properties and functionalities [25].

3.2. Reaction Temperature

The reaction temperature is a critical parameter that significantly influences the nucleation, growth kinetics, phase composition, and crystallinity of ZnO nanoparticles. Elevated reaction temperatures typically accelerate nucleation and growth rates, resulting in smaller particle sizes and enhanced crystallinity. Nonetheless, excessively high temperatures may also trigger thermally induced phase transformations, such as the formation of metastable phases or the aggregation of nanoparticles [57]. For example, in the hydrothermal synthesis of ZnO nanowires, higher reaction temperatures promote the anisotropic growth of nanowires along specific crystallographic directions, resulting in longer and more uniform nanostructures. Conversely, lower reaction temperatures may favor the formation of nanoparticles with different morphologies, such as nanospheres or nanoplates [58]. Moreover, the reaction temperature can influence the degree of crystallinity and the defects in the ZnO nanoparticles, which in turn affect their optical, electronic, and photocatalytic properties. Higher reaction temperatures promote the formation of well-crystallized ZnO nanoparticles with fewer defects, resulting in enhanced photocatalytic activity and stability [25]. Optimizing the reaction temperature is crucial for controlling the size, morphology, and properties of ZnO nanoparticles for oral cancer applications. By carefully adjusting the reaction temperature to be within a suitable range, researchers can tailor the properties of ZnO nanomaterials to meet the specific requirements of targeted therapy, drug delivery, or imaging in oral cancer treatment [57].

3.3. Growth Conditions

The growth conditions, including the pH, solvent composition, reaction time, and precursor-to-solvent ratio, also play a critical role in determining the properties of ZnO-based nanomaterials. These parameters influence the kinetics of nucleation, growth, and crystal growth, as well as the stability and dispersibility of nanoparticles in the reaction medium [59]. The pH level of the reaction solution impacts the solubility of the zinc ions and the hydrolysis rate of the precursor species, consequently influencing the nucleation and growth kinetics of the ZnO nanoparticles. Generally, alkaline pH conditions accelerate nucleation and growth rates by promoting the hydrolysis of zinc precursor species and the formation of stable nuclei. However, excessively high pH values may result in the generation of undesirable byproducts or phase impurities, such as zinc hydroxides or zinc carbonates [60]. The choice of solvent and solvent composition also influences the solubility of the precursor species, the stability of the reaction intermediates, and the morphology of the ZnO nanoparticles. For the sol–gel synthesis of ZnO nanoparticles, polar solvents like water or alcohols are frequently employed due to their ability to dissolve zinc salts and stabilize precursor solutions. Nonpolar solvents, such as hexane or toluene, may be employed for the synthesis of ZnO nanoparticles via nonaqueous routes, offering advantages such as better control over particle size and reduced agglomeration [61].

Furthermore, the reaction time and precursor-to-solvent ratio dictate the extent of particle growth and aggregation during the synthesis process. Extended reaction durations typically yield larger particle sizes and wider size distributions because of ongoing nucleation and Ostwald ripening. In contrast, shorter reaction times often produce smaller nanoparticles with more uniform morphologies [62]. Through the careful optimization of growth conditions, researchers can customize the size, morphology, crystallinity, and surface characteristics of ZnO nanoparticles to suit particular applications in oral cancer therapy. Fine-tuning these parameters allows for the development of ZnO-based nanomaterials with enhanced therapeutic efficacy, biocompatibility, and targeting specificity, paving the way for precise cancer treatment strategies [63].

4. Surface Functionalization and Modification Strategies

Surface functionalization and modification are essential for customizing the properties of ZnO-based nanomaterials for targeted oral cancer therapy [64]. By modifying the surface chemistry of ZnO nanoparticles, researchers can enhance their biocompatibility, stability, dispersibility, and targeting specificity, consequently, enhancing their therapeutic effectiveness while minimizing off-target effects [10]. In this section, various surface functionalization and modification strategies employed to optimize ZnO nanomaterials for oral cancer applications are explored.

4.1. Ligand Conjugation

Attaching targeting ligands, including antibodies, peptides, or small molecules, onto the surface of ZnO nanoparticles enables specific recognition and binding to cancer cells overexpressing corresponding receptors or biomarkers [65]. This targeted delivery approach enhances the accumulation of ZnO nanoparticles within the tumor microenvironment while reducing the nonspecific uptake by healthy tissues, thereby improving therapeutic outcomes and minimizing side effects [8]. An example includes the development of folate receptor-targeted ZnO nanoparticles designed for delivering anticancer drugs selectively to oral cancer cells that overexpress folate receptors. Folic acid, serving as a high-affinity ligand for folate receptors, can be conjugated onto the surface of ZnO nanoparticles via covalent coupling or surface adsorption methods. Upon systemic administration, folate-functionalized ZnO nanoparticles preferentially accumulate within folate receptor-positive oral cancer cells, leading to the enhanced cellular uptake and cytotoxicity of the encapsulated drugs [66]. Similarly, epidermal growth factor receptor (EGFR)-targeted ZnO nanoparticles have been explored for the precise targeting of EGFR-overexpressing oral cancer cells. Epidermal growth factor (EGF) or anti-EGFR antibodies can be conjugated onto the surface of ZnO nanoparticles to facilitate receptor-mediated endocytosis and intracellular drug delivery. This targeted approach enables the precise localization of therapeutic agents within the tumor tissue, enhancing their therapeutic efficacy while minimizing systemic toxicity [67].

4.2. Polymer Coating

Polymer coating is another effective strategy for the surface modification of ZnO nanoparticles, offering advantages like enhanced stability, biocompatibility, and drug-loading capacity [68]. Biocompatible polymers, such as polyethylene glycol (PEG), polyvinylpyrrolidone (PVP), or chitosan, can be adsorbed or covalently attached onto the surface of ZnO nanoparticles to form a stable coating layer [69]. PEGylation, in particular, has emerged as a widely used surface modification strategy for ZnO nanoparticles due to its ability to impart stealth properties and prolong the circulation time in vivo [70]. ZnO nanoparticles coated with PEG show decreased protein adsorption, opsonization, and clearance via the reticuloendothelial system (RES), resulting in extended systemic circulation and improved tumor accumulation through the enhanced permeability and retention (EPR) effect [71]. Furthermore, polymer coatings can serve as carriers for the therapeutic compounds that are encapsulated and released under controlled conditions, such as chemotherapeutic drugs, nucleic acids, or imaging contrast agents. The hydrophilic nature of polymer coatings enables the efficient loading of hydrophobic drugs via physical encapsulation or chemical conjugation, while the porous structure allows for sustained release kinetics and improved bioavailability [72].

4.3. Surface Charge Modification

Surface charge modification is a versatile approach for tuning the physicochemical properties and biological interactions of ZnO nanoparticles. By altering the surface charge through functionalization with charged molecules or polymers, researchers can modulate the cellular uptake, biodistribution, and pharmacokinetics of ZnO nanomaterials, thereby optimizing their therapeutic efficacy and safety profiles [73]. For example, the cationic surface modification of ZnO nanoparticles can promote electrostatic interactions with negatively charged cell membranes, facilitating cellular internalization and intracellular drug delivery. Quaternary ammonium compounds, such as polyethyleneimine (PEI) or chitosan, can be coated onto the surface of ZnO nanoparticles to impart a positive surface charge and enhance their cellular uptake efficiency [74]. Conversely, the anionic surface modification of ZnO nanoparticles can improve their colloidal stability, reduce nonspecific protein adsorption, and mitigate cytotoxicity [75]. Anionic polymers, such as poly(acrylic acid) (PAA) or poly(sodium 4-styrenesulfonate) (PSS), can be adsorbed onto the surface of ZnO nanoparticles, conferring a negative surface charge and improving their biocompatibility under physiological conditions [76].

4.4. Bioconjugation Techniques

Bioconjugation techniques, such as click chemistry, thiol chemistry, or carbodiimide-mediated coupling, offer precise control over the functionalization of ZnO nanoparticles with biomolecules, including peptides, proteins, nucleic acids, and imaging probes. These techniques enable the site-specific attachment of biomolecules onto the surface of ZnO nanoparticles, preserving their structural integrity and biological activity [77]. Click chemistry, for instance, involves the selective reaction between azide and alkyne functional groups to form covalent bonds under mild physiological conditions. Azide-functionalized biomolecules can be conjugated onto alkyne-modified ZnO nanoparticles via click chemistry, allowing for precise control over the density and orientation of surface-immobilized ligands [78]. Thiol chemistry, on the other hand, exploits the high affinity between thiol (-SH) groups and gold or silver nanoparticles to facilitate thiol-gold or thiol-silver bond formation. Thiol-functionalized biomolecules, such as peptides or antibodies, can be anchored onto gold-coated ZnO nanoparticles through thiol chemistry, enabling the stable and oriented immobilization of targeting ligands for enhanced tumor targeting and imaging [79]. Carbodiimide-mediated coupling entails activating carboxyl (-COOH) groups on biomolecules through carbodiimide reagents, such as *N*-(3-dimethylaminopropyl)-*N*′-ethylcarbodiimide hydrochloride (EDC) and *N*-hydroxysuccinimide (NHS). Activated biomolecules can then be covalently attached to amino (-NH_2) groups on the surface of ZnO nanoparticles via amide bond formation, allowing for the efficient coupling of targeting ligands or therapeutic agents [80].

Surface functionalization and modification strategies offer versatile approaches for tailoring the properties of ZnO-based nanomaterials for targeted oral cancer therapy [81]. Researchers can improve the specificity, efficacy, and safety of ZnO nanomaterials and reduce off-target effects through several methods, including conjugating targeting ligands, applying biocompatible polymer coatings, modifying surface charge, and using bioconjugation techniques.. These surface engineering approaches hold promise for advancing precision cancer therapy and improving patient outcomes in oral cancer treatment [82].

5. The Therapeutic Efficacy of Zinc Oxide-Based Nanomaterials in Oral Cancer

The potential therapeutic effectiveness of ZnO-based nanomaterials in oral cancer shows promise for enhancing precision cancer therapy (Table 3). ZnO nanoparticles possess inherent anticancer properties due to their capability to produce ROS when exposed to light or ultraviolet (UV) radiation, resulting in cytotoxicity induced by oxidative stress in cancer cells. Additionally, ZnO nanoparticles can be functionalized and engineered to enhance their specificity, stability, and biocompatibility for targeted oral cancer therapy [83]. This section explores the therapeutic efficacy of ZnO-based nanomaterials in oral cancer, including their anticancer mechanisms, performance in in vitro and in vivo studies, and clinical potentials..

Table 3. Zinc oxide (ZnO)-based nanomaterials in oral cancer hold promise for advancing precise cancer therapy.

S. No.	Materials	Size	Preparation Method	Characterization Methods	Biological Studies (In Vitro/In Vivo)	Key Findings in Oral Cancer	References
1.	ZnO nanoparticles	~50 nm	Not specified	TEM, XRD, DLS	In vitro	Promoting toxicity in CAL 27 oral cancer cell lines via the activation of PINK1/Parkin-mediated mitophagy.	[84]
2.	ZnO-CR Nanoparticles	100–200 nm	Green synthesis method	SEM, FTIR, XRD	In vitro	Induced apoptosis in KB cells.	[85]
3.	ZnO—reduced graphene oxide (ZnO–rGO) nanocomposite	3–5 nm	Sol–gel process	Powder XRD, UV–Vis spectroscopy, EDX, TEM	In vitro	The ZnO–rGO nanocomposite exhibited high sensitivity and a low detection limit for IL8, demonstrating its potential for non-invasive oral cancer detection.	[86]
4.	ZnO—Piperine Nanoparticles (ZnO-PIP NPs)	50–100 nm	Green synthesis	UV spectroscopy, SEM, XRD, FTIR, EDAX	In vitro	Induction of apoptosis in oral cancer cells via the BCL2/BAX/P53 signaling pathway.	[87]
5.	ZnO-CU Nanoparticles (Curcumin-mediated ZnO NPs)	100–200 nm	Green synthesis	SEM, EDAX, UV spectroscopy, FTIR, XRD	In vitro	Induced apoptosis in oral cancer cells through the BCL2/BAX/P53 pathway.	[88]
6.	ZnO Nanoparticles (CV-ZnONPs)	30–45 nm	Green synthesis	UV–Vis spectrophotometry, XRD, TEM, EDX, FT-IR, PL	In vitro	Inhibited KB cell viability, decreased MMP, enhanced ROS levels, induced apoptotic cell death, altered nuclear morphology, increased caspase activity.	[89]
7.	ZnO Nanoparticles	50–100 nm	Synthesized using a precipitation method	TEM, XRD, FTIR	In vitro	ZnO-NPs induced growth inhibition and apoptosis in gingival squamous cell carcinoma (GSCC) cells but not in normal cells.	[90]
8.	ZnO-CA Nanoparticles	100–200 nm	Chemical synthesis	SEM, FTIR, XRD	In vitro	ZnO-CA NPs exhibit dose-dependent anticancer activity against Human Oral Epidermal Carcinoma KB cells.	[91]
9.	ZnO Nanoparticles	30–80 nm	Green synthesis	UV-VIS spectral analysis, EDX analysis, XRD pattern analysis, FTIR analysis, SEM analysis	In vitro	Potent antifungal effect against Candida albicans, synergistic effect with nystatin, cytotoxic to oral cancer cells but non-toxic to normal cells.	[92]

5.1. Anticancer Mechanisms

The anticancer mechanisms of ZnO nanoparticles involve multiple pathways, including ROS generation, mitochondrial dysfunction, apoptosis induction, and cell cycle arrest [90]. Upon irradiation with light or UV radiation, ZnO nanoparticles absorb photons and become photoexcited, resulting in the generation of reactive oxygen species (ROS) like hydroxyl radicals (•OH) and superoxide ions ($O2\bullet^-$) via photocatalytic reactions. The buildup of ROS triggers oxidative harm to cellular elements such as lipids, proteins, and DNA, resulting in mitochondrial dysfunction, membrane permeabilization, and ultimately, apoptotic cell death [93]. Furthermore, ZnO nanoparticles can disrupt the intracellular signaling pathways involved in cell proliferation, survival, and metastasis, thereby inhibiting tumor growth and progression. Studies have demonstrated that ZnO nanoparticles downregulate the expression of anti-apoptotic proteins like Bcl-2 while upregulating pro-apoptotic proteins such as Bax and caspases. This process results in mitochondrial membrane depolarization and caspase-mediated apoptosis in cancer cells [94]. Additionally, ZnO nanoparticles can prompt cell cycle arrest at different checkpoints, including G1/S and G2/M phases, by regulating the expression of cell cycle regulatory proteins like cyclins and cyclin-dependent kinases (CDKs). Consequently, this modulation prevents uncontrolled cell proliferation and inhibits tumor growth [95].

Akhtar et al. (2012) investigated the cytotoxic effects of ZnO NPs on human hepatocellular carcinoma (HepG2), human lung adenocarcinoma (A549), and human bronchial epithelial (BEAS-2B) cells, as well as primary rat astrocytes and hepatocytes, and revealed that ZnO NPs selectively killed cancer cells without affecting normal cells. Further studies on HepG2 cells showed that ZnO NPs upregulated both the mRNA and the protein levels of the tumor suppressor gene p53 and the apoptotic gene bax while downregulating the anti-apoptotic gene bcl-2. Additionally, ZnO NPs induced caspase-3 enzyme activity, DNA fragmentation, reactive oxygen species (ROS) generation, and oxidative stress. This study's findings demonstrate that ZnO NPs likely induce apoptosis in cancer cells via the ROS-mediated p53 pathway, which is common among anticancer drugs [96].

5.2. In Vitro Studies

Multiple in vitro investigations have showcased the anticancer potential of ZnO-based nanomaterials against various oral cancer cell lines, encompassing squamous cell carcinoma (SCC) and mucoepidermoid carcinoma (MEC) cells. These studies have documented the dose-dependent cytotoxicity of ZnO nanoparticles against oral cancer cells, marked by reduced cell viability, proliferation, migration, and invasion, alongside heightened apoptosis and cell cycle arrest. Additionally, ZnO nanoparticles have been shown to exhibit selectivity towards cancer cells over normal cells, indicating their potential as targeted therapeutics for oral cancer [97]. The functionalization of ZnO nanoparticles with targeting ligands, such as folate or epidermal growth factor (EGF), further enhances their cytotoxicity and selectivity towards oral cancer cells by facilitating receptor-mediated endocytosis and intracellular drug delivery [98]. Moreover, combination therapies involving ZnO nanoparticles and conventional chemotherapeutic drugs, such as cisplatin or doxorubicin, have demonstrated synergistic effects on oral cancer cell viability, and these findings suggest the potential for combination approaches to surmount drug resistance and enhance treatment outcomes [66].

Wang et al. (2018) conducted a study to investigate the potential therapeutic efficacy of ZnO NPs in the treatment of oral cancer, namely CAL 27 human tongue cancer cells. Their research demonstrates a dose-dependent decrease in cell viability following ZnO NP treatment, which is attributable to ROS production and mitochondrial damage. Surprisingly, they discover the role of PINK1/Parkin-mediated mitophagy in this cytotoxicity, implying a new mechanism for ZnO NP-induced toxicity. These findings open the door for the further exploration of ZnO NPs as a prospective option for oral cancer therapy, warranting future in vivo studies for clinical translation [84].

Marunganathan et al. (2024) found that marine-derived κ-carrageenan-coated zinc oxide nanoparticles (ZnO-CR NPs) can effectively carry drugs and induce apoptosis in oral cancer cells. The study demonstrates that ZnO-CR NPs have synergistic antibacterial activity against dental infections, as well as a dose-dependent anticancer effect on KB cells. Structural analysis reveals ZnO-CR NPs' remarkable antibacterial and antioxidant activities, indicating a potential for dental applications. Molecular docking analysis reveals the mechanisms behind their antibacterial action. These findings imply that ZnO-CR NPs are unique tools for tackling oral infections and oral cancer, presenting a viable way to tackle antimicrobial resistance [85].

Verma and Singh (2019) investigate the multifunctional characteristics of a ZnO-rGO nanocomposite. This nanocomposite demonstrates promising potential in non-invasive oral cancer detection through an electrochemical immunosensing approach. The synthesized ZnO–rGO nanocomposite exhibited excellent sensitivity and a low detection limit for interleukin-8 (IL8), a biomarker associated with oral cancer. These findings suggest a significant stride toward developing effective diagnostic tools for oral cancer, potentially revolutionizing early detection and treatment outcomes [86].

Shaik et al.'s 2024 study's focus on oral cancer underscores the pressing need for innovative therapeutic strategies in combating this disease. Oral cancer presents considerable hurdles due to its complicated etiology and limited treatment options. By using ZnO-PIP NPs to target oral cancer cells, the work opens up a viable therapy option. The capacity of ZnO-PIP NPs to cause apoptosis in oral cancer cells via the BCL2/BAX/P53-signaling pathway has enormous potential for suppressing tumor growth and improving patient outcomes. This approach not only addresses the tumor directly but also complements traditional treatments by targeting dental pathogens, potentially contributing to cancer development or progression. However, while these findings are promising, further research, particularly in vivo studies and clinical trials are essential for assessing the safety and efficacy of ZnO-PIP NPs for potential clinical applications in oral cancer therapy [87].

Tayyeb et al. (2024) investigate the manufacturing and therapeutic potential of curcumin-mediated zinc oxide nanoparticles (ZnO-CU NPs) for oral health, specifically in the treatment of oral cancer. The study provides a multifunctional strategy for tackling oral health concerns by combining zinc oxide nanoparticles' intrinsic antibacterial characteristics with curcumin's anticancer effects. The comprehensive characterization of ZnO-CU NPs confirms their structural integrity and functional properties, laying a solid foundation for further investigation. Notably, the study elucidates the complex mechanisms behind ZnO-CU NPs' antioxidant, antibacterial, and anticancer actions, highlighting their potential as integrated therapeutic agents. While the results are intriguing, more in vivo investigations and clinical trials are required to confirm their safety and efficacy for therapeutic use. This research signifies a significant step towards advancing oral healthcare through innovative nanomedicine approaches, with potential implications for improving treatment outcomes and the quality of life for patients with oral cancer [88].

Shanmugam et al. (2022) present important information about the therapeutic potential of zinc oxide nanoparticles (ZnONPs) in oral cancer treatment. Their study focuses on the prospective anticancer benefits of ZnONPs generated from natural sources. The discussion underscores the importance of apoptosis induction as a key strategy in cancer treatment, emphasizing the unique biochemical and morphological changes associated with apoptotic cell death. The study demonstrates that the formulated CV-ZnONPs effectively triggered apoptosis in oral cancer KB cells through multiple pathways, including ROS accumulation, mitochondrial membrane potential disruption, and the activation of caspases. These findings underscore the potential of CV-ZnONPs as a novel anticancer agent against oral cancer, offering a promising avenue for future research and their development in cancer therapeutics [89].

Wang et al. (2020) investigated the processes driving ZnO-NP-induced apoptosis in GSCC cells, focusing on mitochondrial dysfunction and the p70S6K-signaling pathway. The results indicate that ZnO-NPs have selective cytotoxicity against GSCC cells while sparing normal cells, making them a promising candidate for oral cancer therapy. This comprehensive analysis provides vital insights into the potential of ZnO-NPs as a novel anti-tumor agent for treating GSCC [90].

The research by Ravikumar et al. sheds light on the promising potential of zinc oxide nanoparticles (ZnO NPs) functionalized with cinnamic acid (CA) for addressing various challenges in oral health, particularly in combating oral cancer and dental pathogens. By combining the unique properties of ZnO NPs with the therapeutic attributes of CA, the synthesized ZnO-CA NPs exhibit remarkable antioxidant, antimicrobial, and anticancer activities. The synergistic effects observed underscore the importance of hybrid approaches in nanoparticle-based therapies. Moreover, the molecular docking results provide valuable insights into the mechanisms underlying the interaction between CA and dental pathogen receptors, paving the way for targeted therapeutic interventions. This research signifies a significant step towards the development of innovative dental treatments with broad-spectrum efficacy and tailored applications [91].

The study presents a compelling approach to combat Candida albicans, a major cause of oral candidiasis, using green-synthesized zinc nanoparticles (ZnNPs) derived from Lavandula angustifolia extract. By combining ZnNPs with nystatin, a potent antifungal drug, synergistic effects were observed, enhancing the inhibition and mortality of C. albicans. The study underscores the potential of using nanotechnology for augmenting traditional antifungal therapies, offering a promising avenue for combating oral infections. Additionally, the selective cytotoxicity of ZnNPs towards cancerous cells highlights their therapeutic potential in oral cancer treatment, warranting further investigation into their mechanisms and toxicity profiles [92].

5.3. In Vivo Studies

In vivo studies have provided further evidence of the therapeutic efficacy of ZnO-based nanomaterials in oral cancer using animal models, such as xenograft or orthotopic tumor models. ZnO nanoparticles have been shown to inhibit tumor growth, reduce tumor volumes and weights, and prolong survival in oral cancer-bearing mice following systemic or local administration. The histological analysis of tumor tissues has revealed extensive apoptosis, reduced proliferation, and disrupted angiogenesis in response to ZnO nanoparticle treatment, indicating their potential as effective therapeutics for oral cancer [12]. Furthermore, ZnO nanoparticles have good pharmacokinetic and biodistribution patterns in vivo, with their preferential accumulation in tumor tissues due to the increased permeability and retention (EPR) effect. Surface functionalization with targeting ligands increases tumor selectivity and accumulation while reducing off-target effects and systemic toxicity. Additionally, ZnO nanoparticles have been shown to induce minimal acute or chronic toxicity in vital organs, such as the liver, kidneys, and lungs, highlighting their biocompatibility and safety for systemic administration [99].

5.4. Clinical Potential

The therapeutic efficacy of ZnO-based nanomaterials in oral cancer holds significant clinical potential for improving patient outcomes and overcoming challenges associated with conventional treatment modalities. Nanotechnology-based approaches offer several advantages over traditional therapies, including enhanced tumor targeting, reduced systemic toxicity, and improved patient compliance. The clinical translation of ZnO-based nanomaterials for oral cancer therapy requires rigorous preclinical evaluation, optimization of formulation and delivery strategies, and compliance with regulatory guidelines for safety and efficacy [100]. Furthermore, the development of multifunctional ZnO-based nanoplatforms, capable of simultaneous imaging, drug delivery, and therapeutic monitoring, holds promise for personalized and precise cancer therapy. Incorporating imaging modalities like fluorescence, magnetic resonance imaging (MRI), or positron emission tomography (PET) facilitates the real-time visualization of tumor growth, metastasis, and treatment response, facilitating early diagnosis and personalized treatment planning [64].

In the study conducted by Vishal et al. (2021), the efficacy of zinc oxide (ZnO) eugenol paste as a dressing material for raw wounds following wide excision of oral potentially malignant disorders (PMDs) is investigated. The combination of zinc's wound healing properties and eugenol's antiseptic effects presents a promising option. The results indicate good hemostasis, pain relief, granulation, and epithelialization, with excellent adherence to the wound. Notably, no allergic reactions were observed. Although it is not a replacement for skin grafts, ZnO eugenol paste demonstrates utility as a cost-effective, easy-to-use dressing material for oral surgical wounds, particularly in resource-limited settings. Further research on a larger scale could provide valuable insights [101].

ZnO-based nanomaterials represent a promising therapeutic approach for targeted oral cancer therapy, offering multifaceted anticancer mechanisms, selective cytotoxicity towards cancer cells, and favorable pharmacokinetics and safety profiles in preclinical studies. Further research is warranted to elucidate the molecular mechanisms underlying the therapeutic efficacy of ZnO nanoparticles, optimize formulation and delivery strategies, and translate preclinical findings into clinical applications for the benefit of patients with oral cancer [64].

6. Challenges in the Fabrication of ZnO-Based Nanomaterials for Oral Cancer Therapy

While ZnO-based nanomaterials hold great promise for targeted oral cancer therapy, several challenges need to be addressed to realize their full potential. Additionally, exploring future perspectives and research directions is essential for advancing the development and clinical translation of ZnO-based nanotherapeutics [11]. Biocompatibility and Toxicity: Despite their biocompatibility in many preclinical studies, there are still concerns regarding the long-term biocompatibility and potential toxicity of ZnO nanoparticles, particularly upon systemic administration. The accurate assessment of the biocompatibility profile, including acute and chronic toxicity, immunogenicity, and biodistribution, is essential for ensuring the safety of ZnO-based nanotherapeutics in clinical settings [102]. Drug Loading and Release: The efficient loading and controlled release of therapeutic agents from ZnO nanoparticles pose significant challenges due to their high surface area and reactivity. Strategies for improving the drug-loading capacity, stability, and release kinetics while minimizing premature drug leakage and burst release need to be developed for effective drug delivery and sustained therapeutic efficacy [103]. Specificity and Targeting: Achieving the selective targeting and accumulation of ZnO nanoparticles within oral cancer tissues while minimizing off-target effects remains a major challenge. Strategies for enhancing tumor specificity, such as surface functionalizations with targeting ligands or stimuli-responsive moieties, need to be optimized to overcome biological barriers and improve tumor penetration and retention [104]. Regulatory Approval: The regulatory approval and clinical translation of ZnO-based nanotherapeutics for oral cancer therapy require comprehensive preclinical evaluation, including pharmacokinetic studies, toxicity assessments, and efficacy validation in relevant animal models. Meeting regulatory requirements for safety, efficacy, and manufacturing standards is essential for advancing ZnO-based nanotherapeutics from the bench to the bedside [105].

7. Future Perspectives

The development of multifunctional ZnO-based nanoplatforms capable of simultaneous imaging, drug delivery, and therapeutic monitoring holds promise for personalized and precision cancer therapy. The integration of imaging modalities, such as fluorescence, MRI or PET, enables the real-time visualization of tumor growth, metastasis, and treatment response, facilitating early diagnosis and treatment optimization [14]. Combining ZnO-based nanotherapeutics with conventional chemotherapy, radiotherapy, or immunotherapy offers synergistic effects and enhanced therapeutic outcomes in oral cancer treatment. Combination therapies can overcome drug resistance, minimize systemic toxicity, and improve treatment efficacy through complementary mechanisms of action, such as ROS generation, DNA damage, or immune modulation [106]. Advancements in targeted drug delivery systems, such as ligand-mediated targeting, stimuli-responsive release, and nanocarrier-based delivery, offer opportunities for enhancing the specificity, efficacy, and safety of ZnO-based nanotherapeutics in oral cancer therapy. The rational design of targeted delivery systems tailored to the unique biological characteristics of oral cancer tissues can improve tumor penetration, cellular uptake, and the therapeutic index while minimizing off-target effects [107]. Theranostic approaches combining therapeutic and diagnostic capabilities within a single nanoplatform enable the real-time monitoring of treatment response and disease progression, facilitating personalized treatment planning and optimization. The integration of imaging probes, biomarkers, and therapeutic agents into ZnO-based nanotherapeutics enables noninvasive imaging, targeted therapy, and therapeutic monitoring, paving the way for personalized and precise cancer therapy [108]. Biomimetic nanomaterials inspired by natural systems offer unique advantages for oral cancer therapy, including enhanced biocompatibility, targeting specificity, and therapeutic efficacy. Mimicking biological structures, functions, and interactions, such as cell membranes, extracellular vesicles, or tumor microenvironments, enables precise control over nanomaterial properties and behaviors, facilitating improved tumor targeting, penetration, and therapeutic outcomes [109]. Addressing the key challenges and exploring future perspectives in the field of ZnO-based nanomaterials for oral cancer therapy is essential for advancing the development and clinical translation of nanotherapeutics. By overcoming technical hurdles, optimizing formulation and delivery strategies, and harnessing innovative approaches, ZnO-based nanotherapeutics hold great promise for improving patient outcomes and revolutionizing the treatment of oral cancer in the future.

8. Conclusions

The development of ZnO-based nanomaterials shows great potential for advancing precise cancer therapy, particularly in treating oral cancer. With their unique properties and versatile surface engineering strategies, ZnO-based nanotherapeutics offer a multifunctional platform for targeted drug delivery and imaging. Synthesis methods like sol–gel and hydrothermal synthesis enable precise control over nanoparticle properties, while surface functionalization enhances the specificity and stability for oral cancer treatment. In vitro and in vivo studies demonstrate ZnO-based nanomaterials' ability to induce cytotoxicity and apoptosis in oral cancer cells with minimal off-target effects. However, challenges such as biocompatibility and regulatory approval remain. Future directions include developing multifunctional nanoplatforms and combination therapies to improve treatment outcomes. In conclusion, ZnO-based nanotherapeutics represent a promising avenue for personalized and effective oral cancer treatment. Collaborative efforts are crucial for translating these advancements into clinical practice, potentially revolutionizing cancer management and saving lives.

Funding: This study was funded by the National Natural Science Foundation of China (31801563), a Special Support Plan for High-Level Talents in Shaanxi Province, the Foundation of Shaanxi Sanqin Scholars Innovation Team.

Institutional Review Board Statement: Not applicable.

Informed Consent Statement: Not applicable.

Data Availability Statement: No new data were created.

Conflicts of Interest: The authors declare no conflicts of interest.

References

1. Wu, B.; Zhang, T.; Dai, N.; Luo, D.; Wang, X.; Qiao, C.; Liu, J. Global research trends in tongue cancer from 2000 to 2022: Bibliometric and visualized analysis. *Clin. Oral Investig.* **2024**, *28*, 130. [CrossRef] [PubMed]
2. Gavas, S.; Quazi, S.; Karpiński, T.M. Nanoparticles for cancer therapy: Current progress and challenges. *Nanoscale Res. Lett.* **2021**, *16*, 173. [CrossRef] [PubMed]
3. Chehelgerdi, M.; Chehelgerdi, M.; Allela, O.Q.B.; Pecho, R.D.C.; Jayasankar, N.; Rao, D.P.; Thamaraikani, T.; Vasanthan, M.; Viktor, P.; Lakshmaiya, N. Progressing nanotechnology to improve targeted cancer treatment: Overcoming hurdles in its clinical implementation. *Mol. Cancer* **2023**, *22*, 169. [CrossRef] [PubMed]
4. Song, W.; Zhang, M.; Huang, X.; Chen, B.; Ding, Y.; Zhang, Y.; Yu, D.; Kim, I. Smart l-borneol-loaded hierarchical hollow polymer nanospheres with antipollution and antibacterial capabilities. *Mater. Today Chem.* **2022**, *26*, 101252. [CrossRef]
5. Yu, Z.; Gao, L.; Chen, K.; Zhang, W.; Zhang, Q.; Li, Q.; Hu, K. Nanoparticles: A new approach to upgrade cancer diagnosis and treatment. *Nanoscale Res. Lett.* **2021**, *16*, 88. [CrossRef] [PubMed]
6. Liao, Q.; Kim, E.J.; Tang, Y.; Xu, H.; Yu, D.G.; Song, W.; Kim, B.J. Rational design of hyper-crosslinked polymers for biomedical applications. *J. Polym. Sci.* **2024**, *62*, 1517–1535. [CrossRef]
7. Mohamed, K.; Benitto, J.J.; Vijaya, J.J.; Bououdina, M. Recent advances in ZnO-based nanostructures for the photocatalytic degradation of hazardous, non-biodegradable medicines. *Crystals* **2023**, *13*, 329. [CrossRef]
8. Anjum, S.; Hashim, M.; Malik, S.A.; Khan, M.; Lorenzo, J.M.; Abbasi, B.H.; Hano, C. Recent advances in zinc oxide nanoparticles (ZnO NPs) for cancer diagnosis, target drug delivery, and treatment. *Cancers* **2021**, *13*, 4570. [CrossRef] [PubMed]
9. Rafique, M.S.; Rafique, M.; Tahir, M.B.; Hajra, S.; Nawaz, T.; Shafiq, F. Synthesis methods of nanostructures. In *Nanotechnology and Photocatalysis for Environmental Applications*; Elsevier: Amsterdam, The Netherlands, 2020; pp. 45–56.
10. Fatima, H.; Jin, Z.Y.; Shao, Z.; Chen, X.J. Recent advances in ZnO-based photosensitizers: Synthesis, modification, and applications in photodynamic cancer therapy. *J. Colloid Interface Sci.* **2022**, *621*, 440–463. [CrossRef]
11. Chawla, U.; Dahiya, D.; Kumar, Y.; Bala, A.; Genwa, M.; Agasti, N.; Tandon, S.; Singh, S.P.; Meena, P. A Review on ZnO-based Targeted Drug Delivery System. *Lett. Drug Des. Discov.* **2024**, *21*, 397–420. [CrossRef]

12. Lama, S.; Merlin-Zhang, O.; Yang, C. In vitro and in vivo models for evaluating the oral toxicity of nanomedicines. *Nanomaterials* **2020**, *10*, 2177. [CrossRef] [PubMed]
13. Pei, J.; Yan, Y.; Jayaraman, S.; Rajagopal, P.; Natarajan, P.M.; Umapathy, V.R.; Gopathy, S.; Roy, J.R.; Sadagopan, J.C.; Thalamati, D. A review on advancements in the application of starch-based nanomaterials in biomedicine: Precision drug delivery and cancer therapy. *Int. J. Biol. Macromol.* **2024**, *265*, 130746. [CrossRef] [PubMed]
14. Vagena, I.-A.; Gatou, M.-A.; Theocharous, G.; Pantelis, P.; Gazouli, M.; Pippa, N.; Gorgoulis, V.G.; Pavlatou, E.A.; Lagopati, N. Functionalized ZnO-Based Nanocomposites for Diverse Biological Applications: Current Trends and Future Perspectives. *Nanomaterials* **2024**, *14*, 397. [CrossRef] [PubMed]
15. Jiang, Z.; Liu, B.; Yu, L.; Tong, Y.; Yan, M.; Zhang, R.; Han, W.; Hao, Y.; Shangguan, L.; Zhang, S. Research progresses in preparation methods and applications of zinc oxide nanoparticles. *J. Alloys Compd.* **2023**, *956*, 170316. [CrossRef]
16. Choi, S.C.; Lee, D.K.; Sohn, S.H. Effects of experimental configuration on the morphology of two-dimensional ZnO nanostructures synthesized by thermal chemical-vapor deposition. *Crystals* **2020**, *10*, 517. [CrossRef]
17. Li, Y.; Huang, B.; Liu, Y.; Lan, L.; Ji, Z. Sb_2Se_3/CdS/ZnO photodetectors based on physical vapor deposition for color imaging applications. *Opt. Lett.* **2023**, *48*, 2583–2586. [CrossRef] [PubMed]
18. Haider, A.J.; Jabbar, A.A.; Ali, G.A. A review of pure and doped ZnO nanostructure production and its optical properties using pulsed laser deposition technique. *J. Phys. Conf. Ser.* **2021**, *1795*, 012015. [CrossRef]
19. Ait hssi, A.; Amaterz, E.; Labchir, N.; Atourki, L.; Bouderbala, I.Y.; Elfanaoui, A.; Benlhachemi, A.; Ihlal, A.; Bouabid, K. Electrodeposited ZnO nanorods as efficient photoanodes for the degradation of rhodamine B. *Phys. Status Solidi (A)* **2020**, *217*, 2000349. [CrossRef]
20. Stachowicz, M.; Sajkowski, J.; Pietrzyk, M.; Faye, D.N.; Magalhaes, S.; Alves, E.; Reszka, A.; Pieniążek, A.; Kozanecki, A. Investigation of interdiffusion in thin films of ZnO/ZnCdO grown by molecular beam epitaxy. *Thin Solid Films* **2023**, *781*, 140003. [CrossRef]
21. Li, Z.; Yu, X.; Zhu, Y.; Liu, S.; Wen, X.; Lu, H.; Wang, C.; Li, X.; Li, M.-Y.; Yang, Y. High performance ZnO quantum dot (QD)/magnetron sputtered ZnO homojunction ultraviolet photodetectors. *Appl. Surf. Sci.* **2022**, *582*, 152352. [CrossRef]
22. Ali, R.S.; Sharba, K.S.; Jabbar, A.M.; Chiad, S.S.; Abass, K.H.; HabubiP, N.F. Characterization of ZnO thin film/p-Si fabricated by vacuum evaporation method for solar cell applications. *Neuroquantology* **2020**, *18*, 26. [CrossRef]
23. Millán Ordóñez, E.; Mota, N.; Guil-López, R.; Garcia Pawelec, B.; Fierro, J.L.G.; Navarro Yerga, R.M. Direct synthesis of dimethyl ether on bifunctional catalysts based on Cu–ZnO (Al) and supported $H_3PW_{12}O_{40}$: Effect of physical mixing on bifunctional interactions and activity. *Ind. Eng. Chem. Res.* **2021**, *60*, 18853–18869. [CrossRef]
24. Marín Ramírez, O.A.; Real, S.C.; Vega, N.C.; Tirado, M.C.; Comedi, D.M. ZnO Nanostructures Synthesized by Vapor Transport and Liquid Phase Synthesis Techniques: Growth and Properties. *Sci. Rev.* **2020**, *1*, 6–23.
25. Arya, S.; Mahajan, P.; Mahajan, S.; Khosla, A.; Datt, R.; Gupta, V.; Young, S.-J.; Oruganti, S.K. Influence of processing parameters to control morphology and optical properties of Sol-Gel synthesized ZnO nanoparticles. *ECS J. Solid State Sci. Technol.* **2021**, *10*, 023002. [CrossRef]
26. Ghodrati, M.; Mousavi-Kamazani, M.; Zinatloo-Ajabshir, S. $Zn_3V_3O_8$ nanostructures: Facile hydrothermal/solvothermal synthesis, characterization, and electrochemical hydrogen storage. *Ceram. Int.* **2020**, *46*, 28894–28902. [CrossRef]
27. Bekele, B.; Degefa, A.; Tesgera, F.; Jule, L.T.; Shanmugam, R.; Priyanka Dwarampudi, L.; Nagaprasad, N.; Ramasamy, K. Green versus chemical precipitation methods of preparing zinc oxide nanoparticles and investigation of antimicrobial properties. *J. Nanomater.* **2021**, *2021*, 9210817. [CrossRef]
28. Zhang, X.; Han, Y.; Liu, W.; Pan, N.; Li, D.; Chai, J. A novel synthesis of hexagonal cylinder-like ZnO with an excellent performance by a surfactant-free microemulsion-hydrothermal method. *J. Ind. Eng. Chem.* **2021**, *97*, 326–336. [CrossRef]
29. Shkir, M.; Palanivel, B.; Khan, A.; Kumar, M.; Chang, J.-H.; Mani, A.; AlFaify, S. Enhanced photocatalytic activities of facile auto-combustion synthesized ZnO nanoparticles for wastewater treatment: An impact of Ni doping. *Chemosphere* **2022**, *291*, 132687. [CrossRef] [PubMed]
30. Huo, D.; Chen, B.; Li, M.; Meng, G.; Lei, Y.; Zhu, C. Template-assisted fabrication of Ag-nanoparticles@ ZnO-nanorods array as recyclable 3D surface enhanced Raman scattering substrate for rapid detection of trace pesticides. *Nanotechnology* **2021**, *32*, 145302. [CrossRef]
31. Yalcin, M. Microwave-assisted synthesis of ZnO nanoflakes: Structural, optical and dielectric characterization. *Mater. Res. Express* **2020**, *7*, 055019. [CrossRef]
32. Al-Wasidi, A.S.; Naglah, A.; Kalmouch, A.; Adam, A.M.A.; Refat, M.; Moustafa, G. Preparation of Cr_2O_3, MnO_2, Fe_2O_3, NiO, CuO, and ZnO oxides using their glycine complexes as precursors for in situ thermal decomposition. *Egypt. J. Chem.* **2020**, *63*, 1109–1118.
33. Abdulrahman, A.F.; Abd-Alghafour, N. Synthesis and characterization of ZnO nanoflowers by using simple spray pyrolysis technique. *Solid-State Electron.* **2022**, *189*, 108225. [CrossRef]
34. Raha, S.; Ahmaruzzaman, M. ZnO nanostructured materials and their potential applications: Progress, challenges and perspectives. *Nanoscale Adv.* **2022**, *4*, 1868–1925. [CrossRef] [PubMed]
35. Kumar, J.A.; Krithiga, T.; Manigandan, S.; Sathish, S.; Renita, A.A.; Prakash, P.; Prasad, B.N.; Kumar, T.P.; Rajasimman, M.; Hosseini-Bandegharaei, A. A focus to green synthesis of metal/metal based oxide nanoparticles: Various mechanisms and applications towards ecological approach. *J. Clean. Prod.* **2021**, *324*, 129198. [CrossRef]

36. Haghighat, M.; Alijani, H.Q.; Ghasemi, M.; Khosravi, S.; Borhani, F.; Sharifi, F.; Iravani, S.; Najafi, K.; Khatami, M. Cytotoxicity properties of plant-mediated synthesized K-doped ZnO nanostructures. *Bioprocess Biosyst. Eng.* **2022**, *45*, 97–105. [CrossRef] [PubMed]
37. Suba, S.; Vijayakumar, S.; Vidhya, E.; Punitha, V.; Nilavukkarasi, M. Microbial mediated synthesis of ZnO nanoparticles derived from *Lactobacillus* spp: Characterizations, antimicrobial and biocompatibility efficiencies. *Sens. Int.* **2021**, *2*, 100104. [CrossRef]
38. Waqif, H.; Munir, N.; Farrukh, M.A.; Hasnain, M.; Sohail, M.; Abideen, Z. Algal macromolecular mediated synthesis of nanoparticles for their application against citrus canker for food security. *Int. J. Biol. Macromol.* **2024**, *263*, 130259. [CrossRef] [PubMed]
39. Balčiūnaitienė, A.; Štreimikytė, P.; Puzerytė, V.; Viškelis, J.; Štreimikytė-Mockeliūnė, Ž.; Maželienė, Ž.; Sakalauskienė, V.; Viškelis, P. Antimicrobial activities against opportunistic pathogenic bacteria using green synthesized silver nanoparticles in Plant and Lichen Enzyme-Assisted Extracts. *Plants* **2022**, *11*, 1833. [CrossRef] [PubMed]
40. Barani, M.; Masoudi, M.; Mashreghi, M.; Makhdoumi, A.; Eshghi, H. Cell-free extract assisted synthesis of ZnO nanoparticles using aquatic bacterial strains: Biological activities and toxicological evaluation. *Int. J. Pharm.* **2021**, *606*, 120878. [CrossRef] [PubMed]
41. Singh, K.; Singh, G.; Singh, J. Sustainable synthesis of biogenic ZnO NPs for mitigation of emerging pollutants and pathogens. *Environ. Res.* **2023**, *219*, 114952. [CrossRef]
42. Pomastowski, P.; Król-Górniak, A.; Railean-Plugaru, V.; Buszewski, B. Zinc oxide nanocomposites—Extracellular synthesis, physicochemical characterization and antibacterial potential. *Materials* **2020**, *13*, 4347. [CrossRef] [PubMed]
43. Murali, M.; Gowtham, H.; Shilpa, N.; Singh, S.B.; Aiyaz, M.; Sayyed, R.; Shivamallu, C.; Achar, R.R.; Silina, E.; Stupin, V. Zinc oxide nanoparticles prepared through microbial mediated synthesis for therapeutic applications: A possible alternative for plants. *Front. Microbiol.* **2023**, *14*, 1227951. [CrossRef] [PubMed]
44. Aadnan, I.; Zegaoui, O.; Daou, I.; da Silva, J.C.E. Synthesis and physicochemical characterization of a ZnO-Chitosan hybrid-biocomposite used as an environmentally friendly photocatalyst under UV-A and visible light irradiations. *J. Environ. Chem. Eng.* **2020**, *8*, 104260. [CrossRef]
45. Aldeen, T.S.; Mohamed, H.E.A.; Maaza, M. ZnO nanoparticles prepared via a green synthesis approach: Physical properties, photocatalytic and antibacterial activity. *J. Phys. Chem. Solids* **2022**, *160*, 110313. [CrossRef]
46. Akintelu, S.A.; Folorunso, A.S. A review on green synthesis of zinc oxide nanoparticles using plant extracts and its biomedical applications. *BioNanoScience* **2020**, *10*, 848–863. [CrossRef]
47. Gorup, L.F.; Amorin, L.H.; Camargo, E.R.; Sequinel, T.; Cincotto, F.H.; Biasotto, G.; Ramesar, N.; La Porta, F.d.A. Methods for design and fabrication of nanosensors: The case of ZnO-based nanosensor. In *Nanosensors for Smart Cities*; Elsevier: Amsterdam, The Netherlands, 2020; pp. 9–30.
48. Wojnarowicz, J.; Chudoba, T.; Lojkowski, W. A review of microwave synthesis of zinc oxide nanomaterials: Reactants, process parameters and morphologies. *Nanomaterials* **2020**, *10*, 1086. [CrossRef]
49. Sağlam, H.K.; Sarıtaş, S.; Ertugrul, M. Effect of Various Precursors on ZnO Thin Films by USP Technique. *Erzincan Univ. J. Sci. Technol.* **2021**, *14*, 926–935. [CrossRef]
50. Droepenu, E.K.; Wee, B.S.; Chin, S.F.; Kok, K.Y.; Maligan, M.F. Zinc oxide nanoparticles synthesis methods and its effect on morphology: A review. *Biointerface Res. Appl. Chem.* **2022**, *12*, 4261–4292.
51. Abdullah, J.A.A.; Guerrero, A.; Romero, A. Efficient and Sustainable Synthesis of Zinc Salt-Dependent Polycrystal Zinc Oxide Nanoparticles: Comprehensive Assessment of Physicochemical and Functional Properties. *Appl. Sci.* **2024**, *14*, 1815. [CrossRef]
52. Akhtar, H.; Alhamoudi, F.H.; Marshal, J.; Ashton, T.; Darr, J.A.; Rehman, I.U.; Chaudhry, A.A.; Reilly, G. Synthesis of cerium, zirconium, and copper doped zinc oxide nanoparticles as potential biomaterials for tissue engineering applications. *Heliyon* **2024**, *10*, e29150. [CrossRef]
53. Saha, J.K.; Bukke, R.N.; Mude, N.N.; Jang, J. Significant improvement of spray pyrolyzed ZnO thin film by precursor optimization for high mobility thin film transistors. *Sci. Rep.* **2020**, *10*, 8999. [CrossRef]
54. Szczesny, R.; Scigala, A.; Derkowska-Zielinska, B.; Skowronski, L.; Cassagne, C.; Boudebs, G.; Viter, R.; Szłyk, E. Synthesis, optical, and morphological studies of ZnO powders and thin films fabricated by wet chemical methods. *Materials* **2020**, *13*, 2559. [CrossRef] [PubMed]
55. Aspoukeh, P.K.; Barzinjy, A.A.; Hamad, S.M. A novel approach to the green synthesis of zinc oxide nanorods using Thymus kotschyanus plant extract: Effect of ammonium hydroxide and precursor concentration. *Nano Express* **2023**, *4*, 045001. [CrossRef]
56. Thakur, S.; Mandal, S.K. Precursor-and time-dependent morphological evolution of ZnO nanostructures for comparative photocatalytic activity and adsorption dynamics with methylene blue dye. *ACS Omega* **2020**, *5*, 16670–16680. [CrossRef]
57. Shaba, E.Y.; Jacob, J.O.; Tijani, J.O.; Suleiman, M.A.T. A critical review of synthesis parameters affecting the properties of zinc oxide nanoparticle and its application in wastewater treatment. *Appl. Water Sci.* **2021**, *11*, 48. [CrossRef]
58. Oh, D.K.; Choi, H.; Shin, H.; Kim, K.; Kim, M.; Ok, J.G. Tailoring zinc oxide nanowire architectures collectively by catalytic vapor-liquid-solid growth, catalyst-free vapor-solid growth, and low-temperature hydrothermal growth. *Ceram. Int.* **2021**, *47*, 2131–2143. [CrossRef]
59. Chang, C.; Rad, S.; Gan, L.; Li, Z.; Dai, J.; Shahab, A. Review of the sol–gel method in preparing nano TiO_2 for advanced oxidation process. *Nanotechnol. Rev.* **2023**, *12*, 20230150. [CrossRef]

60. Govender, K.; Boyle, D.S.; Kenway, P.B.; O'Brien, P. Understanding the factors that govern the deposition and morphology of thin films of ZnO from aqueous solution. *J. Mater. Chem.* **2004**, *14*, 2575–2591. [CrossRef]
61. Boyle, T.J.; Bunge, S.D.; Andrews, N.L.; Matzen, L.E.; Sieg, K.; Rodriguez, M.A.; Headley, T.J. Precursor structural influences on the final ZnO nanoparticle morphology from a novel family of structurally characterized zinc alkoxy alkyl precursors. *Chem. Mater.* **2004**, *16*, 3279–3288. [CrossRef]
62. Yusoff, A.H.; Salimi, M.N.; Jamlos, M.F. A review: Synthetic strategy control of magnetite nanoparticles production. *Adv. Nano Res.* **2018**, *6*, 1.
63. Cojocaru, L.; Olivier, C.; Toupance, T.; Sellier, E.; Hirsch, L. Size and shape fine-tuning of SnO_2 nanoparticles for highly efficient and stable dye-sensitized solar cells. *J. Mater. Chem. A* **2013**, *1*, 13789–13799. [CrossRef]
64. Weng, Z.; Xu, Y.; Gao, J.; Wang, X. Research progress of stimuli-responsive ZnO-based nanomaterials in biomedical applications. *Biomater. Sci.* **2023**, *11*, 76–95. [CrossRef] [PubMed]
65. Rasmussen, J.W.; Martinez, E.; Louka, P.; Wingett, D.G. Zinc oxide nanoparticles for selective destruction of tumor cells and potential for drug delivery applications. *Expert Opin. Drug Deliv.* **2010**, *7*, 1063–1077. [CrossRef]
66. Kunjiappan, S.; Pavadai, P.; Vellaichamy, S.; Ram Kumar Pandian, S.; Ravishankar, V.; Palanisamy, P.; Govindaraj, S.; Srinivasan, G.; Premanand, A.; Sankaranarayanan, M. Surface receptor-mediated targeted drug delivery systems for enhanced cancer treatment: A state-of-the-art review. *Drug Dev. Res.* **2021**, *82*, 309–340. [CrossRef]
67. Vyas, K.; Rathod, M.; Patel, M.M. Insight on nano drug delivery systems with targeted therapy in treatment of oral cancer. *Nanomed. Nanotechnol. Biol. Med.* **2023**, *49*, 102662. [CrossRef] [PubMed]
68. Amgoth, C.; Phan, C.; Banavoth, M.; Rompivalasa, S.; Tang, G. Polymer properties: Functionalization and surface modified nanoparticles. In *Role of Novel Drug Delivery Vehicles in Nanobiomedicine*; IntechOpen: London, UK, 2019.
69. Rafeeq, H.; Hussain, A.; Ambreen, A.; Waqas, M.; Bilal, M.; Iqbal, H.M. Functionalized nanoparticles and their environmental remediation potential: A review. *J. Nanostructure Chem.* **2022**, *12*, 1007–1031. [CrossRef]
70. Batool, M.; Khurshid, S.; Daoush, W.M.; Siddique, S.A.; Nadeem, T. Green synthesis and biomedical applications of ZnO nanoparticles: Role of PEGylated-ZnO nanoparticles as doxorubicin drug carrier against MDA-MB-231 (TNBC) cells line. *Crystals* **2021**, *11*, 344. [CrossRef]
71. Bao, J.; Zhang, Q.; Duan, T.; Hu, R.; Tang, J. The fate of nanoparticles in vivo and the strategy of designing stealth nanoparticle for drug delivery. *Curr. Drug Targets* **2021**, *22*, 922–946. [CrossRef]
72. Caldorera-Moore, M.E.; Liechty, W.B.; Peppas, N.A. Responsive theranostic systems: Integration of diagnostic imaging agents and responsive controlled release drug delivery carriers. *Acc. Chem. Res.* **2011**, *44*, 1061–1070. [CrossRef]
73. Canta, M.; Cauda, V. The investigation of the parameters affecting the ZnO nanoparticle cytotoxicity behaviour: A tutorial review. *Biomater. Sci.* **2020**, *8*, 6157–6174. [CrossRef]
74. Wingett, D.; Louka, P.; Anders, C.B.; Zhang, J.; Punnoose, A. A role of ZnO nanoparticle electrostatic properties in cancer cell cytotoxicity. *Nanotechnol. Sci. Appl.* **2016**, *9*, 29–45. [CrossRef]
75. Srivastav, A.K.; Dhiman, N.; Khan, H.; Srivastav, A.K.; Yadav, S.K.; Prakash, J.; Arjaria, N.; Singh, D.; Yadav, S.; Patnaik, S. Impact of surface-engineered ZnO nanoparticles on protein corona configuration and their interactions with biological system. *J. Pharm. Sci.* **2019**, *108*, 1872–1889. [CrossRef] [PubMed]
76. Guo, H.; Sun, P.; Liang, Y.; Ma, Y.; Qin, Z.; Cui, S. In-situ fabrication of polyelectrolyte-CSH superhydrophilic coatings via layer-by-layer assembly. *Chem. Eng. J.* **2014**, *253*, 198–206. [CrossRef]
77. Sapsford, K.E.; Algar, W.R.; Berti, L.; Gemmill, K.B.; Casey, B.J.; Oh, E.; Stewart, M.H.; Medintz, I.L. Functionalizing nanoparticles with biological molecules: Developing chemistries that facilitate nanotechnology. *Chem. Rev.* **2013**, *113*, 1904–2074.
78. Lee, C.-M.; Jeong, H.-J.; Kim, D.W.; Sohn, M.-H.; Lim, S.T. The effect of fluorination of zinc oxide nanoparticles on evaluation of their biodistribution after oral administration. *Nanotechnology* **2012**, *23*, 205102. [CrossRef] [PubMed]
79. Yakimova, R.; Selegård, L.; Khranovskyy, V.; Pearce, R.; Lloyd Spetz, A.; Uvdal, K. ZnO materials and surface tailoring for biosensing. *Front. Biosci. (Elite Ed.)* **2012**, *4*, 254–278. [CrossRef]
80. Cozzens, Y. Functionalization of Gold and Zinc Oxide Nanoparticles with Thiol-Containing Biomolecules and Polymers. Doctoral Dissertation, University of Massachusetts Lowell, Lowell, MA, USA, 2023.
81. Zhang, Y.; R Nayak, T.; Hong, H.; Cai, W. Biomedical applications of zinc oxide nanomaterials. *Curr. Mol. Med.* **2013**, *13*, 1633–1645. [CrossRef]
82. Kumar, S.G.; Rao, K.K. Zinc oxide based photocatalysis: Tailoring surface-bulk structure and related interfacial charge carrier dynamics for better environmental applications. *Rsc Adv.* **2015**, *5*, 3306–3351. [CrossRef]
83. Singh, T.A.; Das, J.; Sil, P.C. Zinc oxide nanoparticles: A comprehensive review on its synthesis, anticancer and drug delivery applications as well as health risks. *Adv. Colloid Interface Sci.* **2020**, *286*, 102317. [CrossRef] [PubMed]
84. Wang, J.; Gao, S.; Wang, S.; Xu, Z.; Wei, L. Zinc oxide nanoparticles induce toxicity in CAL 27 oral cancer cell lines by activating PINK1/Parkin-mediated mitophagy. *Int. J. Nanomed.* **2018**, *13*, 3441–3450. [CrossRef]
85. Marunganathan, V.; Kumar, M.S.K.; Kari, Z.A.; Giri, J.; Shaik, M.R.; Shaik, B.; Guru, A. Marine-derived κ-carrageenan-coated zinc oxide nanoparticles for targeted drug delivery and apoptosis induction in oral cancer. *Mol. Biol. Rep.* **2024**, *51*, 89. [CrossRef] [PubMed]
86. Verma, S.; Singh, S. Non-invasive oral cancer detection from saliva using zinc oxide-reduced graphene oxide nanocomposite based bioelectrode. *MRS Commun.* **2019**, *9*, 1227–1234. [CrossRef]

87. Shaik, M.R.; Kandaswamy, K.; Guru, A.; Khan, H.; Giri, J.; Mallik, S.; Shah, M.A.; Arockiaraj, J. Targeted piperine-coated zinc oxide nanoparticle induces the biofilm inhibition of dental pathogens and apoptosis of oral cancer through the BCL-2/BAX/P53 signaling pathway. *BMC* **2024**. *preprint*. [CrossRef]
88. Tayyeb, J.Z.; Priya, M.; Guru, A.; Kishore Kumar, M.S.; Giri, J.; Garg, A.; Agrawal, R.; Mat, K.B.; Arockiaraj, J. Multifunctional curcumin mediated zinc oxide nanoparticle enhancing biofilm inhibition and targeting apoptotic specific pathway in oral squamous carcinoma cells. *Mol. Biol. Rep.* **2024**, *51*, 423. [CrossRef] [PubMed]
89. Shanmugam, K.; Sellappan, S.; Alahmadi, T.A.; Almoallim, H.S.; Natarajan, N.; Veeraraghavan, V.P. Green synthesized zinc oxide nanoparticles from Cinnamomum verum bark extract inhibited cell growth and induced caspase-mediated apoptosis in oral cancer KB cells. *J. Drug Deliv. Sci. Technol.* **2022**, *74*, 103577. [CrossRef]
90. Wang, S.-W.; Lee, C.-H.; Lin, M.-S.; Chi, C.-W.; Chen, Y.-J.; Wang, G.-S.; Liao, K.-W.; Chiu, L.-P.; Wu, S.-H.; Huang, D.-M. ZnO nanoparticles induced caspase-dependent apoptosis in gingival squamous cell carcinoma through mitochondrial dysfunction and p70S6K signaling pathway. *Int. J. Mol. Sci.* **2020**, *21*, 1612. [CrossRef] [PubMed]
91. Ravikumar, O.; Marunganathan, V.; Kumar, M.S.K.; Mohan, M.; Shaik, M.R.; Shaik, B.; Guru, A.; Mat, K. Zinc oxide nanoparticles functionalized with cinnamic acid for targeting dental pathogens receptor and modulating apoptotic genes in human oral epidermal carcinoma KB cells. *Mol. Biol. Rep.* **2024**, *51*, 352. [CrossRef] [PubMed]
92. Nasiri, S.; Mahmoudvand, H.; Shakibaei, M.; Mousavi, S.A.H.; Sepahvand, A. Antifungal effects of zinc nanoparticles green synthesized by Lavandula angustifolia extract, alone and combined with nystatin against Candida albicans, a major cause of oral candidiasis. *J. HerbMed Pharmacol.* **2022**, *11*, 540–545. [CrossRef]
93. Sirelkhatim, A.; Mahmud, S.; Seeni, A.; Kaus, N.H.M. Preferential cytotoxicity of ZnO nanoparticle towards cervical cancer cells induced by ROS-mediated apoptosis and cell cycle arrest for cancer therapy. *J. Nanoparticle Res.* **2016**, *18*, 219. [CrossRef]
94. He, G.; Nie, J.-J.; Liu, X.; Ding, Z.; Luo, P.; Liu, Y.; Zhang, B.-W.; Wang, R.; Liu, X.; Hai, Y. Zinc oxide nanoparticles inhibit osteosarcoma metastasis by downregulating β-catenin via HIF-1α/BNIP3/LC3B-mediated mitophagy pathway. *Bioact. Mater.* **2023**, *19*, 690–702. [CrossRef]
95. Hou, J.; Liu, H.; Zhang, S.; Liu, X.; Hayat, T.; Alsaedi, A.; Wang, X. Mechanism of toxic effects of Nano-ZnO on cell cycle of zebrafish (*Danio rerio*). *Chemosphere* **2019**, *229*, 206–213. [CrossRef] [PubMed]
96. Akhtar, M.J.; Ahamed, M.; Kumar, S.; Khan, M.M.; Ahmad, J.; Alrokayan, S.A. Zinc oxide nanoparticles selectively induce apoptosis in human cancer cells through reactive oxygen species. *Int. J. Nanomed.* **2012**, *7*, 845–857.
97. Al-darwesh, M.Y.; Ibrahim, S.S.; Mohammed, M.A. A Review on Plant Extract Mediated Green Synthesis of Zinc oxide Nanoparticles and Their biomedical Applications. *Results Chem.* **2024**, *7*, 101368. [CrossRef]
98. Xie, X.; Zhang, Y.; Li, F.; Lv, T.; Li, Z.; Chen, H.; Jia, L.; Gao, Y. Challenges and opportunities from basic cancer biology for nanomedicine for targeted drug delivery. *Curr. Cancer Drug Targets* **2019**, *19*, 257–276. [CrossRef] [PubMed]
99. Mishra, P.K.; Mishra, H.; Ekielski, A.; Talegaonkar, S.; Vaidya, B. Zinc oxide nanoparticles: A promising nanomaterial for biomedical applications. *Drug Discov. Today* **2017**, *22*, 1825–1834. [CrossRef] [PubMed]
100. León-Buitimea, A.; Garza-Cárdenas, C.R.; Román-García, M.F.; Ramírez-Díaz, C.A.; Ulloa-Ramírez, M.; Morones-Ramírez, J.R. Nanomaterials-based combinatorial therapy as a strategy to combat antibiotic resistance. *Antibiotics* **2022**, *11*, 794. [CrossRef] [PubMed]
101. Khaitan, T.; Prajapati, V. Zinc oxide eugenol paste as a dressing material on surgical raw wounds after wide excision of oral potentially malignant disorders: A prospective controlled clinical trial. *Indian J. Dent. Sci.* **2021**, *13*, 98–102. [CrossRef]
102. Rosenberg, M.; Visnapuu, M.; Vija, H.; Kisand, V.; Kasemets, K.; Kahru, A.; Ivask, A. Selective antibiofilm properties and biocompatibility of nano-ZnO and nano-ZnO/Ag coated surfaces. *Sci. Rep.* **2020**, *10*, 13478. [CrossRef] [PubMed]
103. Gholamali, I.; Yadollahi, M. Doxorubicin-loaded carboxymethyl cellulose/Starch/ZnO nanocomposite hydrogel beads as an anticancer drug carrier agent. *Int. J. Biol. Macromol.* **2020**, *160*, 724–735. [CrossRef]
104. Zhou, Q.; Zhang, L.; Li, Y.; Wang, J.; He, X.; Zhang, J.; Qiao, Y.; Wu, H.; Zhu, L. Targeting and sensitizing MDR cancer by an MMP2 and pH dual-responsive ZnO-based nanomedicine. *Cancer Nanotechnol.* **2023**, *14*, 56. [CrossRef]
105. Khabir, Z.; Holmes, A.M.; Lai, Y.-J.; Liang, L.; Deva, A.; Polikarpov, M.A.; Roberts, M.S.; Zvyagin, A.V. Human epidermal zinc concentrations after topical application of ZnO nanoparticles in sunscreens. *Int. J. Mol. Sci.* **2021**, *22*, 12372. [CrossRef] [PubMed]
106. Ortiz-Casas, B.; Galdamez-Martinez, A.; Gutierrez-Flores, J.; Ibañez, A.B.; Panda, P.K.; Santana, G.; de la Vega, H.A.; Suar, M.; Rodelo, C.G.; Kaushik, A. Bio-acceptable 0D and 1D ZnO nanostructures for cancer diagnostics and treatment. *Mater. Today* **2021**, *50*, 533–569. [CrossRef]
107. Cevaal, P.M.; Ali, A.; Czuba-Wojnilowicz, E.; Symons, J.; Lewin, S.R.; Cortez-Jugo, C.; Caruso, F. In vivo T cell-targeting nanoparticle drug delivery systems: Considerations for rational design. *ACS Nano* **2021**, *15*, 3736–3753. [CrossRef] [PubMed]
108. Liu, Y.; Zeng, S.; Ji, W.; Yao, H.; Lin, L.; Cui, H.; Santos, H.A.; Pan, G. Emerging theranostic nanomaterials in diabetes and its complications. *Adv. Sci.* **2022**, *9*, 2102466. [CrossRef]
109. Xu, X.; Li, T.; Jin, K. Bioinspired and biomimetic nanomedicines for targeted cancer therapy. *Pharmaceutics* **2022**, *14*, 1109. [CrossRef]

molecules

MDPI

Review

Advancements in Nanosystems for Ocular Drug Delivery: A Focus on Pediatric Retinoblastoma

Kevin Y. Wu [1], Xingao C. Wang [2], Maude Anderson [1] and Simon D. Tran [3,*]

1 Department of Surgery, Division of Ophthalmology, University of Sherbrooke, Sherbrooke, QC J1G 2E8, Canada; yang.wu@usherbrooke.ca (K.Y.W.)
2 Faculty of Medicine and Health Sciences, McGill University, Montreal, QC H3T 1J4, Canada
3 Faculty of Dental Medicine and Oral Health Sciences, McGill University, Montreal, QC H3A 1G1, Canada
* Correspondence: simon.tran@mcgill.ca

Abstract: The eye's complex anatomical structures present formidable barriers to effective drug delivery across a range of ocular diseases, from anterior to posterior segment pathologies. Emerging as a promising solution to these challenges, nanotechnology-based platforms—including but not limited to liposomes, dendrimers, and micelles—have shown the potential to revolutionize ophthalmic therapeutics. These nanocarriers enhance drug bioavailability, increase residence time in targeted ocular tissues, and offer precise, localized delivery, minimizing systemic side effects. Focusing on pediatric ophthalmology, particularly on retinoblastoma, this review delves into the recent advancements in functionalized nanosystems for drug delivery. Covering the literature from 2017 to 2023, it comprehensively examines these nanocarriers' potential impact on transforming the treatment landscape for retinoblastoma. The review highlights the critical role of these platforms in overcoming the unique pediatric eye barriers, thus enhancing treatment efficacy. It underscores the necessity for ongoing research to realize the full clinical potential of these innovative drug delivery systems in pediatric ophthalmology.

Keywords: retinoblastoma; drug delivery systems (DDS); nanosystems; nanoparticles; nanotechnology; nanomedicine; ocular drug delivery; pediatric ocular disease; retinoblastoma

1. Introduction

In the realm of pediatric oncology, retinoblastoma emerges as the foremost intraocular malignancy, presenting unique challenges in its treatment due to the delicate context of its pediatric patient base and the intricacies of ocular drug delivery. Conventional treatment modalities, including enucleation, chemotherapy, and radiotherapy, while effective to varying degrees, are fraught with limitations, such as systemic toxicity, recurrence, and long-term side effects, highlighting the urgent need for more targeted and personalized therapeutic strategies. In this context, the burgeoning field of nanotechnology offers a promising horizon. This review article delves into the current landscape of retinoblastoma treatment challenges and showcases the revolutionary potential of nanosystems in enhancing ocular drug delivery. Through a comprehensive exploration of various nanoparticle types—including gold, mesoporous silica, iron, polymeric, and lipid nanoparticles—this article elucidates their application in overcoming the biological barriers to drug delivery in the eye, potentially offering targeted therapy with reduced side effects and improved efficacy. Covering the literature from 2017 to 2023, this article comprehensively examines these nanocarriers' potential impact on transforming the treatment landscape for pediatric ocular diseases.

2. Overview of Retinoblastoma

2.1. Epidemiology

Retinoblastoma is recognized as the most prevalent primary intraocular malignancy among children, securing its position as the second most common of such tumors across all age groups, only surpassed by uveal melanoma. This malignancy manifests with a frequency ranging from 1 in every 14,000 to 20,000 live births, translating to an estimated 250–300 new cases emerging annually within the United States alone. It exhibits no preference regarding gender or ethnicity, affecting both sexes and all races indiscriminately. Notably, in 30–40% of instances, retinoblastoma presents bilaterally [1]. A significant majority, approximately 90%, of retinoblastoma cases are identified in children younger than three years of age.

The age at diagnosis of retinoblastoma is intricately linked to both the presence of a family history of the disease and its bilateral or unilateral presentation. Children with a known familial history of retinoblastoma are typically diagnosed at an average age of 8 months. In contrast, those affected by the disease in both eyes, or bilaterally, are usually diagnosed at around 12 months of age. Meanwhile, patients exhibiting unilateral disease, where the tumor is confined to one eye, are often diagnosed at a later stage, around 24 months [1].

This variation in diagnosis timing highlights the influence of genetic predispositions and the scope of the disease's manifestation. Furthermore, the incidence of retinoblastoma on a global scale exhibits a stark variation, with up to a fiftyfold difference primarily attributed to the variability in birth rates across different regions. Registries have recorded the highest incidences of retinoblastoma in African countries, indicating a geographical disparity in the prevalence of this condition [2].

2.2. Etiological Insights and Risk Factors

Retinoblastoma emerges due to detrimental alterations in the RB1 gene, specifically located on the long arm of chromosome 13 at the 13q14 locus [3]. The malignancy develops when mutations occur in both copies of the RB1 gene. In bilateral cases, which comprise a minority of occurrences, there is a 98% likelihood of the mutations being of germline origin. While familial retinoblastoma is rare, accounting for 5% of all cases, the vast majority of cases, or 95%, are sporadic. Within these sporadic cases, 60% are unilateral with no germline mutation detected, leaving the remainder exhibiting germline mutations and the potential for multiple tumor formations.

Heritable retinoblastoma is characterized by a mutation in one RB1 gene allele across all body cells. The disease progresses to malignancy when the remaining allele undergoes mutation, potentially due to environmental factors. This condition results in bilateral and multifocal tumors, significantly increasing the risk of secondary non-ocular cancers (e.g., pineoblastoma, osteosarcoma, soft tissue sarcoma, melanoma) [4]. The base risk of developing a secondary cancer is 6%, with this risk increasing fivefold if external beam radiation therapy is applied to the primary tumor.

Conversely, non-heritable retinoblastoma, which usually presents unilaterally, does not follow a pattern of genetic transmission and thus does not elevate the risk of secondary non-ocular cancers. Identified in patients with no family history of the disease, this type implicates a 1% risk for both the siblings and offspring of affected individuals. Significantly, non-heritable retinoblastomas constitute approximately 90% of unilateral cases [4].

2.3. Diagnostic Approaches and Clinical Presentation

2.3.1. Initial Assessment and Clinical Signs

Diagnosis of retinoblastoma primarily relies on clinical assessment. Clinical signs and symptoms at the point of diagnosis vary depending on the tumor's size and position. Leukocoria (a white reflection from the pupil) and strabismus (misalignment of the eyes) are the most frequently observed initial indicators of the disease [5]. Although less common, other symptoms, such as iris heterochromia, spontaneous hyphema, pseudo-hypopyon, and signs of ocular inflammation, may also be present (Figure 1). On occasion, smaller tumors might be detected during routine eye examinations, with complaints regarding vision being rare, largely because the condition predominantly affects children of pre-school age [6].

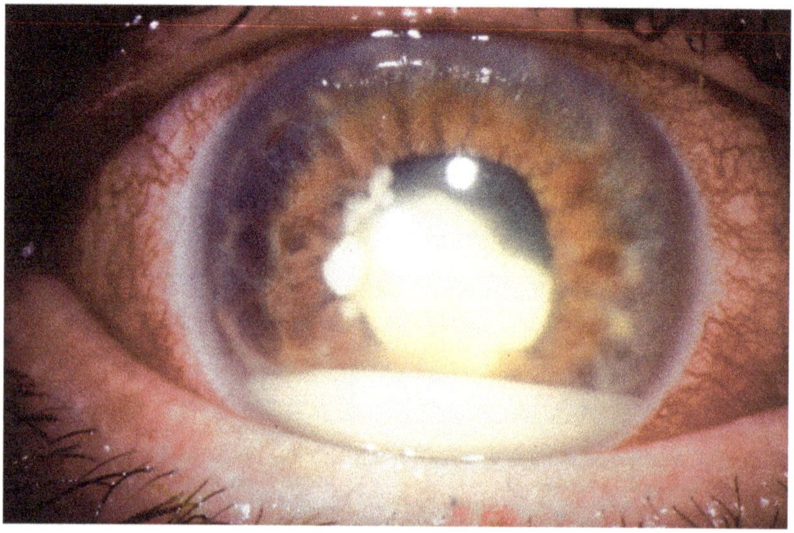

Figure 1. Manifestation of retinoblastoma accompanied by ocular inflammation and pseudo-hypopyon in the anterior chamber. Image credit: Prof. Clare Gilbert, International Centre for Eye Health (ICEH), London School of Hygiene & Tropical Medicine (www.iceh.org.uk, accessed on 24 February 2024). This work is licensed under a Creative Commons Attribution-NonCommercial-NoDerivatives 4.0 International License.

2.3.2. Development and Variants

Retinoblastoma emerges as a translucent, gray-to-white tumor within the retina, supported by enlarged, twisted vessels. As it progresses, the tumor calcifies, adopting a distinctive chalky appearance. It exhibits two primary growth patterns: exophytic, developing beneath the retina and potentially causing widespread retinal detachment, and endophytic, growing on the retinal surface toward the vitreous cavity. Endophytic tumors may obscure blood vessels and are prone to producing vitreous seeds, which can spread within the eye, potentially forming new tumors. These seeds can also migrate to the anterior chamber, leading to nodules on the iris or a pseudo-hypopyon. Such cases frequently encounter complications, such as secondary glaucoma and rubeosis iridis. Diffuse infiltrating retinoblastoma, a rarer form identified later in childhood, usually manifests unilaterally and complicates diagnosis due to the obscured retina from dense vitreous cells, often being mistaken for uveitis with an unknown origin [6].

2.3.3. Diagnostic Imaging and Evaluation

MRI is pivotal in diagnosing retinoblastoma due to its superior soft-tissue resolution and non-radiative nature. These modalities help identify the characteristic calcifications and evaluate the optic nerve, orbits, and brain. Systemic metastasis assessments, including bone marrow and lumbar puncture, are generally not recommended unless there are neurological symptoms or signs of extraocular extension [7]. Additionally, examining the parents and siblings for signs of retinoblastoma or retinocytoma is crucial to identify a hereditary predisposition.

2.3.4. Metastasis and Extraocular Extension

In developed countries, it is uncommon for patients with retinoblastoma to have metastasis or intracranial extension at the time of diagnosis. When metastasis does occur, it typically involves the abdominal viscera, brain, bones, lymph nodes, and spinal cord, often as a result of the tumor spreading through the optic nerve or choroid. Growth of the tumor into the orbit can cause proptosis, and its invasion into the anterior chamber can promote lymphatic dissemination, which may be detected through palpable lymph nodes [8].

2.3.5. Classification

The management of retinoblastoma has evolved significantly, with primary local and/or systemic chemotherapy now being preferred over external beam radiotherapy. This shift has led to the widespread adoption of the International Classification System for Intraocular Retinoblastoma globally. Within this framework, the classification of eyes is based on tumor size, the presence of subretinal fluid, and the degree of vitreous and subretinal seeding. The system categorizes eyes from Group A (most salvageable) to Group E (least salvageable) with chemotherapy. Group E encompasses cases with anterior chamber involvement, neovascular glaucoma, vitreous hemorrhage, and/or necrosis, typically deemed unsalvageable [9].

2.4. Prognosis and Management Strategies

In industrialized nations, the prognosis is favorable, with survival rates above 95% for intraocular cases. However, this rate significantly declines to below 50% upon extraocular extension. Thus, the treatment protocols prioritize, in descending order, the preservation of life, the eye, and vision. The contemporary management of intraocular retinoblastoma integrates various modalities, including enucleation, systemic and local chemotherapy, laser and cryotherapy, along with external beam and plaque brachytherapy. For cases exhibiting metastatic spread, a combination of intensive chemotherapy, radiation therapy, and bone marrow transplantation is adopted. A multi-disciplinary team approach, involving ocular oncologists, pediatric ophthalmologists, pediatric oncologists, and radiation oncologists, is essential for optimizing treatment outcomes [10].

3. Challenges in Treating Retinoblastoma

3.1. Enucleation

Enucleation stands as a cornerstone treatment for retinoblastoma, offering a complete surgical removal of the tumor in the majority of cases. This procedure is typically deemed suitable under certain conditions, including when the tumor occupies over half of the eye, when there is suspicion of orbital or optic nerve involvement, when the anterior segment is affected, in the presence of neovascular glaucoma, or when the vision potential of the affected eye is severely compromised. The surgical technique aims to maximize the length of the optic nerve removed, ideally exceeding 10 mm [11].

3.2. Laser and Cryotherapy

The treatment of retinoblastoma frequently involves the use of the 810 nm infrared diode laser, highly regarded for its precision in targeting retinal tumors. This technique can be administered as a standalone treatment or as an adjunct to chemotherapy, offering flexibility in managing the disease [12].

For smaller tumors, with an apical thickness up to 3 mm, cryotherapy is preferred. It employs a triple freeze–thaw technique under direct observation, distinguishing its application based on tumor location: laser photoablation for posterior tumors and cryoablation for anterior ones. Both methods require multiple sessions and continuous monitoring to address tumor recurrence or treatment-related complications effectively [13].

3.3. Radiotherapy

External beam radiation therapy (EBRT) was a widely popular method for treating RB in the past. It is a local treatment delivering external radiation beams to the target tissue. A consequence of this treatment modality is its potential to induce secondary tumors. Wong et al. (1997) found that genetic predisposition to hereditary RB and radiation increase the risk of secondary malignancy [14]. Abramson et al. (1998) suggested that the long-term effect of radiation treatment depends strongly on the age at first exposure to EBRT, and it is thus not recommended before 12 months of age [15]. Though effective, its potential major complications cause this treatment to be of last resort. Yousef et al. (2020) found that EBRT was able to control RB eyes after the failure of combined chemotherapy and focal therapy [16]. Today, this technique is recommended in patients who are not candidates for safer therapeutic modalities [17].

3.4. Chemotherapy

Chemotherapy is a great alternative to EBRT, as it spares the risks of secondary malignancy. Systemic chemotherapy is not shown to be effective when administered alone and can cause important consequences, such as hearing deficits, neutropenia, and infection [18]. Intra-arterial delivery of chemotherapy can cause neutropenia and the need for blood transfusion, although to a lesser extent than systemic delivery. Furthermore, the invasive nature of arterial delivery can result in systemic side effects, such as transient ischemic attacks and strokes [19]. Additionally, vascular effects, such as vitreous hemorrhage, arterial occlusion, and retinal detachment, can occur [16,19]. Although the cause remains unknown, some suggest that it is a drug-specific side effect. Steinle et al. (2012) demonstrated vascular toxicity of melphalan and carboplatin (CRB) [20], and histological changes supporting such toxicity were shown by Tse et al. (2013) [21]. Intra-arterial injections are also limited by the blood–retinal barrier (BRB) and the avascular nature of the vitreous; thus, repeated injections are required to express adequate vitreous drug concentrations [22,23] (Figure 2). Intravitreal drug delivery is the preferred method for treating vitreous seeds. This approach allows for direct delivery of drugs to the vitreous and increased local bioavailability. However, this raises the question of potential toxicity to the eye and surrounding tissues due to high concentrations within the vitreous. Yousef et al. (2021) concluded that aftereffects at standard doses are not uncommon, with 59% developing side effects, with retinal toxicity and cataracts being the leading results [24]. Intravitreal injections also often require multiple injections, increasing the chances of endophthalmitis. Nanoparticles (NPs) as drug delivery systems can address the toxic complications, drug stability, and physiological barriers currently hindering chemotherapy injections. Table 1 provides a summary of treatment types and respective challenges discussed in this section.

Table 1. Retinoblastoma—Current treatment challenges.

Treatment	Modality	Challenges	References
EBRT	N/A	- Secondary tumors - Treatment of last resort	[14–17]
Chemotherapy	Systemic	- Ineffective alone - Systemic toxicity	[18]
	Intra-arterial	- Invasive therapy - Need for equipment and specialists - Vascular side effects among others - Limited by BRB and avascular vitreous	[19–23]
	Intravitreal	- Toxicity to eye and surrounding tissue - Requires repeated injections, endophthalmitis	[24]

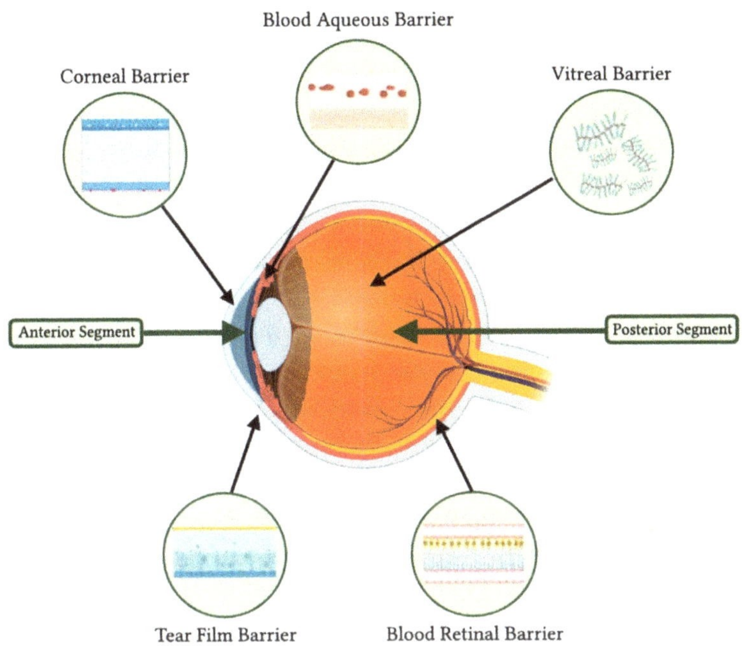

Figure 2. Anatomical and physiological barriers of the eye.

4. Nano-Based Strategies

4.1. Inorganic Nanoparticles

4.1.1. Gold Nanoparticles (GNPs)

GNPs have a range of possible applications, from diagnostic tools to therapeutic delivery, including low toxicity and high surface area to volume ratio, enabling high loading capacity and delivery to the retina [25]. Yan et al. (2021) took advantage of their high surface area to volume ratio to coat a gold(I)-thiol-peptide with polyacryl sulfhydryl imidazole (PSI). PSI coating of the GNPs resulted in a lower Zeta potential at pH 7.4, falling from 37 mV to 28 mV, and the NPs' spherical shape remained unchanged. Peptide-derived molecular glue was embedded to target Murine Double Minute X (MDMX) degradation, which allows for the restoration of p53 and p73, two tumor suppressor genes. Additionally, PSI coating enabled the nanoparticle to be pH-responsive, only releasing its content in a tumor microenvironment, which is normally more acidic than normal tissue [26,27]. In vitro studies on WERI-RB1 cells demonstrated a dose-dependent degradation of MDMX with a DC50 of 154 nM. In a patient-derived xenograft (PDX) model of pancreatic carcinoma measuring 100 ± 25 mm^3, this NP inhibited tumor growth by 85.7% within 10 days, and downregulation of MDMX was seen on histological analysis. Furthermore, no weight change, difference in blood biochemical index, or pathological findings were observed following treatment [26,27]. Kalmodia et al. (2017) loaded GNPs with anti-human double minute 2 (anti-HDM2) and studied their effect on Y79 cells. These GNPs were spherical, 32–122 nm in size, with a Zeta potential of -11.4; the hydrodynamic diameter (HD) and polydispersity index (PI) were 66.72 and 0.303, respectively. Their experiment on Y79 cells showed a statistically significant decrease in cells in the G1 phase following treatment, suggesting a mechanism of G2/M phase arrest and p53-mediated apoptosis [28]. These two studies illustrate the wide variety of structures that GNPs can take to target the same problem of retinoblastoma. Darviot et al. (2019) merged laser treatment and nanoparticles to reduce the energy required to destroy cancerous cell membranes via heat. Two types of GNPs were utilized: citrate-capped 100 nm and 80 nm 50:50 gold–silver. Interestingly, at 250 J cm^{-2}, the laser–GNP interaction resulted in up to 98% cell death in the vitreous phantom of 15 cP, mimicking the vitreous environment, compared to 82% in the culture environment, showing optimistic results for clinical application. However, one limitation is the lack of homogenous attachment of NPs to the cultured cells, since their interaction relies solely on electrostatic attraction [29]. Hence, there is opportunity to explore surface coatings targeting Y79 cells for future enhancement of the treatment modality. Similarly, Moradi et al. (2020) demonstrated the synergistic effect of ultrasonic hyperthermia and GNPs. The fabricated spherical GNPs had a diameter of around 60 nm, with a Z potential of +38.6 mV and a hydrodynamic diameter of 89 nm. In vitro studies on Y79 cells highlighted that cell viability of 50% was achieved after 9 min of hyperthermia alone, whereas it was achieved in 4.5 min with the presence of gold nanoparticles [30]. Moradi et al. (2020) followed up with another study investigating the synergistic effect of 20 Gy brachytherapy, hyperthermia, and GNPs in rabbit eye models inoculated with Y79 cells. These GNPs had similar properties, being spherical, 60 nm in size, with HD of 80 nm and Zeta potential of +38.6 mV. Though this combination therapy caused a significant reduction in tumor size, resulting in tumor growth inhibition of 85%, compared to their individual potentials, it also enhanced inflammation, scarring, and hemorrhage occurrences [31]. Thus, there is a need for investigation into the protocols addressing variable factors, such as the ideal temperature, length of treatment, and heat source, before delving into clinical studies.

4.1.2. Mesoporous Silica Nanoparticles (MSNPs)

MSNPs have been investigated for drug delivery and imaging among others, attributable to their high surface, pore volume, drug-loading capacity, and ease in incorporating surface functionalization [32]. There is a substantial research focus on the efficient targeting of tumor cells. Folic acid receptors are significantly overexpressed in retinoblastoma cells, and targeting such receptors could benefit cellular uptake [33]. Hence, their high drug-loading capacity and availability for surface-targeting properties could benefit chemotherapeutic delivery to retinoblastoma cells. Qu et al. (2018) explored this concept by synthesizing folic acid conjugated MSNPs embedded with topotecan. The addition of surface folic acid (FA) not only had benefits in terms of cellular uptake but also enabled controlled drug release. The original spherical MSNP containing topotecan (TPT) had a size of 110 $\pm$ 2.54 nm and increased to 168.5 $\pm$ 1.65 nm following the addition of FA, but it kept its spherical shape. In vitro release pattern testing using a dialysis protocol highlighted the controlled release of MSNPs with FA receptors, as 60% of TPT was released after 24 h of incubation compared to 80% in MSNPs without FA receptors. In vivo testing in Y79-cell-bearing xenograft tumor models demonstrated the efficiency of folic acid in targeting tumor cells, which allowed for a reduction in tumor volume of ~300 mm^3 compared to ~1000 mm^3 in MNPs without FA receptors, which further supports the idea of increased cellular uptake due to the presence of FA receptors [34]. Using a similar approach of targeting retinoblastoma (RB) cells and in order to address carboplatin (CRB) side effects, such as neurological toxicities and thrombocytopenia, and limitations of physiological barriers, Qu et al. (2017) used MSNPs to effectively deliver the drug. Rather than depending on diffusion, this nanoparticle targeted epithelial cell adhesion molecule (EpCAM) receptors overexpressed in RB cells by attaching EpCAM to the surface of the MSNPs loaded with carboplatin (CRB). The nanoparticles were spherical and had a Zeta potential of -20.1 ± 2.15 mV and a size of ~150 nm. An IC_{50} value of 1.38 μg/mL compared to free CRB IC_{50} value of 3.26 μg/mL demonstrated its significantly higher cytotoxicity attributed to its higher cellular internalization due to ligand targeting. Further, in vitro testing on Y79 cells revealed that free CRB induced 15% apoptosis compared to 40% and 65% in CRB-containing MSNPs and those with EpCAM receptors, respectively [35,36]. Sodagar Taleghani et al. (2019) opted to design a stimuli-responsive and cancer-cell-targeting MSNPs to control and target drug release. Taking advantage of their unique biological need for above-normal glucose uptake and the higher extracellular pH of tumor tissues compared to healthy tissue, the MSNPs loaded with deferasirox and containing pH-responsive polyamidoamine

(PAMAM) dendrimer and decorated with glucuronic acid had a Zeta potential of 5.3 mV. In in vitro studies, at pH 7.4, only 15% of deferasirox was released compared to 66% at pH 4.5, demonstrating the sensitivity of PAMAM dendrimers to pH. The viability of Y79 cells when induced with deferasirox-loaded sugar-decorated nanocarrier was around 39.85 ± 0.45% for a concentration of 200 μg/mL compared to 72.84 ± 1.29% for those without sugar conjugation, highlighting the benefits of sugar conjugation in the uptake of the drug via receptor-mediated endocytosis [37].

4.1.3. Iron Nanoparticles

Iron NPs have a particular characteristic of being of superparamagnetic nature, allowing them to be excellent candidates in biomedical imaging as well as hyperthermic in nature in response to magnetic fields [38]. Demirci et al. (2019) used dextran-coated magnetic NPs in magnetic hyperthermia, where internalized nanoparticles are exposed to a magnetic field and convert the energy into heat, killing tumor cells, which are sensitive to heat. These NPs were not found to be toxic in the absence of a magnetic field and were selectively cytotoxic to Y79 RB cells instead of ARPE-19 cells upon magnetic induction. At a concentration of 0.75 mg/mL, 50% of Y79 cell death occurred compared to ARPE-19 cells, which had a viability of 88%. Moreover, apoptosis began less than 24 h after induction and involved both the mitochondrial cell death pathway and apoptotic gene expression [39]. Seydi et al. (2023) studied superparamagnetic iron oxide nanoparticles (SPIONs) targeting the mitochondria of Y79 RB cells. These SPIONs had an average particle size of 20–40 nm and a bulk density of 1.20 g/cm^3. This resulted in mitochondrial swelling, a collapse in mitochondrial membrane potential (MMP), a decrease in succinate dehydrogenase (SDH), and an increase in caspase-3 and ROS, leading to an overall decline in cell viability and an IC_{50} of 250 nm in RB mitochondria [40]. Although the in vitro results are positive, the exact properties of such nanoparticles remain unknown, such as penetration capability in retinal tissue and the choroid [39]. Hence, it is important for in vivo experiments to explore potential ocular toxicity. Further, although the hyperthermic properties of iron NPs allow them to exert therapeutic effects alone, it would be interesting to explore the possible synergistic effects of hyperthermic reactions and chemotherapeutic drugs loaded in iron NPs.

4.1.4. Silver Nanoparticles

Silver nanoparticles (AgNPs) are alternative vehicles for delivery and have been widely applied in the antimicrobial context due to their broad-spectrum antimicrobial activity. They also have great potential in anti-cancer treatment due to their low toxicity, magnetic properties, and surface area to volume ratio. Importantly, AgNPs alone tend to agglomerate due to their surface charges, hence the importance of surface coating, especially in the context of drug delivery through the vitreous—a size- and charge-sensitive, difficult environment to cross [41]. Turbinaria Ornata are algae containing Laminarin, a polysaccharide with anti-tumor and anti-apoptotic features among other biological activities [42,43]. Remya et al. (2017) first developed a technique for rapidly synthesizing biological AgNPs from Turbinaria Ornata extracted from brown seaweed. Biologically synthesized AgNPs have enhanced therapeutic effects compared to their chemical counterparts while being environmentally friendly and cost-efficient [44–47]. Mixing 10 mL of the natural extract with 90 mL of 1 mM aqueous silver nitrate ($AgNO_3$) yielded polydispersed AgNps with a size of 22–32 nm and a Zeta potential of −28.7 mV. In vitro experimentation demonstrated beneficial cytotoxic and apoptosis effects on Y79 cells with good radical scavenging effects and IC_{50} of 10.5 μg/mL [46]. Remya et al. (2018) followed up with a similar study where the AgNPs were synthesized using 5 mL of laminarin and 95 mL of 1 mM AgNO3, which resulted in 21–34 nm uniform and spherical particles with IC_{50} of 16.45 μg/mL in Y79 cell lines. Furthermore, the mechanism involved breaking DNA double strands, leading to increased sub-G1 apoptotic cell growth and inhibiting proliferation [46,47]. The biosynthesis of these AgNPs using algae allows for an environmentally friendly, cost-effective synthesis method [48].

4.2. Organic Nanoparticles

4.2.1. Polymeric Nanoparticles

Polymeric nanoparticles are composed of various polymers, with the most common being poly(lactic-co-glycolic acid) (PLGA) and polycaprolactone (PCL), which are approved by the FDA [49]. Furthermore, they are biocompatible and degradable, with high stability and solubility. Moreover, their structure allows for enhanced drug accumulation, which is ideal for loading and delivering intact drugs to the retina, enhancing their bioavailability at the site of action [50]. Godse et al. (2021) studied the role of etoposide-loaded, chitosan-coated, and galactose-conjugated PLGA NPs in Y79 cells in vitro. These spherical PLGA NPs had a Zeta potential of +25 mV, which is favorable for diffusion across the vitreous and penetration of the retina, and the size ranged from 150 to 160 nm. Galactose targeted RB cells through their overexpression of sugar receptors, allowing for a cellular uptake of 70.02% compared to 49% in PLGA NPs without galactose in Y79 cells. Chitosan stabilized the NPs, permitting sustained release of the drug for over 32 h compared to a complete release of the free drug after 6 h. The enhanced properties of this nanoparticle permitted increased cellular uptake, cytotoxicity, and apoptosis [51]. Silva et al. (2019) adopted a similar approach, where they evaluated the cytotoxic effects of oleanolic (OA) and ursolic (UA) acids loaded in PLGA NPs and demonstrated decreased drug cytotoxicity when loaded in nanoparticles. These nanoparticles had sizes ranging from 213.55 ± 1.60 nm to 217.98 ± 2.74 nm and Zeta potentials of −27.12 ± 0.27 mV and −26.85 ± 0.49 mV depending on the type of mixture of OA and UA being loaded—natural or synthetic, respectively. In vitro analysis of Y79 cells demonstrated cell viability of 15.43% when exposed to the free synthetic mixture of OA and UA compared to 65.62% with PLGA NPs. Advantageously, in vitro exposure to these nanoparticles in HepG2 and Caco-2, colon and hepatic cells, showed the absence of systemic toxicity, highlighting their potential as oral dosage forms [52]. Zhuang et al. (2021) exposed carboplatin-loaded, sodium alginate (SA) surface-modified PLGA NPs to Y79 cells in vitro, which highlighted the benefits of SA when it comes to cellular uptake and the pace of drug delivery. The PLGA NPs were round, with a mean size of 253.94 ± 66.53 nm and a Zeta potential of around −43.1 ± 8.1 mV. The burst release of CRB was examined at 24 h and was 18.86% ± 4.3% and 40.01% ± 8.2% for PLGA NPs with and without SA, respectively. Analysis of the inhibitory effect on Y79 cell viability showed that PLGA NPs with SA exhibited higher effects at all concentrations and times compared to SA-absent PLGA NPs. Their future incentives include in vivo topical administration of their engineered NP as a treatment comparable to intravitreal drug delivery and its side effects [53]. Based on these studies, there exists an endless possibility of combinations of types of polymers, drugs, and surface modification. The therapeutic results of each variable are yet to be understood. For instance, Sims et al. (2019) tested melphalan-loaded PLGA NPs with various surface modifiers, and only the Tet Methylcytosine Dioxygenase 1 (TET1) and Methoxy Polyethylene Glycol (MPG) groups demonstrated improved efficacy relative to unmodified NPs. MPG-modified NPs had a diameter of 129 ± 38 nm, and TET1 had a diameter of 123 ± 33 nm. Melphalan loading at 1 mg/mL saturated batches in MPG and TET1 NPs showed statistically significant differences: 135.7 ± 7.8 and 212.7 ± 4.5 μg melphalan per NP, respectively. The IC_{50} values of MPG and TET1 were 0.35 ± 0.06 and 0.23 ± 0.04 mg NP/mL, respectively, and they differed in binding patters, with MPG PLGA NPs having the highest level of cell internalization after 1.5 h compared to the TET1-modified group, which only increased after 24 h. These results demonstrate the impact of surface modifications on the changing physiology of NPs [23]. Likewise, when synthesizing a nanoparticle, it is important to consider the trade-offs between positively and negatively charged carriers, respectively, to improve internalization and distribution. Lastly, the size of NPs is an important factor when considering leakage through important biological barriers, which could cause systemic toxicity [51]. Hence, there exists a strong need for investigation into the optimized structures of nanoparticles and their modifiable factors to highlight the ideal combinations specific for treating retinoblastoma. Finally, chitosan-derived nanoparticles are a sub-type of polymeric NPs and have been investigated to overcome the administration challenges with natural chitosan, which is insoluble in neutral media. Comparative studies between N-trimethyl chitosan (TMC) and thiolated chitosan (TC)—the derivatives of chitosan—highlighted the superiority of thiolated chitosan nanoparticles (TCs-NPs). In fact, Delrish et al. (2021) believed that chitosan nanoparticles could address the barriers of effective intravitreal delivery of topotecan hydrochloride (TPH) in treating RB and aimed at comparing the effectiveness between topotecan-loaded N-trimethyl chitosan nanoparticles (TPH-TMCs-NPs) and TPH-TCs-NPs in addressing these obstacles, such as controlled drug delivery and poor cellular uptake. TPH-TMCs-NPs and TPH-TC-NPs were both spherical in shape but had different sizes (39 $\pm$ 3, 25 $\pm$ 2 nm), Zeta potentials (38 $\pm$ 3, 12 $\pm$ 2 mV), and EE (73.34 $\pm$ 2, 85.23 $\pm$ 2%). The difference in these properties reflected different outcomes in xenograft models intravitreally injected with Y79 cells, where TPH-TC-NPs exhibited 90% tumor necrosis compared to TPH-TMCs-NPs (20%) and free TPH (15%) It is hypothesized that TPH-TCs-NPs showed superior cellular uptake and cytotoxicity and allowed for penetration of the vitreous due to their small size, low anionic, and small Zeta potential (12 $\pm$ 2 mV), which allowed them to efficaciously penetrate the vitreous humor compared to the latter, which had a higher Zeta potential [54]. Following this discovery, Delrish et al. (2022) engineered carboxymethyl dextran (CMD)-TMCs-NPs with a surface charge of 29 $\pm$ 4.31 mV and CMD-TC-NPs with a charge of 11 $\pm$ 2.27 mV. The diameters of these chitosan NPs were 42 $\pm$ 4.23 and 34 $\pm$ 3.78 nm, respectively. They assessed the biodistribution of these NPs in xenograft mouse models previously injected with Y79 cells and highlighted once again the effect of surface charge of NPs on post-intravitreal diffusion to the retina. CMD-TMCs-NPs were completely immobilized due to their highly positive charge [55]. Recently, Ghassemi et al. (2023) combined all these findings to synthesize TPH-CMD-TCS-NPs. Combining TPH drug therapy, CMD for improved NP stability, and TCS as a vehicle for delivery, they were spherical in shape, with a size, PDI, Zeta potential, and IC_{50} of 30 $\pm$ 4 nm, 0.24 $\pm$ 0.03, 10 $\pm$ 3 mV, 40.40, respectively. In vivo studies in rabbit xenograft models demonstrated a significant decrease in rabbit tumor volume seven days after injection, highlighted by 91 $\pm$ 2% tumor necrosis. Additionally, no histological retinal deformities were found, suggesting an alternative anti-tumor treatment with low toxicity [56].

4.2.2. Lipid Nanoparticles

Lipid-based NPs (LNPs) are appealing due to their biocompatibility, degradability, scale-up capacity, and possibility of delivering hydrophilic and lipophilic drugs specifically, such as etoposide—a lipophilic medication used as chemotherapy in treating retinoblastoma. There exist numerous kinds of lipid NPs, varying from liposome-based, solid-lipid-based (SLNs) to nanostructured lipid carriers (NCLs), which are composed of a mix of solid and liquid lipids [57]. Ahmad et al. (2019) highlighted the variable features of lipid NPs based on the nature of the lipid matrix, its concentration, and particle size. For example, lipid concentration plays an important role in entrapment efficiency (EE) and particle size. Based on this, they engineered an optimized LNP, with a particle size, polydispersity index (PDI), and EE of 239.43 $\pm$ 2.35 nm, 0.261 $\pm$ 0.001, and 80.96 $\pm$ 2.21%, respectively. In vitro drug release studies comparing free etoposide and etoposide loaded in the optimized lipid NP demonstrated biphasic and slow release in the latter—75.74% $\pm$ 1.56 after 48 h—compared to the near total release of the free drug after 16 h. This finding also supports the sustained vitreous concentration of etoposide following intravitreal administration of the lipid NP in enucleated mouse eyes. The NPs also allowed for sustained release of etoposide for at least seven days compared to a trace amount of the free drug after the second day [58]. Marathe et al. (2022) studied a α-tocopherol succinate (αTS)-based nanostructured lipid carriers (NCLs) to overcome the poor aqueous solubility of paclitaxel (PTX). This study highlighted the importance of considering the solid and liquid lipid ratio depending on the loaded drug and its properties, as this parameter can greatly influence the parameters of NLCs, such as size. Their optimized NLCs had a size, PDI, and Zeta potential of 186.2 ± 3.9 nm, 0.17 ± 0.03, and −33.2 ± 1.3 mV, respectively. Marathe et al. further developed on the importance of variables when constructing a NP by evaluating its stability over 60 days. NLCs containing polyethylene glycol (PEG) NLCs demonstrated higher stability in terms of particle size, PDI, and Zeta potential compared to pure NLCs, suggesting an alteration in the physiochemical properties of NLCs after PEGylation. Drug release reached a maximum of 40% and plateaued until the end of the study at 48 h compared to 67% for the PEG NLCs [59]. Both studies have underlined the potential lipid nanoparticle structural changes possible when altering the variables. When looking at a combination therapy of genetic therapy and drug delivery, Tabatabaei et al. (2019) fabricated spherical, switchable LNPs containing melphalan and miR-181a with a size of 171 ± 4 nm, Zeta potential of 24.5 ± 0.7 mV, and PDI of 0.13 ± 0.04. The switchable LNPs allowed for conformation change and endosomal escape at acidic pH. The EE of melphalan and miR-181a were 93.0% ± 0.2 and 97.5% ± 0.7, respectively. They concluded that the delivery of dual-loaded LNPs containing melphalan and miR-181a resulted in amplified effects compared to both being delivered separately. For instance, LNPs containing miR-181a alone resulted in 37% reduction in Y79 cells compared to 72% when delivering LNPs containing both miR-181a and melphalan in in vivo treatments of mouse vitreous [60]. Conversely, Gibson et al. (2020) manufactured switchable LNPs containing siRNA. Use of the extrusion method yielded LNPs with a size of 162 ± 1 nm, Zeta potential of 31.6 ± 1.0 mV, and PDI of 0.135 ± 0.03. These siRNA LNPs targeting survivin sequential to chemotherapy increased the therapeutic effects of melphalan and carboplatin, with survivin being resistant to the drugs before its downregulation. Further, survivin silencing before chemotherapy allows for retained effectiveness at a lower dose, reducing its potentially toxic effects. Indeed, survivin silencing allowed for melphalan and topotecan IC_{50} to be reduced by 77%. As an illustration, treatment of Y79 cells using 30 μM of CRB and 0.25 μM of topotecan following survivin pre-treatment was necessary for 50% cell viability compared with 191 μM and 0.5 μM, respectively, when used individually in the absence of miR-181a [61]. Finally, still on the topic of synergistic effects, Wang et al. (2023) investigated the co-delivery of melphalan and black phosphorus quantum dots (BPQDs) dually loaded in LNPs for photothermal therapy. These spherical LNPs were 82–180 nm in diameter, with a PDI of 0.15–0.16, EE of 40%, and 43.7% for melphalan and BPQDs, respectively. In vivo studies in mouse xenograft models inoculated with WERI-RB-1 cells revealed that co-loaded LNPs showed an inhibitory effect of 65% compared to melphalan alone (51%) on tumor proliferation. One interesting finding is that free BPQDs were more cytotoxic than those loaded in nanoparticles, which is optimal for mitigating their toxic side effects, such as nephrotoxicity. In fact, BPQDs alone induced the highest inhibitory effect, at 79%, but they showed the highest ki67 levels, which were reduced in co-loaded LNPs [62,63]. As mentioned previously, ongoing research to optimize the formulation of LNPs only or within a combination therapy is needed to better understand the characteristics and changes in the structure and function, which loading of different elements may cause. For example, as previously discussed, Tabatabaei et al. (2019) highlighted that incorporation of miR-181a reduced the surface charge of LNPs from 40.4 ± 8.2 to 24.5 ± 0.7 mV but maintained their cationic properties [60]. Dual loading of elements can also cause incompatibility or tissue toxicity, hence the importance of interaction analysis before delivery. Indeed, Gibson et al. (2020) showed that all drugs have different properties, and the targeting of survivin silencing did not enhance the therapeutic potential of Teniposide compared to other drugs, such as carboplatin, suggesting a different intracellular mechanism of this drug [61].

4.2.3. Protein Nanoparticles

As with lipid nanoparticles, protein NPs can be generated using various building blocks, such as albumin and lipoprotein, and they have advantages in their preparation, where toxic chemicals can be omitted. They are also stable, cost-effective, and have high loading capacity [64]. Moreover, proteins are amphiphilic, allowing for interactions with hydrophilic and hydrophobic drugs, and their abundance in charged groups enables various chemical modifications, such as surface-modified targeting properties [65]. Therefore, their high loading capacity and selective targeting capabilities can allow for optimal cancerous cell uptake. In fact, cancer stem cells—which are found in both primary RB and Y79 cells—have chemoresistant properties, since they induce cell arrest, while chemotherapy targets proliferating cells [66–69]. Narayana et al. (2021) produced lactoferrin protein nanoparticles (LFNPs)—targeting the prominent lactoferrin (LF) receptors in tumor cells due to increased iron demand—to treat retinoblastoma and mitigate chemoresistance to carboplatin (CRB) and etoposide (ETP). LFNPs containing CRB (CRB-LFNPs) and those containing ETP (ETP-LFNPs) had dimensions and EE of 61.2 nm, 60%, and 45.15 nm, 38%. They found that LF-CRB and LF-ETP displayed increased cellular uptake, retention, and cytotoxicity compared to their free drug counterparts and that the release of NP content was highest at pH 6. As an illustration, the analysis of the drug effect on Y79 cell population yielded free CRB IC_{50} of 230.3 compared to 118.2 for CRB-LFNPs. Moreover, the free CRB uptake was 9.99 $\mu g/10^6$, with drug retention at 15.46% after 48 h compared to CRB-LFNPs, where drug uptake and retention were higher (17.38 $\mu g/10^6$ and 54.43%). Similar trends were observed when comparing free ETP and those loaded in LFNPs. Their experiments centered on cancer stem cells (CSCs) due to their characteristic feature of drug resistance. The increased cytotoxicity of these LFNPs on Y79 CSCs offers promising potential in targeting the drug resistance of CSCs. It is worth evaluating the possibility of dual drug loading or sequential NP delivery of both CPT and ETP for potential synergistic properties [65]. The optimal results in vitro may be translated to future in vivo experiments.

4.2.4. Nanomicelles

These nanoparticles are structured with amphiphilic monomers, hydrophobic heads, and hydrophilic tails, permitting high hydrophobic drug loading, stability, and solubility [70]. Curcumin's hydrophobic nature, poor bioavailability, and rapid degradation have pushed for the discovery of curcumin analog alternatives, such as 3,4-difluorobenzylidene curcumin (CDF), to address these issues [71]. Alsaab et al. (2017) constructed amphiphilic poly(styrene-co-maleic acid)-conjugated-folic-acid (SMA-FA) CDF nanomicelles to enhance the targeting ability of the hydrophobic drug in the hopes of reducing the therapeutic levels of chemotherapeutic agents, which often lead to toxicity when present at high levels. The spherical nanomicelle had a size, PDI, Zeta potential, and EE of 193.6 $\pm$ 20 nm, 0.175 $\pm$ 0.05, –7.12 $\pm$ 4 mV, and 75.98 $\pm$ 12%, respectively. The targeting formulation allowed for higher therapeutic activity in Y79 cells, as reflected by a smaller IC50 of 1.02 $\pm$ 0.55 μM compared to 4 $\pm$ 1.64 μM for non-targeting NPs (i.e., nanomicelles without folic acid). However, such trend was not found in WERI-RB1 cells due to their lower folate receptor expression. Nonetheless, these targeting nanomicelles result in increased cytotoxicity due to higher internalization of the drug. This delivery method can help address the conventional use of high concentrations of chemotherapeutics due to poor retinal uptake of the free drug [72]. These results could perhaps be translated to natural curcumin, addressing its degradation and bioavailability challenges. Celastrol, a Chinese herbal medicine, is a topic of interest within nanomicelles. This bioactive component has previously shown potential in chronic inflammatory or auto-immune diseases, as well as anti-cancer characteristics [73]. Li et al. (2020) sought to invent a novel method of treating angiogenesis-mediated retinoblastoma using celastrol-loaded polymeric nanomicelle (CNM) and addressing the poor water solubility of the herbal medicine. These CNMs had a spherical shape with a diameter of 48 nm, with a celastrol loading content of 7.36%, and they exhibited controlled release. In vitro studies on chick embryo chorioallantoic membrane assays (CAM) demonstrated positive results, inhibiting vascular formation in a concentration-dependent manner. Following intraperitoneal injection in xenograft mouse models with SO-RB50 cells, similar optimal results were found. Following recurrent administration of 27.2 mg/kg CNMs for 16 days, significant tumor suppression was observed. The average tumor weight was 61.40 ± 20.82 mg compared to the control, while the change in body weight was omitted. CNMs inhibit the vascular endothelial growth factor A (VEGF-A) pathway, which is critical in angiogenesis and prevents endothelial cell migration. This novel therapeutic model demonstrates potential in inhibiting angiogenesis-specific RB, with the opportunity to be studied in other angiogenesis-based ocular pathologies, such as retinopathy of prematurity [74]. Still on the topic of celastrol, Guo et al. (2021) set to design a redox-sensitive nanomicelle (RSNM) for tumor-targeted celastrol delivery. Their reduction-sensitive grafted copolymer poly[thioctic acid-grafted-poly(ethylene glycol)/(benzylamine)] nanomicelles were spherical, with a size of 70 nm and a celastrol loading of 8.51%. RSNMs and drug release occurred in lysosomal reduction environments. The cellular uptake in Y79 cells in vitro was rapid and was observed just 10 min following incubation of RSNMs, with celastrol migration to the nuclear contents of cells within 1 h and proliferation inhibition within 4 h. The controlled release in response to tumor microenvironments is beneficial for apoptosis due to its time-dependent properties. Further analysis concluded that celastrol does this through caspase-9 and caspase-3 activation within RB Y79 cells [75]. Studies comparing these reduction-sensitive nanomicelles and the targeting properties of (SMA-FA)-CDF could offer insights into the benefits and challenges of both enhancers. Furthermore, the revelation of celastrol's effect on apoptotic and VEGF-A pathways highlights its various mechanisms of action, which can be used selectively.

Figure 3 illustrates the common methods of drug delivery, including those discussed in this section, such as intravitreal and topical delivery.

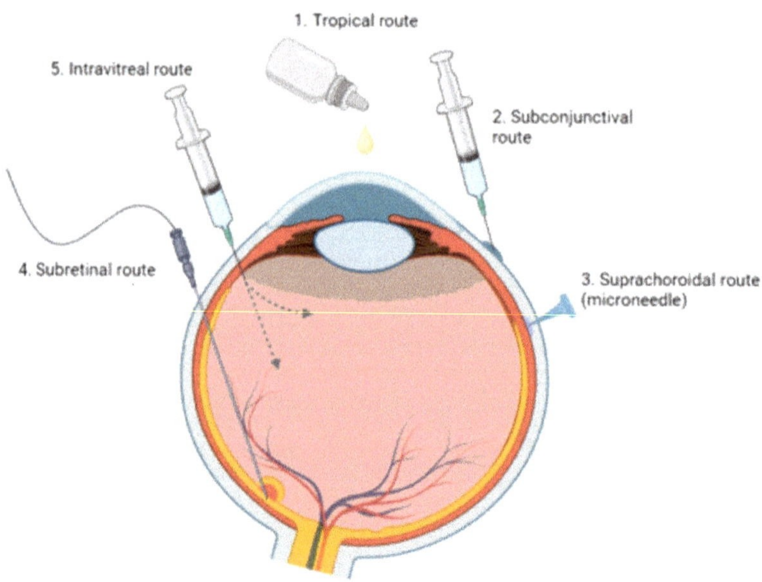

Figure 3. Ophthalmic medication delivery routes. This illustration features five modes of delivery, including topical, subconjunctival, suprachoroidal, subretinal, and intravitreal methods.

5. Clinical Barriers and Future Perspectives

5.1. Trends

5.1.1. Smart Release of Nanoparticle Contents

As mentioned previously, the release of nanoparticle contents can be triggered by an environmental change, such as acidic pH within tumor cells [27,37,60]. This enables a targeted release, diminishing the potential risk of cytotoxicity in healthy cells. Likewise, Long et al. (2021) synthesized a green-light-responsive nanocarrier to overcome the inner blood–retinal barrier, which intravitreally injected drugs face (Figure 2). Clathrin-like trigonal molecules loaded with doxorubicin had a size of 99.04 nm, with a Zeta potential, PDI, and EE of −25.10 mV, 0.10–0.15, and 13.6%. In a constructed in vitro inner BRB model, they compared the amount of DOX found across the endothelial monolayer from DOX-loaded non-irradiated nanoparticles (20%) and irradiated nanoparticles (50%), highlighting the increased extravasation following the release of DOX. This is due to DOX having a smaller size and hydrophobicity, allowing it to cross the layer with ease compared to the NP complex. Additionally, free drug injections in WERI-RB-1-cell-bearing mice caused a 10% loss in body weight due to systemic toxicity, whereas this was not the case within the nanoparticle group following intravitreal injection. This method is unique, as it benefits from the properties of both NPs and DOX for optimal drug delivery. NPs are a vehicle for bringing DOX closer to its site of action, avoiding its rapid elimination via the intravenous route, until it reaches the BRB, where it is too large to cross the barrier. The drug is then freed from its vehicle to arrive at its site of action [76]. This therapeutic element demonstrates great potential even beyond retinoblastoma, as it can be applied to any disease site reachable by the green light but not by NPs. Nonetheless, there remains a need for more research studies on this subject, especially long-term toxicity follow-ups, to ensure safety before clinical experimentations.

5.1.2. Surface Receptor Targeting Nanoparticles

It has been proven that retinoblastoma cells, among other cancerous cells, have modified physical properties and biological demands. Previous studies have synthesized lactoferrin nanoparticles to target the enhanced LF receptors on tumor cells, including Y79 cells. This characteristic is a result of increased iron demand in the rapidly dividing cancerous cells [77]. Folate-coated nanoparticles targeting RB cells through their increased folate receptors have also been widely studied, showing enhanced cellular uptake compared to their unconjugated counterparts [34,72]. Combining RB cells' increased demand for iron and folate receptors, Sadri et al. engineered a nanoparticle with dual-targeting properties conjugated with folic acid and transferrin, which physiologically facilitates uptake in cancer cells. These oleic acid (OA)-coated superparamagnetic iron oxide NPs (SPIONs) were loaded with Vincristine (VCR), were spherical, and had the dimension, Zeta potential, loading capacity, and EE of 82.1 nm, 25.0 mV, 8.7%, and 87.15%. This study was able to highlight increased cellular uptake within Y79 RB cells compared to healthy ARPE-19 in vitro, suggesting the positive effect of dual receptors. This was supported by the IC50 value of the free drug (10.61) compared to that of the SPIONs (4.87) in Y79 cells [78]. However, there is a lack of direct comparison between mono-targeting NPs and dual-targeting NPs to illustrate the extent of their benefits. Finally, RB cells are known to express sugar receptors, with special affinity for galactose and mannose [79]. Although many studies have demonstrated positive effects in terms of the uptake and cytotoxicity of sugar-modified NPs, potential research comparing folate, sugar, and LF receptors can allow for a better understanding of their unique properties. In summary, these various targeting receptors all demonstrated optimistic results in cancerous cell targeting, which in turn increased cellular uptake and cytotoxicity while minimizing toxicity to other untargeted cells due to lower affinity.

5.1.3. Multi-Functional Nanoparticles

Similar to a combination therapy—where systemic chemotherapy in addition to focal therapy is used to treat retinoblastoma—a nanoparticle can be engineered to have more than one mechanism of action at a tumor site. For example, Zou et al. (2022) experimented with tuftsin-loaded carbonized metal–organic framework (CMT) NPs with a Zeta potential of −12.1 mV and a size of 303.1 ± 48.53 nm. These CMT NPs were superparamagnetic in nature following carbonization, enabling tumor targeting under a magnetic field. This is different from the receptor targeting discussed previously, which is mainly used to bring the drug to its site of action and could present an alternative to complex environments lacking target-specific receptors. These NPs showed adequate and stable thermal conversion (27.08%), allowing for photothermal therapy (PTT). The loading of tuftsin enabled immunotherapeutic effects by inducing macrophage typing. The subsequent laser irradiation of CMT NPs allowed for tuftsin stimulation of in vitro macrophages close to the level of free-drug-treated cells. This was reflected by the high levels of positive CD16/32 cells (33.13 ± 0.23%) in the CMT NP group. In vivo inoculation of tumor-bearing mice highlighted the synergistic effect of PTT and immunotherapy compared to laser alone or a combination of laser and NPs in the absence of tuftsin. Laser and CMT NPs combined allowed for a gradual decrease in tumor size and resulted in the highest rate of volume suppression, illustrated by their low and gradually decreasing relative tumor volume curve in relation to their counterparts. In addition, CMT NPs enabled easy follow-up of treatment efficiency by acting as excellent dual-modal imaging contracts for photoacoustic (PA) and T2-weighted MRI imaging, with the PA signal peaking at 4 h in the tumor region and remaining in the tumor-bearing mouse models of Y79 for up to 24 h. In short, these nanoparticles are multi-functional, with both therapeutic and imaging properties [80]. Analogously, Zheng et al. (2022) demonstrated the benefits of selective-loading NPs with dual-function elements, allowing for a nanoparticle capable of synergistic PDT and PTT effects with ultrasound (US)/PA/MRI imaging potential while simultaneously enhancing cellular uptake due to dual-targeting surface receptors. Folate/magnetic dual-target cationic nanoliposomes with a size of 338.63 ± 10.90 nm and Zeta potential of 31.86 ± 3.49 mV were loaded with indocyanine green (ICG), perfluorohexane (PFH), and Fe_3O_4. In vitro studies on Y79 cells comparing mono- and dual-target NPs highlighted that dual-target NPs reached saturation first at 3 h compared to the other groups, which reached saturation of less than 50% by the same time. Importantly, ICG can display both PTT and PDT effects upon stimulation from the same laser, although its PDT effect is mild due to the hypoxic environment of tumors. The incorporation of PFH, which increases O_2 in the hypoxic environment, enhanced the effect of PDT, a therapy dependent on the presence of oxygen. ROS produced by NPs containing PFH was 6.15 times higher than that produced by NPs in the absence of PFH. Furthermore, the in vivo performance of these nanoparticles in Y79-bearing mice showed the most optimal anti-cancer effect ($p < 0.0001$), as the presence of PFH allowed for the synergistic effect of PTT and PDT [81]. Mudigunda et al. (2022) created Palbociclib (PCB) and near-infrared (NIR)-dye-loaded hybrid (PLGA and PCL) polymeric NPs (PNPs) for the combined PCB and PTT effect. The NPs had a size of 176 ± 43.8, PDI of 0.240, and EE of 80 and 81.5 for PCB and IR, respectively. The in vitro effects on Y79 cells were optimistic, where PCB-IR-PNPs demonstrated the highest inhibitory activity, with 86.5 ± 2.3% cell death compared to free PCB and IR groups (62.5 ± 0.4 and 54.8 ± 6.9% viable cells). Finally, no acute (14 days) toxicity was documented [82]. Wu et al. (2018) utilized laser irradiation as a means of triggering gene transfection, and taking advantage of the targeting properties of FA, they built FA-surface-modified, PFP-, ICG-loaded, and plasmid-DNA-carrying LNPs with laser activation of gene therapy and imaging properties. They had a diameter, Zeta potential, and ICG EE of 328.4 ± 5.5 nm, 35.3 ± 1.9 mV, and 92.1 ± 1.3%. The cationic property of NPs allowed for enhanced plasmid binding of 22.7 ± 0.1 μg compared to 1.4 ± 0.4 μg in neutral NPs. The enhancement of gene transfection is believed to result from laser-mediated liquid-to-gas transition of the NPs, causing a cavitation effect and increased cellular permeability. In both in vitro (Y79) and in vivo (Y79) studies, FA-modified cationic LNPs exhibited enhanced therapeutic effects compared to FA-absent or neutral LNPs. In vivo PA imaging was superior in FA-conjugated cationic LNPs at all time points. At 12 h following injection, all PA values decreased, with FA-conjugated LNPs remaining the highest, slightly below 3 a.u. Finally, it is important to note that the in vivo studies were performed on nude mice with right hind limb subcutaneously implanted tumors, which does not reflect the microenvironment and physiological properties of the eye [83]. Compared to the previously discussed experiments, natural elements, such as Moringa oleifera (MO), display similar synergistic potential in PTT and cytotoxic effects, with potential in photoacoustic imaging due to the fluorescent properties of chlorophyll derivatives within MO. Indeed, Mudigunda et al. (2023) prepared MO and IR encapsulated PCL NPs, which were spherical, cationic, and 160–220 nm in size. PPT induced cytotoxicity in Y79 cells in vitro, causing cell death of 50% in the IR group in the absence of MO compared to 80% in the IR+MO group following light induction [84]. Finally, Wang et al. (2020) identified NPs with low intensity focused ultrasound therapy (LIFU), imaging, and immunotherapy potential using muramyl dipeptide (MDP) and perfluorobutane (PFP) encapsulated in magnetic hollow mesoporous gold nanocages conjugated with iron oxide NPs (AuNC−Fe_3O_4/MDP/PFP NPs). The former is an immunomodulator, and the latter provides an ultrasound contrast and synergistic effect with the presence of LIFU. They had a size of 159.3 nm, Zeta potential of −15.8 mV, and EE of 82.60 ± 2.07 and 27.11 ± 1.20 for MDP and Fe_3O_4, respectively. These NPs were found to release MDP rapidly following LIFU irradiation and activated dendritic cells (DCs). Moreover, the NPs were safe and had no toxic effect on the ARPE-19 or Y79 cells in the absence of LIFU at concentrations as high as 400 μg/mL. In vitro cytotoxic studies of LIFU indicated that the presence of PFP is integral to high treatment efficacy due to its role in acoustic energy aggregation following liquid–gas transition. In vivo testing on Y79-subcutaneous-flank-tumor-bearing mice highlighted the superiority of LIFU and AuNC−Fe_3O_4/MDP/PFP NPs, as they resulted in the highest apoptotic index and lowest proliferative index compared to their counterparts. Weight, hematoxylin and eosin (H&E) stain hematology parameters, and blood chemistry failed to detect toxicity [85]. There exist numerous approaches to achieving certain additional functions of NPs—for example, imaging using biological MO, CMT NPs, or ICG. Despite the increasing multi-functionality of NPs, with these complex combinations comes the risk of consequential interactions and potential toxicity to adjacent organs.

5.2. *Barriers of Nanoparticles in Retinoblastoma*

5.2.1. Long-Term Toxicity and Lack of Clinical Studies

Most studies on NPs in retinoblastoma have shown the absence of toxicity within nanoparticle-treated RB cells or tumors despite enhanced therapeutic effects. Histology was the main modality in evaluating toxicity in mouse models, with most reflecting impeccable retinas [56]. Mice were also weighed for potential signs of toxicity, identifying an absence of general weight loss [74,76,82]. Despite this, there is a lack of long-term follow-up for signs of toxicity. In fact, most studies only verify the absence of acute toxicity, which is observed for a few days to weeks. For example, two studies measured weight, blood samples, biochemistry tests, and H&E staining up to 14 days after injection of nanoparticles, but they were not followed up thereafter [85,86]. In vitro studies have also reported findings of an accumulation of CMT NPs and LNPs in the liver and spleen of tumor-bearing mice through fluorescence analysis, although this is hypothesized to be a normal physiological process of NP phagocytosis via the reticuloendothelial system present in both organs [80,87]. This uncertainty perhaps plays a part in hindering the advancement in RB NP research. Indeed, most studies were either performed in vitro on Y79 cells or in vivo in xenografted animal models, with some of the inoculated tumors inoculated in areas other than the eye, moving away from the ideal microenvironment. Long-term in vitro and in vivo follow-up will significantly solidify our understanding of the effects of these novel therapeutics before moving to clinical studies with RB patients.

5.2.2. Exploration of Common Variables

The engineering of unique nanoparticles requires choosing the type of NP, conjugation, loading, embedding, and synthesis method, making the possibility of combinations endless. As mentioned previously, Delrish et al. (2022) demonstrated the impact of a molecular change on the nanoparticle's overall function. Comparing TC (11 ± 2.27 mV) and TMC NPs (29 ± 4.31 mV), TMC NPs were unable to cross the vitreous to the retina due to the methylation of chitosan and overall positive charge, supporting the hypothesis that surface charge is the limiting factor relating to intravitreal injections reaching their designated site of action [55]. With emerging multi-functional NPs, an additional selection of elements with unique properties is added, such as near-infrared (NIR) and MDP for photothermal and immune properties, respectively. The multiple variables playing a role in the synthesis of NPs warrant the development of unique nanoparticles. In return, the focus can easily be weighted toward novel research rather than supporting research, which improves our understanding of already designed nanoparticles and the potential for enhancing their properties. Figure 4 illustrates the ideal properties of a NP for drug delivery [88].

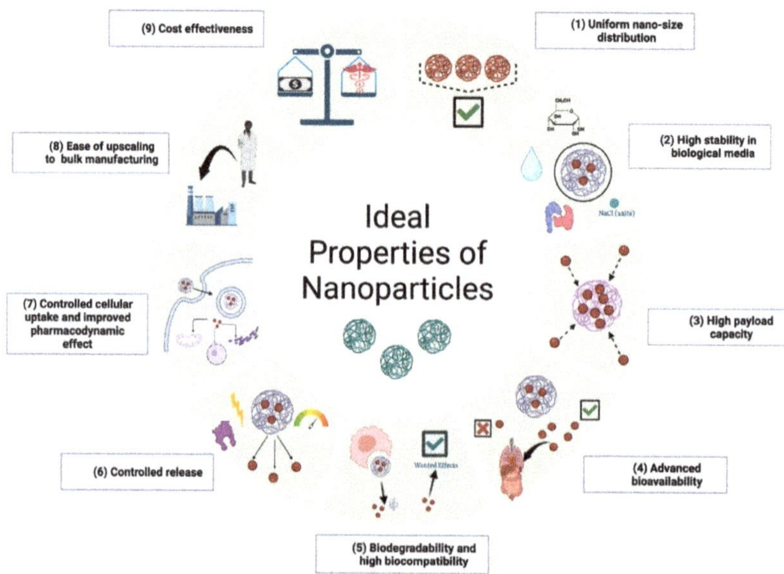

Figure 4. Ideal characteristics of nanostructures as drug delivery systems.

5.3. Future Perspectives

Oncolytic virus (OV) therapy is an emerging method of therapeutics consisting of modifying viruses and transfecting them into tumor cells, with some directly killing the cell while others being able to trigger the host's immune system to fight the cancerous cells, with the potential of treating chemoresistant RB. Popular OVs include herpes virus and adenovirus [89]. Pascual-Pasto (2019) et al. studied the oncolytic adenovirus VCN-01 in targeting chemoresistant RB. This OV targets the altered RB1-E2F pathway causing cancerous cells to dysregulate the cell cycle, leading to uncontrolled proliferation. Through intravitreal injections in mouse Y79 xenograft models, this method induced tumor necrosis and ocular survival and increasing survival following a single intravitreal dose ($p = 0.0002$). Despite this, 2 out of 12 treated mice had detectable viral genome in the plasma 4 h after injection and in the brain tissue. Low systemic dissemination in the liver of rabbit models at day 3 was also observed. Clinical studies on two patients with RB, which was chemo- and radiotherapy-resistant, demonstrated intravitreal inflammation, leading to one participant undergoing enucleation. The second patient demonstrated anti-tumor response, with a reduction in the size and amount of tumoral vitreous seeds, although the size of retinal tumor remained unchanged [90]. Targeting nanoparticles may be able to improve the therapeutic capacity of these OVs and diminish systemic complications, bridging the barrier between OV and RB therapy. Likewise, gene therapy is an emerging therapeutic modality, although the delivery of vectors remains a barrier due to the negative charge, high molecular weight, and hydrophilicity of non-viral vectors in particular [91]. Therefore, Gao et al. (2023) developed an eye drop containing polyamidoamine (PAMAM)—a polyplex—embedded with small interference RNA (siRNA) to achieve gene silencing in orthotopic WERI-RB-1 nude mouse models and overcome the challenges of vector delivery to the posterior segment of the eye. Q8W and N9W-penetratin (89WP)—an absorption enhancer—were added to enhance the efficacy of topical delivery. The spherical particles were 200 nm in size, with a Zeta potential of 30 mV. In vitro experimentation on ARPE-19 and WERI-RB-1 cells highlighted the difficult internalization of free siRNA due to its high molecular weight and other characteristics. Use of PAMAM as a vehicle allowed for 3% and 20% uptake by both cell lines, respectively. The addition of 89WP increased the uptake in WERI-RB-1 cells by 90%. In vivo studies showed similar trends, namely that the polyplex reached the retina 2 h after treatment and remained there for 6 h, spotlighting the benefit of 89WP PAMAM in ocular delivery of non-viral vectors [92]. Their findings pave the way for analysis of various types of nanoparticles (e.g., gold, iron, mesoporous silica NPs) for delivering gene therapy to find appropriate NPs, which can effectively package, load, and compress siRNA [93]. Specifically, nucleic-acid-based NPs are also a point of discussion. Although not explored extensively in retinoblastoma, Wang et al. (2024) recently experimented with spherical nucleic acid (SNA) NPs to deliver siRNA. These SNA NPs with a dense DNA shell contain aptamers, targeting disialoganglioside (GD2) positive RB cells, and are loaded with siRNA and the inhibitor NVP-CGM097. These structures were 20 nm in diameter, and their loading efficiency ranged from 38.09 to 39.76%. The SNA NPs were also stable at room temperature for over 72 h. The in vitro binding capacity in Y79 and WERI-RB-1 cells was 89.2 and 87.4%, and the synergistic effect of siRNA targeting mouse double minute 2 homolog (MDM2)-mRNA transcription and NVP-CGM097 targeting MDM2 resulted in an inhibitory effect of 80.76% in Y79 cells, which was less than melphalan at 90.37%. However, in vivo studies on Y79 and WERI-RB-1 xenograft nude mouse models demonstrated that the SNA NPs caused less retinal damage than melphalan. Retinal thickness was noticeably reduced by melphalan, and the thickness only recovered on day 21 compared to a milder reduction and rapid recovery on day 14 in the SNA NP groups [94]. Compared to siRNA, DNA therapeutic agents are more stable and have a higher degradation resistance, making them potential candidates for RB treatment [95]. On the topic of nucleic acid NPs, Hu et al. (2024) developed aptamer-modified manganese dioxide (MnO_2) nanosponge cores (hMNs), absorbing two DNAzyme agents. Aptamer was added for targeting properties toward nucleolin-overexpressed RB, shown by the increased uptake of the NPs in Y79 cells in vitro compared to healthy APRE-19 cells. The NPs were spherical, with a diameter of 200 nm and Zeta potential of -17.50 ± 2.00 mV. In vivo injection into Y79 xenograft nude mouse tumors illustrated the enhanced effect of aptamer. On day 14, the tumor volume of aptamer-modified NPs was 210.80 ± 17.84 mm^3 compared to 338.68 ± 58.17 mm^3 in the NP group without aptamer and 565.95 ± 47.63 mm^3 in the control group [96]. To conclude, there is potential for DNA in aiding the construction of nanoparticles and for DNAzyme therapy, but there remains a need for concrete experiments evaluating the aforementioned DNA and siRNA. Additionally, our understanding of the role of DNA in engineering NPs for retinoblastoma remains unclear, with few studies focusing on its potential effect.

Moving away from therapeutics, the conventional monitoring of disease consists of a mix of fundus and histological examinations, and imaging, among others, which are limited by cost and resources. Liu et al. synthesized NPs using trisodium citrate dihydrate and ferric chloride hexahydrate for an RB monitoring platform via machine learning of aqueous humor metabolic fingerprinting using NP-enhanced laser desorption/ionization, demonstrating the potential of NPs beyond therapeutic application in retinoblastoma [97].

Table 2 summarizes the characteristics, features, and stage of research of the nanoparticles discussed in Sections 4 and 5.

Table 2. Nanoparticles in retinoblastoma.

Nanocarrier	Function	Characteristics	Observations	Stage	Reference
GNPs	Target MDMX degradation	- Peptide-derived MG loaded - PSI coated	- PSI optimized blood circulation time - PH-dependent internalization optimal in cancer cells - Clearable through mononuclear phagocytic system - Absence of acute toxicity, no changes in weight, biochemical index of blood, or pathological findings	WERI-RB-1 cells in vitro, intravitreal orthotopic xenograft retinoblastoma mouse model in vivo, PDX model of pancreatic carcinoma in vivo	[27]
	Inhibit p53-HDM2	- Anti-HDM2 peptide loaded	- Cell arrest at G2M phase and increased apoptosis - Optimal cell internalization - NPs increased the stability and avoided degradation of the peptide	Y79 cells in vitro	[28]
	Laser-induced cell disruption	N/A	- NPs bubble when exposed to heat, causing cell membrane disruption - In vitro NPs attachment to cells is heterogenous - Vitreous body advantageous for treatment - Absent regeneration at 40 J cm^{-2} or more - Successful irradiation of cells and cell aggregates	Y79 cells in vitro and vitreous phantom	[29]
	Ultrasonic hyperthermia	N/A	- Ultrasonic waves allow for focused targeting - Cytotoxicity is proportional to hyperthermia time - Acoustic cavitation effect - Synergistic effect present	Y79 cells in vitro	[30]
	Ultrasound hyperthermia	- Evaluation of the synergistic effect of brachytherapy, ultrasound hyperthermia, and gold nanoparticles	- Combination group showed greatest inhibition of tumor growth - Combination group showed more adverse effects - Retinal gliosis and scarring were found - Need for therapeutic planning	RB-induced rabbit cells in vivo	[31]

Table 2. *Cont.*

Nanocarrier	Function	Characteristics	Observations	Stage	Reference
GNPs	Imaging, LIFU, and immunotherapy	- MDP, PFP loaded	- Fe_3O_4 magnetic and T2 enhancing properties - MDPs promote Dc maturation and recognition of tumor cells - Biosafe and compatible in vitro and in vivo	Y79 and ARPE-19 cells in vivo, Y79-tumor-bearing mice in flanks in vivo	[85]
MSNPs	Enhance topotecan	- Topotecan loaded - Folic acid conjugated	- Folic-acid conjugate allows for increased uptake in RB cells - Enhanced anti-cancer effects due to increased uptake in vitro and in vivo - Controlled drug release	Y79 cells in vitro, Y79-cell-bearing xenograft tumor model in vivo	[34]
	Target malignant cells	- Carboplatin loaded - EpCAM conjugated	- Sustained drug release - Endocytosis pathway - Higher anti-cancer effect and apoptosis	Y79 in vitro	[36]
	N/A	- Glucuronic acid conjugated - Polyamidoamine dendrimer conjugated - Deferasirox loaded	- PH-dependent release - High loading efficiency and controlled delivery - Sugar-modified surface allows for improved cellular uptake	Y79 in vitro	[37]
Iron NPs	Magnetic hyperthermia using iron NPs	- Dextran coated	- Minimal cytotoxicity of NPs in absence of magnetic hyperthermia - Apoptosis through intrinsic and extrinsic pathways - Diffuse in Y79 cells but localized to lysosomes and endosomes in ARPE-19 cells	Y79 and ARPE-19 cells in vitro	[39]
SPIONs	Target mitochondria	N/A	- Decreased SDH activity - Increased MMP and mitochondrial swelling - SPIONs decline cell viability and increase caspase-3 activity	Y79 cells in vitro	[40]

Table 2. *Cont.*

Nanocarrier	Function	Characteristics	Observations	Stage	Reference
SPIONs	Chemo-hyperthermia therapy	- VCR loaded - FA and TF conjugated - Pluronic coated	- Toxicity in Y79 higher, indicating receptor targeting - NPs enhance ROS production upon AMF - Increased half-life compared to free drug - Low toxicity and good biocompatibility - Magnetic	Y79 and ARPE-19 cells in vitro	[78]
AgNPs	N/A	- Laminarin loaded	- Cytotoxicity in a dose-dependent manner - IC50 16.45 µg/mL - Apoptosis through extensive double strand breaks - Good scavenging activity, dependent on concentration of the AgNPs	Y79 cells in vitro	[47]
	N/A	- Laminarin loaded	- IC_{50} 10.5 µg/mL - Cytotoxicity depends on size and dose concentration - Causes morphological cell changes - Promising free radical scavenging effect	Y79 cells in vitro	[46]
PLGA NPs	Treatment with galactose conjugated ENPs	- Galactose conjugated - Chitosan coated - Etoposide loaded	- Sustained release up to 32 h - Greater cytotoxicity and apoptosis compared to free drug - Toxicity against HepG2 and Caco-2 reduced once loaded - Pure PLGA NPs non-toxic	Y79 cells in vitro	[51]
	Evaluate difference in NP loading vs. free	- OA and UA loaded	- NPs reduce drug toxicity at high concentrations - NPs only display significant cytotoxicity in Y79 cells - Lower IC50 in free drugs as compared to NPs	Y79, HepG2, Caco-2 cells in vitro	[52]

Table 2. *Cont.*

Nanocarrier	Function	Characteristics	Observations	Stage	Reference
PLGA NPs	Effects of these NPs on RB	- Carboplatin loaded - Sodium alginate surface modified	- Slow and sustained delivery with presence of SA - SA allowed for increased cellular uptake for unknown reasons - Intraocular toxicity is unknown - Potential for topical delivery	Y79 cells	[53]
PLGA NPs	Compare various surface-modified PLGAs	- Melphalan loaded - MGP, PEG, TET1, Avidin-Palm surface modified	- Adapted synthesis of PLGA NPs allowed for increased drug loading - Efficacy based on drug and NP concentration - Surface-modified MPG showed similar efficacy to free melphalan - Cell internalization increases with time, but a significant number of NPs associated with cell surface	Y79 cells in vitro	[23]
PCL NPs	Photothermal potential	- MO and NIR loaded	- PTT efficiency proportional to intensity of NIR light - NIR light facilitates NP release - Imaging properties of MO - Synergistic effect via downregulation of HSP70	Y79 cells in vitro	[84]
TMC and TC Nps	Biodistribution of intravitreal injection	- Thiole and methyl conjugated - CMD loaded	- Higher affinity of CMD-TCs-NPs for retina - TMS-derived NPs are immobilized in vitreous	Y79 cells in vitro	[55]
	Delivery of TPH	- TPH loaded	- Drug release GSH-sensitive in vitro - Increased cytotoxicity after loading - TPH-TCs-NPs show highest cytotoxicity due to thiol group percentage in vitro and in vivo - Enhanced cellular necrosis by TPH-TCs-NPs	BSS and FBS media in vitro, in vitro RB xenograft mouse model in vivo	[54]

Table 2. *Cont.*

Nanocarrier	Function	Characteristics	Observations	Stage	Reference
TC-NPs	Intravitreal delivery	- TPH and CMD loaded	- Improved apoptosis compared to free drug - Suppression of RB tumor growth in NP treated rabbits - No retinal damage observed on histology	Y79 cells in vitro, xenograft RB rabbit models in vivo	[56]
SLN	Posterior eye delivery optimization	- Etoposide loaded	- Particle size, PDI, % entrapment efficiency affect therapeutic potential of SLN - Biphasic release with initial burst, then sustained release - Reduced toxicity of retina and blood plasma concentration compared to free drug	In vitro and rat eye in vivo	[58]
NLC	Stable delivery of PTX	- PTX loaded - α-tocopherol succinate based - PEG conjugated	- Maximum drug release of 40% - No difference in properties following sterilization - Properties of lipids and nanoparticles affect therapeutic properties - PEG increased physical stability of NPs	In vitro	[59]
LNPs	PTT	- BPQDs and melphalan loaded	- Upregulates ki67 expression - Cellular uptake within 20 min - Early and increased apoptosis - BPQDs-based NPs inhibit cell proliferation and killing - Photothermal efficiency related to concentration power and time - LNP reduces cytotoxicity of free BPQDs	RB cells in vitro, orthotopic xenograft of WERIRB-1 cells in mice in vivo	[63]
Switchable LNPs	Combination therapy	- Melphalan and miR-181a loaded	- Increased bioavailability of drug following encapsulation - MiR-181a decreases MAPK1 and Bcl-2 and enhances BAX - Combined loading has enhanced effects compared to co-delivery of separate entities - Switchable lipids change conformation at acidic pH	Primary RB cells and Y79 in vitro, xenograft RB models in rat in vivo	[60]

Table 2. *Cont.*

Nanocarrier	Function	Characteristics	Observations	Stage	Reference
Switchable LNPs	Sensitize cancer cells to chemotherapy	- siRNA loaded	- Switchable lipids change conformation at acidic pH - Survivin silencing reduces therapeutic dose of drugs, except teniposide - siRNA sequence specific to survivin - Potential benefits of using drug-loaded LNPs instead of free drug after silencing for enhanced effects	13 cell lines, including Y79 RB cells in vitro	[61]
LFNPs	Evaluate efficacy of novel NP in chemoresistance	- CPT or EPT loaded	- Concentration of free drugs higher than drug-loaded NPs - Cytotoxicity of drug-loaded NPs higher than free drug - NPs increase drug uptake, retention	Y79 CSCs in vitro	[65]
Nanomicelles	Evaluate the potential of CDF in RB therapy	- CDF loaded - Folic-acid conjugated	- Selective cytotoxicity to RB cells compared to ARPE-19 cells - Nanomicelles in absence of drug show insignificant toxicity - Free CDF faces similar hurdles as curcumin in terms of solubility and degradation - Targeting NPs showed lower IC_{50} compared to non-targeting counterparts	Y79, WERI-RB, ARPE-19 cells in vitro	[72]
CNMs	Evaluate Celastrol potential in angiogenesis	- Celastrol loaded	- CNMs inhibit HUVECs migration in dose-dependent manner - Blocking VEGF-A pathway - Decrease tumor volume and weight - No influence on mouse body weight - Histology staining shows decreased vascularization	HUVECs and SO-RB 50 in vitro and xenograft mouse model in vivo	[74]
RSNMs	N/A	- Celastrol loaded	- Activation of caspase-related proteins - Cellular uptake seen in under 10 min - Slow diffusion from cell to its nuclear contents - Apoptosis was time-dependent	Y79 cells in vitro	[75]

Table 2. *Cont.*

Nanocarrier	Function	Characteristics	Observations	Stage	Reference
CMT NPs	Dual-mode image-guided laser/immune co-therapy	- Tuftsin coated	- Good thermal conversion ability - Low cost compared to gold NPs - Tuftsin is macrophage-specific - Concentration of NPs increases under magnetic field - PA signals remained after 24 h; potential in image-guided tumor therapy - Negative enhancement of T2WI MRI imaging - Successful PPT in vivo, decreasing tumor volume - Tuftsin induces macrophage typing - Absence of toxicity using CMT	Y79, ARPE-19, Ana-1 in vitro, Y79-tumor-bearing mice in vivo	[80]
LNPs	Dual-target cationic	- Folate conjugated - Spions, PFH, ICG loaded	- Folate magnetic dual target increased cellular uptake - Synergistic effect of ICG on PDT and PTT - Excellent biosafety - PFH allows for oxygen reserve, enhancing PDT effect	Y79 and ARPE-19 cells in vitro, Y79-tumor-bearing mice in vivo	[81]
	Multi-functional LNPs	- Folate conjugated - DOX, ICG, PFP loaded	- PFP enhances drug release through microbubbles induced via laser irradiation - FA-DOX-ICG-PFP-LNPs +laser irradiation showed the lowest cell viability and synergistic effect - Strong intake of NPs in liver and spleen, no histological abnormalities	Y79 and HUVECs in vitro, xenograft mouse models in vivo	[86]
	Multi-functionality, including gene therapy	- FA conjugated - PFP, ICG, TK-GFP plasmid loaded	- PA/US contrast following irradiation - Synergistic effect of electrostatic absorption and folate targeting on internalization - Cationic property of NPs allows for plasmid binding - Subcutaneous mouse tissue in vivo rather than eye	Y79 cells in vitro, nude mouse limbs in vivo	[83]

Table 2. *Cont.*

Nanocarrier	Function	Characteristics	Observations	Stage	Reference
PNPs	PCB and PTT combination therapy	- PLGA and PCL embedded - PCB and NIR loaded	- Time-dependent increase in temperature allowing for controlled drug release - Adequate photoacoustic imaging properties - Synergistic cytotoxicity - Absence of behavioral toxicity, mortality, or body weight decrease	Y79 cells in vivo, mouse models in vivo	[82]
Clathrin-like NPs	Overcome BRB	- Dox loaded	- Cellular uptake increased following light irradiation in vitro and in vivo - Minimal eye irritation and no structural damage - Unnoticeable systemic toxicity - Free drug treatment caused body weight decrease of 10%, whereas absent in loaded NPs	HUVECs and WERI-RB-1 cells in vitro, and orthotopic retinoblastoma tumor mouse model in vivo	[76]
N/A	VCN-01 therapy	N/A	- VCN-01 cytotoxic against RB cells in vitro - Intravitreal injection, slight and short-term leakage into blood - 2/12 mice had detectable viral genome in plasma 4 h after injection - Clinically feasible with anti-cancer effects on vitreous seeds - Local vitreous inflammation	Y79 and primary RB cultures in vitro, mouse, rabbit, and human in vivo	[90]
PAMAM	Non-viral gene therapy	- siRNA loaded	- Enters cells through clathrin-mediated endocytosis - Topical administration reaches the posterior segment of the eye within 2 h - Elimination within 6 h	ARPE-19 and WERI-RB-1 cells in vitro	[92]

Table 2. *Cont.*

Nanocarrier	Function	Characteristics	Observations	Stage	Reference
SNA NPs	siRNA delivery	- siRNA, NVP-CGM097, aptamer loaded	- Synergistic effect of loaded components on MDM2 pathway - Melphalan showed in vitro superiority in cell killing - Both SNA NPs and melphalan reduced pupil leukosis, a sign of anti-tumor effect - Melphalan exerted more toxic effect on retinal thickness compared to NPs	Y79 and WERI-RB-1 cells in vitro and in vivo in nude mouse xenograft models	[94]
MNO_2 and DNAzymes NPs	Dual-gene therapy	Aptamer surface modified	- DNAzymes target two separate mRNAs - Effective delivery to cells within 4 h - Potential for dual-mode imaging - Aptamer increases cellular uptake in vitro and in vivo - Absence of toxicity in vivo due to absent body weight change - Increased H&E staining tumor cell necrosis compared to control	ARPE-19, Y79 cells, Y79-tumor-bearing mice	[96]

6. Conclusions

This review highlights the significant challenges in treating pediatric retinoblastoma and the emerging potential of nanotechnology in revolutionizing ocular drug delivery. Retinoblastoma, a leading intraocular cancer in children, presents challenges, such as anatomical barriers, drug instability, the risk of secondary tumors, and systemic toxicity from conventional treatments, such as chemotherapy and radiotherapy. Nanosystems, including gold, mesoporous silica, polymeric, and lipid nanoparticles, offer promising in vitro and in vivo solutions in animal models. Through these studies, it is clear that in order to target RB cells, the nanoparticles need to be small in size, stable, with a high drug loading capacity, and non-toxic to non-cancerous cells. Some of the studies discussed have also highlighted the preferential cationic property of NPs in favoring movement along the vitreous environment; this is particularly important in the context of retinoblastoma, as the most effective site of action is found behind the vitreous. Moreover, it is beneficial for these nanoparticles to be highly modifiable, allowing for targeted delivery. This can be achieved in many ways, including NP surface receptors targeting upregulated elements within tumor cells or pH sensitivity to tumor microenvironment. Although the addition of functional elements to a NP, such as PTT and imaging, can be beneficial, they are not necessary at the moment. Focusing on engineering simple mono-functional nanoparticles with the goal of treating retinoblastoma, enhancing current in vivo models to simulate the microenvironment of the eye, allowing long-term toxicity follow-ups, and then undergoing clinical trials to further their advancement are the next steps in the near future.

Despite its potential, the application of nanotechnology in treating retinoblastoma is still in its early stages, with hurdles such as long-term toxicity and limited clinical data. Future research is crucial to overcoming these barriers, improving simple nanoparticle design, and advancement toward clinical trials. By addressing these challenges, nanotechnology holds the promise of transforming retinoblastoma treatment, enhancing patient outcomes, and preserving vision with minimal adverse effects.

Author Contributions: Conceptualization, K.Y.W.; writing—original draft preparation, K.Y.W. and X.C.W.; writing—review and editing, K.Y.W., X.C.W. and M.A.; supervision, M.A. and S.D.T. All authors have read and agreed to the published version of the manuscript.

Funding: This research received no external funding.

Institutional Review Board Statement: Not applicable.

Informed Consent Statement: Not applicable.

Data Availability Statement: Not applicable.

Conflicts of Interest: The authors declare no conflicts of interest.

References

1. Mattosinho, C.C.D.S.; Moura, A.T.M.S.; Oigman, G.; Ferman, S.E.; Grigorovski, N. Time to Diagnosis of Retinoblastoma in Latin America: A Systematic Review. *Pediatr. Hematol. Oncol.* **2019**, *36*, 55–72. [CrossRef]
2. Alkatan, H.M.; Al Marek, F.; Elkhamary, S. Demographics of Pediatric Orbital Lesions: A Tertiary Eye Center Experience in Saudi Arabia. *J. Epidemiol. Glob. Health* **2019**, *9*, 3–10. [CrossRef]
3. Zahn, J.; Chan, M.P.; Wang, G.; Patel, R.M.; Andea, A.A.; Bresler, S.C.; Harms, P.W. Altered Rb, P16, and P53 Expression Is Specific for Porocarcinoma Relative to Poroma. *J. Cutan. Pathol.* **2019**, *46*, 659–664. [CrossRef] [PubMed]
4. House, R.J.; Hsu, S.T.; Thomas, A.S.; Finn, A.P.; Toth, C.A.; Materin, M.A.; Vajzovic, L. Vascular Findings in a Small Retinoblastoma Tumor Using OCT Angiography. *Ophthalmol. Retin.* **2019**, *3*, 194–195. [CrossRef] [PubMed]
5. Kletke, S.N.; Feng, Z.X.; Hazrati, L.-N.; Gallie, B.L.; Soliman, S.E. Clinical Predictors at Diagnosis of Low-Risk Histopathology in Unilateral Advanced Retinoblastoma. *Ophthalmology* **2019**, *126*, 1306–1314. [CrossRef] [PubMed]
6. Ishaq, H.; Patel, B.C. Retinoblastoma. In *StatPearls*; StatPearls Publishing: Treasure Island, FL, USA, 2024.
7. Retinoblastoma: Diagnosis and Management—The UK Perspective—PubMed. Available online: https://pubmed.ncbi.nlm.nih.gov/25940424/ (accessed on 20 March 2024).
8. Darwich, R.; Ghazawi, F.M.; Rahme, E.; Alghazawi, N.; Burnier, J.V.; Sasseville, D.; Burnier, M.N.; Litvinov, I.V. Retinoblastoma Incidence Trends in Canada: A National Comprehensive Population-Based Study. *J. Pediatr. Ophthalmol. Strabismus* **2019**, *56*, 124–130. [CrossRef] [PubMed]

9. Fabian, I.D.; Reddy, A.; Sagoo, M.S. Classification and Staging of Retinoblastoma. *Community Eye Health* **2018**, *31*, 11. [PubMed]
10. Schefler, A.C.; Kim, R.S. Recent Advancements in the Management of Retinoblastoma and Uveal Melanoma. *F1000Research* **2018**, *7*, 476. [CrossRef] [PubMed]
11. Pelton, R.W.; Patel, B.C. Superomedial Lid Crease Approach to the Medial Intraconal Space: A New Technique for Access to the Optic Nerve and Central Space. *Ophthalmic Plast. Reconstr. Surg.* **2001**, *17*, 241–253. [CrossRef]
12. Chawla, B.; Jain, A.; Azad, R. Conservative Treatment Modalities in Retinoblastoma. *Indian J. Ophthalmol.* **2013**, *61*, 479–485. [CrossRef]
13. Abramson, D.H.; Ellsworth, R.M.; Rozakis, G.W. Cryotherapy for Retinoblastoma. *Arch. Ophthalmol.* **1982**, *100*, 1253–1256. [CrossRef] [PubMed]
14. Wong, F.L. Cancer Incidence after Retinoblastoma. Radiation Dose and Sarcoma Risk. *JAMA J. Am. Med. Assoc.* **1997**, *278*, 1262–1267. [CrossRef] [PubMed]
15. Abramson, D.H.; Frank, C.M. Second Nonocular Tumors in Survivors of Bilateral Retinoblastoma. *Ophthalmology* **1998**, *105*, 573–580. [CrossRef] [PubMed]
16. Yousef, Y.A.; Mohammad, M.; Jaradat, I.; Shatnawi, R.; Banat, S.; Mehyar, M.; Al-Nawaiseh, I. The Role of External Beam Radiation Therapy for Retinoblastoma after Failure of Combined Chemoreduction and Focal Consolidation Therapy. *Ophthalmic Genet.* **2020**, *41*, 20–25. [CrossRef] [PubMed]
17. Kim, J.-Y.; Park, Y. Treatment of Retinoblastoma: The Role of External Beam Radiotherapy. *Yonsei Med. J.* **2015**, *56*, 1478. [CrossRef] [PubMed]
18. Rizzuti, A.E. The Adverse Events of Chemotherapy for Retinoblastoma: What Are They? Do We Know? *Arch. Ophthalmol.* **2008**, *126*, 862. [CrossRef] [PubMed]
19. Manjandavida, F.; Stathopoulos, C.; Zhang, J.; Honavar, S.; Shields, C. Intra-Arterial Chemotherapy in Retinoblastoma—A Paradigm Change. *Indian J. Ophthalmol.* **2019**, *67*, 740. [CrossRef] [PubMed]
20. Steinle, J.J.; Zhang, Q.; Thompson, K.E.; Toutounchian, J.; Yates, C.R.; Soderland, C.; Wang, F.; Stewart, C.F.; Haik, B.G.; Williams, J.S.; et al. Intra-Ophthalmic Artery Chemotherapy Triggers Vascular Toxicity through Endothelial Cell Inflammation and Leukostasis. *Investig. Ophthalmol. Vis. Sci.* **2012**, *53*, 2439. [CrossRef] [PubMed]
21. Tse, B.C.; Steinle, J.J.; Johnson, D.; Haik, B.G.; Wilson, M.W. Superselective Intraophthalmic Artery Chemotherapy in a Nonhuman Primate Model: Histopathologic Findings. *JAMA Ophthalmol.* **2013**, *131*, 903. [CrossRef]
22. Kalita, D.; Shome, D.; Jain, V.G.; Chadha, K.; Bellare, J.R. In Vivo Intraocular Distribution and Safety of Periocular Nanoparticle Carboplatin for Treatment of Advanced Retinoblastoma in Humans. *Am. J. Ophthalmol.* **2014**, *157*, 1109–1115. [CrossRef]
23. Sims, L.B.; Tyo, K.M.; Stocke, S.; Mahmoud, M.Y.; Ramasubramanian, A.; Steinbach-Rankins, J.M. Surface-Modified Melphalan Nanoparticles for Intravitreal Chemotherapy of Retinoblastoma. *Investig. Ophthalmol. Vis. Sci.* **2019**, *60*, 1696. [CrossRef] [PubMed]
24. Yousef, Y.A.; Al Jboor, M.; Mohammad, M.; Mehyar, M.; Toro, M.D.; Nazzal, R.; Alzureikat, Q.H.; Rejdak, M.; Elfalah, M.; Sultan, I.; et al. Safety and Efficacy of Intravitreal Chemotherapy (Melphalan) to Treat Vitreous Seeds in Retinoblastoma. *Front. Pharmacol.* **2021**, *12*, 696787. [CrossRef] [PubMed]
25. Hammami, I.; Alabdallah, N.M.; Jomaa, A.A.; Kamoun, M. Gold Nanoparticles: Synthesis Properties and Applications. *J. King Saud. Univ.-Sci.* **2021**, *33*, 101560. [CrossRef]
26. Boedtkjer, E.; Pedersen, S.F. The Acidic Tumor Microenvironment as a Driver of Cancer. *Annu. Rev. Physiol.* **2020**, *82*, 103–126. [CrossRef] [PubMed]
27. Yan, S.; Yan, J.; Liu, D.; Li, X.; Kang, Q.; You, W.; Zhang, J.; Wang, L.; Tian, Z.; Lu, W.; et al. A Nano-Predator of Pathological MDMX Construct by Clearable Supramolecular Gold(I)-Thiol-Peptide Complexes Achieves Safe and Potent Anti-Tumor Activity. *Theranostics* **2021**, *11*, 6833–6846. [CrossRef] [PubMed]
28. Kalmodia, S.; Parameswaran, S.; Ganapathy, K.; Yang, W.; Barrow, C.J.; Kanwar, J.R.; Roy, K.; Vasudevan, M.; Kulkarni, K.; Elchuri, S.V.; et al. Characterization and Molecular Mechanism of Peptide-Conjugated Gold Nanoparticle Inhibiting P53-HDM2 Interaction in Retinoblastoma. *Mol. Ther.-Nucleic Acids* **2017**, *9*, 349–364. [CrossRef] [PubMed]
29. Darviot, C.; Hardy, P.; Meunier, M. Laser-induced Plasmon-mediated Treatment of Retinoblastoma in Viscous Vitreous Phantom. *J. Biophotonics* **2019**, *12*, e201900193. [CrossRef] [PubMed]
30. Moradi, S.; Mokhtari-Dizaji, M.; Ghassemi, F.; Sheibani, S.; Amoli, F.A. The Effect of Ultrasound Hyperthermia with Gold Nanoparticles on Retinoblastoma Y79 Cells. *Gold Bull.* **2020**, *53*, 111–120. [CrossRef]
31. Moradi, S.; Mokhtari-Dizaji, M.; Ghassemi, F.; Sheibani, S.; Asadi Amoli, F. Increasing the Efficiency of the Retinoblastoma Brachytherapy Protocol with Ultrasonic Hyperthermia and Gold Nanoparticles: A Rabbit Model. *Int. J. Radiat. Biol.* **2020**, *96*, 1614–1627. [CrossRef]
32. Niculescu, V.-C. Mesoporous Silica Nanoparticles for Bio-Applications. *Front. Mater.* **2020**, *7*, 36. [CrossRef]
33. Leamon, C. Folate-Targeted Chemotherapy. *Adv. Drug Deliv. Rev.* **2004**, *56*, 1127–1141. [CrossRef] [PubMed]
34. Qu, W.; Meng, B.; Yu, Y.; Wang, S. Folic Acid-Conjugated Mesoporous Silica Nanoparticles for Enhanced Therapeutic Efficacy of Topotecan in Retina Cancers. *Int. J. Nanomed.* **2018**, *13*, 4379–4389. [CrossRef] [PubMed]
35. Mitra, M.; Kandalam, M.; Verma, R.S.; UmaMaheswari, K.; Krishnakumar, S. Genome-Wide Changes Accompanying the Knockdown of Ep-CAM in Retinoblastoma. *Mol. Vis.* **2010**, *16*, 828–842. [PubMed]

36. Qu, W.; Meng, B.; Yu, Y.; Wang, S. EpCAM Antibody-Conjugated Mesoporous Silica Nanoparticles to Enhance the Anticancer Efficacy of Carboplatin in Retinoblastoma. *Mater. Sci. Eng. C* **2017**, *76*, 646–651. [CrossRef]
37. Sodagar Taleghani, A.; Ebrahimnejad, P.; Heidarinasab, A.; Akbarzadeh, A. Sugar-Conjugated Dendritic Mesoporous Silica Nanoparticles as pH-Responsive Nanocarriers for Tumor Targeting and Controlled Release of Deferasirox. *Mater. Sci. Eng. C* **2019**, *98*, 358–368. [CrossRef] [PubMed]
38. Pucci, C.; Degl'Innocenti, A.; Belenli Gümüş, M.; Ciofani, G. Superparamagnetic Iron Oxide Nanoparticles for Magnetic Hyperthermia: Recent Advancements, Molecular Effects, and Future Directions in the Omics Era. *Biomater. Sci.* **2022**, *10*, 2103–2121. [CrossRef] [PubMed]
39. Demirci, H.; Slimani, N.; Pawar, M.; Kumon, R.E.; Vaishnava, P.; Besirli, C.G. Magnetic Hyperthermia in Y79 Retinoblastoma and ARPE-19 Retinal Epithelial Cells: Tumor Selective Apoptotic Activity of Iron Oxide Nanoparticle. *Trans. Vis. Sci. Technol.* **2019**, *8*, 18. [CrossRef] [PubMed]
40. Seydi, E.; Tahmasebi, G.; Arjmand, A.; Pourahmad, J. Toxicity of Superparamagnetic Iron Oxide Nanoparticles on Retinoblastoma Mitochondria. *Cutan. Ocul. Toxicol.* **2023**, *43*, 69–74. [CrossRef]
41. Ali, A.; Zafar, H.; Zia, M.; Ul Haq, I.; Phull, A.R.; Ali, J.S.; Hussain, A. Synthesis, Characterization, Applications, and Challenges of Iron Oxide Nanoparticles. *Nanotechnol. Sci. Appl.* **2016**, *9*, 49–67. [CrossRef]
42. Kuda, T.; Yano, T.; Matsuda, N.; Nishizawa, M. Inhibitory Effects of Laminaran and Low Molecular Alginate against the Putrefactive Compounds Produced by Intestinal Microflora in Vitro and in Rats. *Food Chem.* **2005**, *91*, 745–749. [CrossRef]
43. Kim, K.-H.; Kim, Y.-W.; Kim, H.B.; Lee, B.J.; Lee, D.S. Anti-Apoptotic Activity of Laminarin Polysaccharides and Their Enzymatically Hydrolyzed Oligosaccharides from Laminaria Japonica. *Biotechnol. Lett.* **2006**, *28*, 439–446. [CrossRef] [PubMed]
44. Barwal, I.; Ranjan, P.; Kateriya, S.; Yadav, S.C. Cellular Oxido-Reductive Proteins of Chlamydomonas Reinhardtii Control the Biosynthesis of Silver Nanoparticles. *J. Nanobiotechnol.* **2011**, *9*, 56. [CrossRef] [PubMed]
45. Buzea, C.; Pacheco, I.I.; Robbie, K. Nanomaterials and Nanoparticles: Sources and Toxicity. *Biointerphases* **2007**, *2*, MR17–MR71. [CrossRef] [PubMed]
46. Remya, R.R.; Radhika Rajasree, S.R.; Aranganathan, L.; Suman, T.Y.; Gayathri, S. Enhanced Cytotoxic Activity of AgNPs on Retinoblastoma Y79 Cell Lines Synthesised Using Marine Seaweed *Turbinaria ornata*. *IET Nanobiotechnol.* **2017**, *11*, 18–23. [CrossRef] [PubMed]
47. Remya, R.R.; Rajasree, S.R.R.; Suman, T.Y.; Aranganathan, L.; Gayathri, S.; Gobalakrishnan, M.; Karthih, M.G. Laminarin Based AgNPs Using Brown Seaweed *Turbinaria ornata* and Its Induction of Apoptosis in Human Retinoblastoma Y79 Cancer Cell Lines. *Mater. Res. Express* **2018**, *5*, 035403. [CrossRef]
48. Davis, T.A.; Volesky, B.; Mucci, A. A Review of the Biochemistry of Heavy Metal Biosorption by Brown Algae. *Water Res.* **2003**, *37*, 4311–4330. [CrossRef] [PubMed]
49. Zielińska, A.; Carreiró, F.; Oliveira, A.M.; Neves, A.; Pires, B.; Venkatesh, D.N.; Durazzo, A.; Lucarini, M.; Eder, P.; Silva, A.M.; et al. Polymeric Nanoparticles: Production, Characterization, Toxicology and Ecotoxicology. *Molecules* **2020**, *25*, 3731. [CrossRef] [PubMed]
50. Nagati, V.; Tenugu, S.; Pasupulati, A.K. Stability of Therapeutic Nano-Drugs during Storage and Transportation as Well as after Ingestion in the Human Body. In *Advances in Nanotechnology-Based Drug Delivery Systems*; Elsevier: Amsterdam, The Netherlands, 2022; pp. 83–102. ISBN 978-0-323-88450-1.
51. Godse, R.; Rathod, M.; De, A.; Shinde, U. Intravitreal Galactose Conjugated Polymeric Nanoparticles of Etoposide for Retinoblastoma. *J. Drug Deliv. Sci. Technol.* **2021**, *61*, 102259. [CrossRef]
52. Silva, A.M.; Alvarado, H.L.; Abrego, G.; Martins-Gomes, C.; Garduño-Ramirez, M.L.; García, M.L.; Calpena, A.C.; Souto, E.B. In Vitro Cytotoxicity of Oleanolic/Ursolic Acids-Loaded in PLGA Nanoparticles in Different Cell Lines. *Pharmaceutics* **2019**, *11*, 362. [CrossRef]
53. Zhuang, H.; Xu, Y.-N.; Zheng, H.-H.; Huan, Y.-R.; Zheng, N.-X.; Lin, L.; Zhang, W.-Z.; Xu, W. Carboplatin-Loaded Surface Modified-PLGA Nanoparticles Confer Sustained Inhibitory Effect against Retinoblastoma Cell In Vitro. *Arq. Bras. Oftalmol.* **2021**, *85*, 450–458. [CrossRef]
54. Delrish, E.; Jabbarvand, M.; Ghassemi, F.; Amoli, F.A.; Atyabi, F.; Lashay, A.; Soleimani, M.; Aghajanpour, L.; Dinarvand, R. Efficacy of Topotecan Nanoparticles for Intravitreal Chemotherapy of Retinoblastoma. *Exp. Eye Res.* **2021**, *204*, 108423. [CrossRef] [PubMed]
55. Delrish, E.; Ghassemi, F.; Jabbarvand, M.; Lashay, A.; Atyabi, F.; Soleimani, M.; Dinarvand, R. Biodistribution of Cy5-Labeled Thiolated and Methylated Chitosan-Carboxymethyl Dextran Nanoparticles in an Animal Model of Retinoblastoma. *J. Ophthalmic Vis. Res.* **2022**, *17*, 58–68. [CrossRef] [PubMed]
56. Ghassemi, F.; Delrish, E.; Jabbarvand, M.; Lashay, A.; Asadi Amoli, F.; Atyabi, F.; Sadat Mirzazadeh Tekie, F.; Dinarvand, R.; Heidari Keshel, S.; Soleimani, M. The Antitumor Effect of Topotecan Loaded Thiolated Chitosan-Dextran Nanoparticles for Intravitreal Chemotherapy: A Xenograft Retinoblastoma Model. *J. Ophthalmic Vis. Res.* **2023**, *18*, 68–80. [CrossRef] [PubMed]
57. Viegas, C.; Patrício, A.B.; Prata, J.M.; Nadhman, A.; Chintamaneni, P.K.; Fonte, P. Solid Lipid Nanoparticles vs. Nanostructured Lipid Carriers: A Comparative Review. *Pharmaceutics* **2023**, *15*, 1593. [CrossRef]
58. Ahmad, I.; Pandit, J.; Sultana, Y.; Mishra, A.K.; Hazari, P.P.; Aqil, M. Optimization by Design of Etoposide Loaded Solid Lipid Nanoparticles for Ocular Delivery: Characterization, Pharmacokinetic and Deposition Study. *Mater. Sci. Eng. C* **2019**, *100*, 959–970. [CrossRef] [PubMed]

59. Marathe, S.; Shadambikar, G.; Mehraj, T.; Sulochana, S.P.; Dudhipala, N.; Majumdar, S. Development of α-Tocopherol Succinate-Based Nanostructured Lipid Carriers for Delivery of Paclitaxel. *Pharmaceutics* **2022**, *14*, 1034. [CrossRef] [PubMed]
60. Tabatabaei, S.N.; Derbali, R.M.; Yang, C.; Superstein, R.; Hamel, P.; Chain, J.L.; Hardy, P. Co-Delivery of miR-181a and Melphalan by Lipid Nanoparticles for Treatment of Seeded Retinoblastoma. *J. Control. Release* **2019**, *298*, 177–185. [CrossRef] [PubMed]
61. Passos Gibson, V.; Derbali, R.M.; Phan, H.T.; Tahiri, H.; Allen, C.; Hardy, P.; Chain, J.L. Survivin Silencing Improved the Cytotoxicity of Carboplatin and Melphalan in Y79 and Primary Retinoblastoma Cells. *Int. J. Pharm.* **2020**, *589*, 119824. [CrossRef] [PubMed]
62. He, C.; Ruan, F.; Jiang, S.; Zeng, J.; Yin, H.; Liu, R.; Zhang, Y.; Huang, L.; Wang, C.; Ma, S.; et al. Black Phosphorus Quantum Dots Cause Nephrotoxicity in Organoids, Mice, and Human Cells. *Small* **2020**, *16*, 2001371. [CrossRef]
63. Wang, S.; Wei, P.; Zhang, Y.; Zhang, S. Lipid-Nanoparticles-Based Co-Delivery of Black Phosphorus Quantum Dots and Melphalan by Photothermal Therapy Combined with Chemotherapy for Retinoblastoma. *Polym. Test.* **2023**, *129*, 108292. [CrossRef]
64. Hong, S.; Choi, D.W.; Kim, H.N.; Park, C.G.; Lee, W.; Park, H.H. Protein-Based Nanoparticles as Drug Delivery Systems. *Pharmaceutics* **2020**, *12*, 604. [CrossRef] [PubMed]
65. Narayana, R.V.L.; Jana, P.; Tomar, N.; Prabhu, V.; Nair, R.M.; Manukonda, R.; Kaliki, S.; Coupland, S.E.; Alexander, J.; Kalirai, H.; et al. Carboplatin- and Etoposide-Loaded Lactoferrin Protein Nanoparticles for Targeting Cancer Stem Cells in Retinoblastoma In Vitro. *Investig. Ophthalmol. Vis. Sci.* **2021**, *62*, 13. [CrossRef] [PubMed]
66. Nair, R.M.; Balla, M.M.; Khan, I.; Kalathur, R.K.R.; Kondaiah, P.; Vemuganti, G.K. In Vitro Characterization of CD133lo Cancer Stem Cells in Retinoblastoma Y79 Cell Line. *BMC Cancer* **2017**, *17*, 779. [CrossRef] [PubMed]
67. Balla, M.M.S.; Vemuganti, G.K.; Kannabiran, C.; Honavar, S.G.; Murthy, R. Phenotypic Characterization of Retinoblastoma for the Presence of Putative Cancer Stem-like Cell Markers by Flow Cytometry. *Investig. Ophthalmol. Vis. Sci.* **2009**, *50*, 1506. [CrossRef] [PubMed]
68. Zeuner, A. The Secret Life of Quiescent Cancer Stem Cells. *Mol. Cell. Oncol.* **2015**, *2*, e968067. [CrossRef]
69. Abdullah, L.N.; Chow, E.K. Mechanisms of Chemoresistance in Cancer Stem Cells. *Clin. Transl. Med.* **2013**, *2*, e3. [CrossRef] [PubMed]
70. Trinh, H.M.; Joseph, M.; Cholkar, K.; Mitra, R.; Mitra, A.K. Nanomicelles in Diagnosis and Drug Delivery. In *Emerging Nanotechnologies for Diagnostics, Drug Delivery and Medical Devices*; Elsevier: Amsterdam, The Netherlands, 2017; pp. 45–58, ISBN 978-0-323-42978-8.
71. Anand, P.; Kunnumakkara, A.B.; Newman, R.A.; Aggarwal, B.B. Bioavailability of Curcumin: Problems and Promises. *Mol. Pharm.* **2007**, *4*, 807–818. [CrossRef] [PubMed]
72. Alsaab, H.; Alzhrani, R.; Kesharwani, P.; Sau, S.; Boddu, S.; Iyer, A. Folate Decorated Nanomicelles Loaded with a Potent Curcumin Analogue for Targeting Retinoblastoma. *Pharmaceutics* **2017**, *9*, 15. [CrossRef]
73. Cascão, R.; Fonseca, J.E.; Moita, L.F. Celastrol: A Spectrum of Treatment Opportunities in Chronic Diseases. *Front. Med.* **2017**, *4*, 69. [CrossRef]
74. Li, Z.; Guo, Z.; Chu, D.; Feng, H.; Zhang, J.; Zhu, L.; Li, J. Effectively Suppressed Angiogenesis-Mediated Retinoblastoma Growth Using Celastrol Nanomicelles. *Drug Deliv.* **2020**, *27*, 358–366. [CrossRef]
75. Guo, Z.; Shi, L.; Feng, H.; Yang, F.; Li, Z.; Zhang, J.; Jin, L.; Li, J. Reduction-Sensitive Nanomicelles: Delivery Celastrol for Retinoblastoma Cells Effective Apoptosis. *Chin. Chem. Lett.* **2021**, *32*, 1046–1050. [CrossRef]
76. Long, K.; Yang, Y.; Lv, W.; Jiang, K.; Li, Y.; Lo, A.C.Y.; Lam, W.C.; Zhan, C.; Wang, W. Green Light-Triggered Intraocular Drug Release for Intravenous Chemotherapy of Retinoblastoma. *Adv. Sci.* **2021**, *8*, 2101754. [CrossRef] [PubMed]
77. Kanwar, J.R.; Samarasinghe, R.M.; Sehgal, R. Nano-Lactoferrin in Diagnostic, Imaging and Targeted Delivery for Cancer and Infectious Diseases. *J. Cancer Sci. Ther.* **2012**, *4*, 31–42. [CrossRef]
78. Sadri, E.; Khoee, S.; Moayeri, S.; Haji Ali, B.; Pirhajati Mahabadi, V.; Shirvalilou, S.; Khoei, S. Enhanced Anti-Tumor Activity of Transferrin/Folate Dual-Targeting Magnetic Nanoparticles Using Chemo-Thermo Therapy on Retinoblastoma Cancer Cells Y79. *Sci. Rep.* **2023**, *13*, 22358. [CrossRef] [PubMed]
79. Griegel, S.; Rajewsky, M.F.; Ciesiolka, T.; Gabius, H.J. Endogenous Sugar Receptor (Lectin) Profiles of Human Retinoblastoma and Retinoblast Cell Lines Analyzed by Cytological Markers, Affinity Chromatography and Neoglycoprotein-Targeted Photolysis. *Anticancer Res.* **1989**, *9*, 723–730. [PubMed]
80. Zou, H.; Li, M.; Li, X.; Zheng, W.; Kuang, H.; Wang, M.; Zhang, W.; Ran, H.; Ma, H.; Zhou, X. Multimodal Imaging and Photothermal Synergistic Immunotherapy of Retinoblastoma with Tuftsin-Loaded Carbonized MOF Nanoparticles. *Drug Deliv.* **2022**, *29*, 1785–1799. [CrossRef] [PubMed]
81. Zheng, W.; Li, X.; Zou, H.; Xu, Y.; Li, P.; Zhou, X.; Wu, M. Dual-Target Multifunctional Superparamagnetic Cationic Nanoliposomes for Multimodal Imaging-Guided Synergistic Photothermal/Photodynamic Therapy of Retinoblastoma. *Int. J. Nanomed.* **2022**, *17*, 3217–3237. [CrossRef] [PubMed]
82. Mudigunda, S.V.; Pemmaraju, D.B.; Paradkar, S.; Puppala, E.R.; Gawali, B.; Upadhyayula, S.M.; Vegi Gangamodi, N.; Rengan, A.K. Multifunctional Polymeric Nanoparticles for Chemo/Phototheranostics of Retinoblastoma. *ACS Biomater. Sci. Eng.* **2022**, *8*, 151–160. [CrossRef] [PubMed]
83. Wu, M.; Xiong, H.; Zou, H.; Li, M.; Li, P.; Zhou, Y.; Xu, Y.; Jian, J.; Liu, F.; Zhao, H.; et al. A Laser-Activated Multifunctional Targeted Nanoagent for Imaging and Gene Therapy in a Mouse Xenograft Model with Retinoblastoma Y79 Cells. *Acta Biomater.* **2018**, *70*, 211–226. [CrossRef]

84. Mudigunda, S.V.; Pemmaraju, D.B.; Sankaranarayanan, S.A.; Rengan, A.K. Bioactive Polymeric Nanoparticles of Moringa Oleifera Induced Phyto-Photothermal Sensitization for the Enhanced Therapy of Retinoblastoma. *Pharmaceutics* **2023**, *15*, 475. [CrossRef]
85. Wang, M.; Yang, Q.; Li, M.; Zou, H.; Wang, Z.; Ran, H.; Zheng, Y.; Jian, J.; Zhou, Y.; Luo, Y.; et al. Multifunctional Nanoparticles for Multimodal Imaging-Guided Low-Intensity Focused Ultrasound/Immunosynergistic Retinoblastoma Therapy. *ACS Appl. Mater. Interfaces* **2020**, *12*, 5642–5657. [CrossRef] [PubMed]
86. Li, M.; Bian, X.; Chen, X.; Fan, N.; Zou, H.; Bao, Y.; Zhou, Y. Multifunctional Liposome for Photoacoustic/Ultrasound Imaging-Guided Chemo/Photothermal Retinoblastoma Therapy. *Drug Deliv.* **2022**, *29*, 519–533. [CrossRef] [PubMed]
87. Overchuk, M.; Zheng, G. Overcoming Obstacles in the Tumor Microenvironment: Recent Advancements in Nanoparticle Delivery for Cancer Theranostics. *Biomaterials* **2018**, *156*, 217–237. [CrossRef] [PubMed]
88. Bodratti, A.M.; Alexandridis, P. Amphiphilic Block Copolymers in Drug Delivery: Advances in Formulation Structure and Performance. *Expert Opin. Drug Deliv.* **2018**, *15*, 1085–1104. [CrossRef] [PubMed]
89. Lin, D.; Shen, Y.; Liang, T. Oncolytic Virotherapy: Basic Principles, Recent Advances and Future Directions. *Signal Transduct. Target. Ther.* **2023**, *8*, 156. [CrossRef] [PubMed]
90. Pascual-Pasto, G.; Bazan-Peregrino, M.; Olaciregui, N.G.; Restrepo-Perdomo, C.A.; Mato-Berciano, A.; Ottaviani, D.; Weber, K.; Correa, G.; Paco, S.; Vila-Ubach, M.; et al. Therapeutic Targeting of the RB1 Pathway in Retinoblastoma with the Oncolytic Adenovirus VCN-01. *Sci. Transl. Med.* **2019**, *11*, eaat9321. [CrossRef] [PubMed]
91. Wang, Y.; Ji, X.; Ruan, M.; Liu, W.; Song, R.; Dai, J.; Xue, W. Worm-Like Biomimetic Nanoerythrocyte Carrying siRNA for Melanoma Gene Therapy. *Small* **2018**, *14*, 1803002. [CrossRef] [PubMed]
92. Gao, X.; Fan, X.; Jiang, K.; Hu, Y.; Liu, Y.; Lu, W.; Wei, G. Intraocular siRNA Delivery Mediated by Penetratin Derivative to Silence Orthotopic Retinoblastoma Gene. *Pharmaceutics* **2023**, *15*, 745. [CrossRef] [PubMed]
93. Dong, Y.; Siegwart, D.J.; Anderson, D.G. Strategies, Design, and Chemistry in siRNA Delivery Systems. *Adv. Drug Deliv. Rev.* **2019**, *144*, 133–147. [CrossRef]
94. Wang, S.; Zhao, Y.; Yao, F.; Wei, P.; Ma, L.; Zhang, S. An Anti-GD2 Aptamer-Based Bifunctional Spherical Nucleic Acid Nanoplatform for Synergistic Therapy Targeting MDM2 for Retinoblastoma. *Biomed. Pharmacother.* **2024**, *174*, 116437. [CrossRef]
95. Su, J.; Sun, C.; Du, J.; Xing, X.; Wang, F.; Dong, H. RNA-Cleaving DNAzyme-Based Amplification Strategies for Biosensing and Therapy. *Adv. Healthc. Mater.* **2023**, *12*, 2300367. [CrossRef] [PubMed]
96. Hu, X.; Zhang, D.; Huang, L.; Zeng, Z.; Su, Y.; Chen, S.; Lin, X.; Hong, S. Construction of a Functional Nucleic Acid-Based Artificial Vesicle-Encapsulated Composite Nanoparticle and Its Application in Retinoblastoma-Targeted Theranostics. *ACS Biomater. Sci. Eng.* **2024**, *10*, 1830–1842. [CrossRef] [PubMed]
97. Liu, W.; Luo, Y.; Dai, J.; Yang, L.; Huang, L.; Wang, R.; Chen, W.; Huang, Y.; Sun, S.; Cao, J.; et al. Monitoring Retinoblastoma by Machine Learning of Aqueous Humor Metabolic Fingerprinting. *Small Methods* **2022**, *6*, 2101220. [CrossRef] [PubMed]

molecules

MDPI

Review

Calcium Phosphate-Based Nanomaterials: Preparation, Multifunction, and Application for Bone Tissue Engineering

Xin Chen [1], Huizhang Li [1], Yinhua Ma [1,*] and Yingying Jiang [2,*]

[1] Department of Orthopedics, Jiading District Central Hospital Affiliated Shanghai University of Medicine & Health Sciences, Shanghai 201800, China; chenxin930@163.com (X.C.); eric164@126.com (H.L.)
[2] Institute of Translational Medicine, Shanghai University, Shanghai 200444, China
* Correspondence: myh760117@sina.com (Y.M.); yjiang8@shu.edu.cn (Y.J.)

Abstract: Calcium phosphate is the main inorganic component of bone. Calcium phosphate-based biomaterials have demonstrated great potential in bone tissue engineering due to their superior biocompatibility, pH-responsive degradability, excellent osteoinductivity, and similar components to bone. Calcium phosphate nanomaterials have gained more and more attention for their enhanced bioactivity and better integration with host tissues. Additionally, they can also be easily functionalized with metal ions, bioactive molecules/proteins, as well as therapeutic drugs; thus, calcium phosphate-based biomaterials have been widely used in many other fields, such as drug delivery, cancer therapy, and as nanoprobes in bioimaging. Thus, the preparation methods of calcium phosphate nanomaterials were systematically reviewed, and the multifunction strategies of calcium phosphate-based biomaterials have also been comprehensively summarized. Finally, the applications and perspectives of functionalized calcium phosphate biomaterials in bone tissue engineering, including bone defect repair, bone regeneration, and drug delivery, were illustrated and discussed by presenting typical examples.

Keywords: calcium phosphate; nanomaterials; bone tissue engineering; multifunction; drug delivery; bioimaging

1. Introduction

Nowadays, over two million bone grafts are needed for bone defects [1,2], which are caused by trauma, infection, and tumors, since the size of the defect is far larger than the self-healing capability of bone tissue. Autologous bone grafts are still considered the gold standard to achieve bone defect repair [3,4]. Allografts also show excellent bioactivity, but the drawbacks are still obvious, including possible disease transmission, immune rejection, second injury, and donor site morbidity [5]. Thus, various bone substitutes have been made to solve the limitation of bone repair caused by the autologous bone, such as inorganic implants or organic implants. Usually, inorganic implants used for bone defects tend to be peri-implantitis [6], be non-degradable [7], and lack osteoinductivity [8], which bring about the continuous inhibition of bone regeneration and cause the absence of strong and effective mechanical support from newborn bone. Thus, patients may suffer a lot from default treatment.

Bone tissue engineering is a promising approach for the regeneration and repair of damaged bone tissues. Biomaterial-based approaches have emerged as an alternative to these traditional methods. Biomaterials can provide a scaffold for cell adhesion, proliferation, and differentiation, and they can also release growth factors and other bioactive molecules to promote bone regeneration. Biomaterials used for bone tissue engineering should have properties such as biocompatibility, biodegradability, osteoconductivity, and osteoinductivity. Biomaterials can be classified into the following four categories based on their composition: calcium phosphate-based biomaterials, metallic biomaterials, polymeric biomaterials, and composite biomaterials. Among these, calcium phosphate-based biomaterials have received the most attention due to their excellent biocompatibility, bioactivity, and similarity to the mineral component of bone [9,10].

Compared to conventional calcium phosphate-based graft materials, calcium phosphate nanomaterials offer several distinct advantages and show unique properties for bone tissue engineering, including enhanced bioactivity, tailored physical and chemical properties, controlled drug delivery, better integration with host tissue, and ease of fabrication and scalability. Specifically, these biomaterials have a high surface area to volume ratio, which provides more space for cell adhesion and proliferation and also promotes cell differentiation [11,12], as well as loading more therapeutic ingredients [13,14]. Additionally, the nano-sized particles can enhance the mechanical properties and show a profile of controlled drug release.

Thus, calcium phosphate nanomaterials have attracted more and more attention, and various preparation strategies have been developed to satisfy clinical requirements. The preparation methods include wet chemical precipitation, solvothermal synthesis, the sol-gel method, microwave-assisted method, sonochemical synthesis, the enzyme-assisted method, as well as spray drying and electrospinning. Among these, the precipitation method is the most commonly used method for the preparation of nano-calcium phosphate-based biomaterials, while the other methods also have their advantages, which are further discussed in the following section.

Furthermore, calcium phosphate-based nanomaterials can be tailored by adjusting their size, shape, and surface chemistry. Functionalized calcium phosphates are endowed with osteogenic properties, angiogenic properties, antimicrobial properties, bioimaging capabilities, and so on. Herein, calcium phosphate-based nanomaterials showed great potential in bone regeneration, antitumor therapy, and drug delivery. Thus, the review is intended to give a comprehensive summary of the preparation, multifunctionality, and application of nano calcium phosphate-based biomaterials for bone tissue engineering, and it also addresses the attention of readers and provides inspiration for the design of bioactive materials for bone tissue engineering.

2. Synthesis Strategies for Calcium Phosphate-Based Nanomaterials

Recently, lots of synthesis methods have been developed to prepare calcium phosphate nanomaterials, such as wet chemical precipitation, solvothermal synthesis, the sol-gel method, the microwave-assisted method, sonochemical synthesis, the enzyme-assisted method, as well as spray drying and electrospinning. This section gives a thorough introduction of the above-mentioned synthesis methods due to their unique advantages for the fabrication of calcium phosphate-based nanomaterials.

2.1. Wet Chemical Precipitation

Wet chemical precipitation is thought to be the simplest method to prepare calcium phosphate nanomaterials, including amorphous calcium phosphate, which is the first solid phases of calcium phosphate, as well as hydroxyapatite, by providing mixed aqueous solutions of calcium ions and phosphate ions. As shown in Figure 1, the preparation of calcium phosphate-based nanomaterials usually involves the dispersion of the starting materials, typically calcium and phosphate precursors, in an aqueous solution, followed by a reaction between them to form a precipitate. The reaction is typically carried out under controlled conditions, such as fixed pH values and reaction times, to obtain the desired properties of the final biomaterials. After the reaction, the precipitate is washed with water or other solvents to remove impurities and obtain the final compound. The specific method used for the preparation of calcium phosphate-based nanomaterials may vary depending on the desired properties and application of the biomaterials.

The wet chemical precipitation method is a relatively simple and widely used method for the preparation of calcium phosphate-based nanomaterials [1]. However, there are some limitations and drawbacks to this method. For instance, the reaction time required for the precipitation process can be quite long, which may result in an incomplete reaction or the formation of impurities [15]. In addition, the resulting compound may not have optimal properties or functionality for certain applications. To overcome these limitations, researchers have explored various modification strategies. For example, the addition of dopants such as magnesium, cerium, and silicon can improve the functionality of the resulting biomaterials [16]. Surfactants, polymers, proteins, and bioactive molecules have been used to regulate the formation of CaP nanomaterials to regulate their components and phase. For example, in the presence of special medium, mimicking the situation of biomineralization in vivo, proteins and calcium ions can generate a kind of nanoparticle, which leads to a sustained release profile and increased bioactivity [17]. Additionally, microwaves and ultrasounds have also been introduced to improve reaction efficiency.

Moreover, precursor concentration, pH value, reaction temperature, mixing and stirring, and solvent influence the structure, morphology, and properties of nano calcium phosphate obtained through wet chemical precipitation [18,19]. Higher precursor concentrations can lead to larger particle sizes and increased crystallinity, while lower concentrations may result in smaller and more amorphous particles [20]. The optimization of precursor concentrations helps to achieve desired particle properties. The pH value of the reaction solution influences the solubility of calcium and phosphate ions and also affects the precipitation kinetics. Varying the pH can lead to different crystalline phases and morphologies of calcium phosphate nanoparticles, and it can also affect the subsequent implications for bioactivity and biocompatibility [21]. Higher temperatures during the precipitation process generally promote faster crystal growth, leading to larger particles with enhanced crystallinity. Conversely, lower temperatures tend to favor the formation of amorphous or poorly crystalline particles [22]. The method and intensity of mixing or stirring have an impact on particle size distribution, agglomeration, and homogeneity. Proper mixing promotes the uniform dispersion of precursors, resulting in more homogeneous nanoparticles. The solvent being in wet chemical precipitation can also affect the reaction kinetics [23], solubility of precursors, and crystal growth.

Overall, though the wet chemical precipitation method has its limitations, it remains an important and widely used method for the preparation of calcium phosphate-based nanomaterials. Researchers continue to explore and optimize this synthesis method to enrich the functionality of CaP nanomaterials for bone tissue engineering.

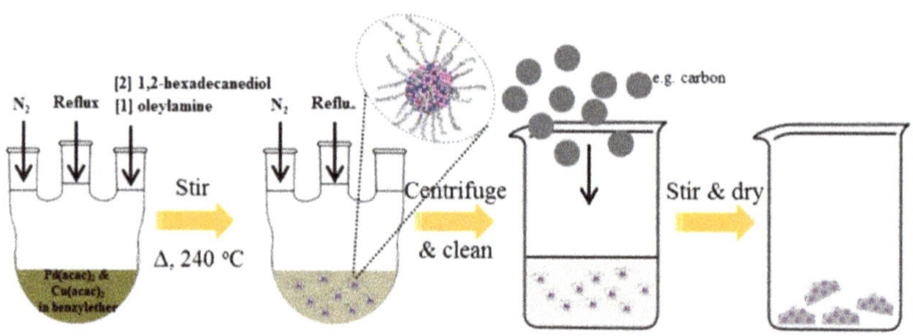

Figure 1. Schematic representation of wet chemical precipitation for the preparation of calcium phosphate-based biomaterial. Reprinted with permission from Ref. [24], Copyright 2019, American Chemical Society (Washington, DC, USA).

2.2. Solvothermal Synthesis

The solvothermal synthesis method is a variation of the hydrothermal method, where organic solvents are used instead of water. This method allows for the use of higher temperatures and pressures, which can increase the solubility of the reactants and promote more rapid reaction rates (Figure 2) [25,26].

In a typical solvothermal synthesis procedure, the starting materials are mixed in a solvent using magnetic stirring. The mixture is then loaded into a sealed container, such as an autoclave, and heated to a high temperature for a fixed period of time. The pressure inside the container is also increased, which can further enhance the solubility of the reactants and accelerate the reaction. After the reaction is complete, the resulting product is typically washed with water or alcohol to remove any impurities or residual reactants. Finally, the product is vacuum-dried to remove any remaining solvent, and the final product can be obtained. Temperature and pressure, reaction time, precursor concentration, solvent, additives, and catalysts influence the structure, morphology, and properties of nano calcium phosphate obtained through solvothermal synthesis. Solvothermal synthesis involves heating the reaction mixture at elevated temperatures and pressures within a sealed autoclave. Temperature and pressure conditions have a significant effect on crystal growth, phase formation, and particle size distribution. Higher temperatures and pressures generally promote faster crystal growth, resulting in larger particles with enhanced crystallinity [27]. Longer reaction times allow for more extensive crystal growth, leading to larger particles, while prolonged reaction times may also result in increased agglomeration or phase transformation [28]. Higher precursor concentrations can lead to the formation of larger particles with increased crystallinity, but at excessively high concentrations, particle agglomeration may occur [29]. Different solvents have varying solubility properties, which affect the precursor dissolution and subsequent precipitation processes. Additional additives or catalysts can also be introduced in solvothermal synthesis to modify the particle characteristics [30]. For example, surfactants or templates can be employed to control particle size or morphology. Catalytic agents may be used to enhance the reaction rate or promote specific crystal phases.

The solvothermal synthesis method has been used to prepare a variety of calcium phosphate-based nanoparticles with controlled size, morphology, and composition. This method allows for greater control over the reaction conditions and can result in the production of biomaterials with improved properties and functionality compared to those obtained by other methods [31]. One of the main benefits of the solvothermal synthesis method is its ability to dissolve almost any material in the solvent, which can be heated and pressurized to its melting point. This allows for the synthesis of highly ordered nanostructures with controlled size, morphology, and composition. For example, the solvothermal method has been used to synthesize highly ordered arrays of microtubes made from a calcium chloride ($CaCl_2$) powder precursor, which can form a block of three-dimensional structure. In addition, the solvothermal method has also been used to transform unstable di-tert-butyl phosphate into a stable precursor for calcium phosphate ceramic biomaterials using different calcium sources [32].

However, the solvothermal method does have some challenges; one of the major weaknesses is the difficulty in controlling the morphology and structure of the resulting nanostructures. This is due to multiple variables, such as the type, volume ratio, and concentration of the starting materials, as well as the reaction conditions, such as temperature and pressure [33]. Furthermore, the use of organic solvents can also pose some challenges, such as the need for appropriate safety precautions and the potential for toxicity [34]. Despite these challenges, the solvothermal method remains an important technique for the synthesis of CaP nanoparticles with tailored properties and functionality for bone tissue engineering and other applications.

2.3. Sol-Gel Method

As shown in Figure 3, the sol-gel method is another wet-chemical method for the synthesis of calcium phosphate-based nanoparticles. It is a relatively new procedure that does not require high temperature to help the compound reaction [35]. The sol-gel method typically involves several stages, including hydrolysis and polycondensation, gelation, drying, and crystallization. In the first step, inorganic materials, such as chlorides, nitrates, and sulfides, or metal alkoxides are dissolved in an acidic or alkaline solution and are stirred for a long time to obtain precursors. Metal alkoxides are then added to the precursors for polymerization, which leads to the development of a gel. Finally, the gel is converted into solid materials by freeze-drying or drying with high temperature [36,37] and can be used for coating scaffolds without any other drying.

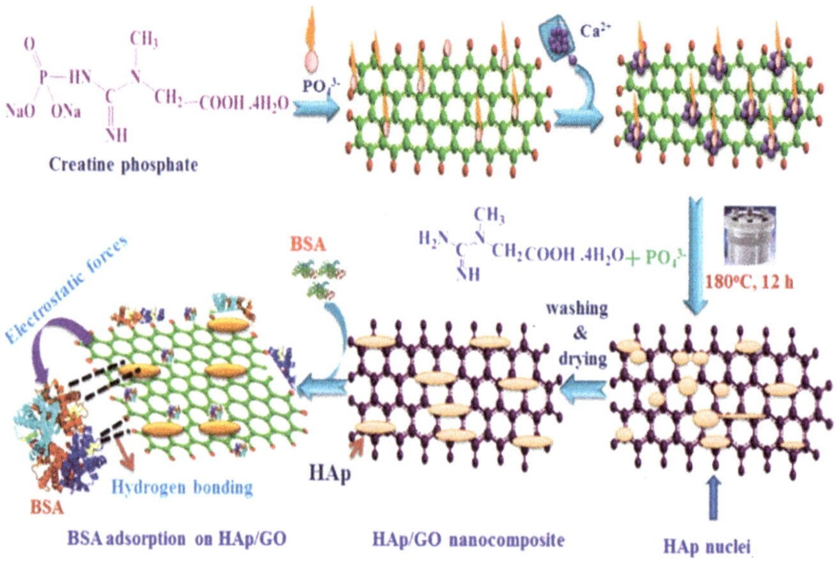

Figure 2. Schematic representation of solvothermal synthesis for the preparation of calcium phosphate-based biomaterial. Reprinted with permission from Ref. [31], Copyright 2016, Royal Society of Chemistry (London, UK).

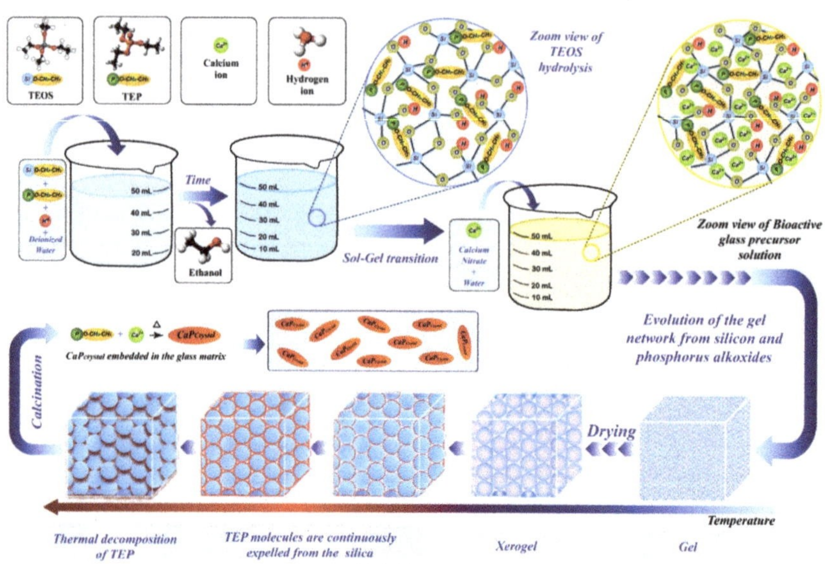

Figure 3. Schematic representation of the classical sol-gel procedure for the preparation of calcium phosphate-based bio-material. Reprinted with permission from Ref. [35], Copyright 2020, Elsevier (Amsterdam, The Netherlands).

Precursor composition, pH and solvent, hydrolysis and condensation ratios, drying methods, and annealing and heat treatment contribute to the regulation of the structure, morphology, and properties of nano calcium phosphate obtained through the sol-gel method [38]. Different precursors, such as inorganic salts or alkoxides, can lead to variations in the stoichiometry, crystallinity, and phase composition of the nanoparticles [39]. Varying the pH can affect the hydrolysis and condensation reactions, which, in turn, influence the particle size, surface charge, and morphology. The hydrolysis of the precursor and polycondensation of the resolved chemical products are the most significant steps in this synthesis [40]. Through this process, a wide range of diameters of nanoparticles can be synthesized by varying the ratio of materials [41]. These steps also affect the features of the final composites, such as specific surface area and microporosity, which can be influenced by using different reagents, various ratios of raw materials, or different temperature ranges [36,42,43]. Different drying techniques, such as freeze-drying or high-temperature drying, can lead to variations in the particle size distribution, agglomeration, and phase composition. Annealing can induce phase transformations, crystal growth, and improved crystallinity. The temperature and duration of heat treatment can be optimized to achieve desired properties, such as enhanced crystallinity, improved stability, and controlled release behavior.

Though there are still big challenges, the sol-gel method is still widely used due to its ability to produce CaP nanomaterials with high purity, good crystallinity, and controllable morphologies, making it suitable for various biomedical applications, including bone tissue engineering.

2.4. Microwave-Assisted Method

Microwave-assisted synthesis is a method of heating and accelerating the chemical reaction between materials to obtain CaP particles [44,45]. As shown in Figure 4 [45], the process involves dissolving soluble materials in a solvent, adjusting the pH value of the mixture, subjecting the mixture to microwave irradiation at a fixed temperature and time, and finally isolating the product through centrifugation, cleaning, and drying [46,47].

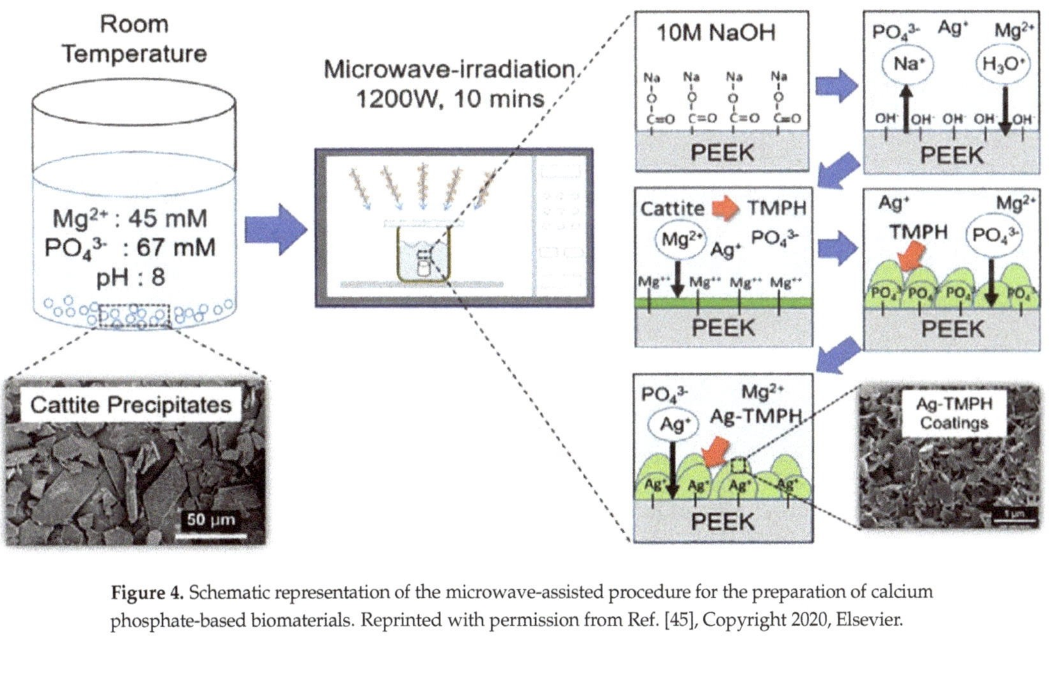

Figure 4. Schematic representation of the microwave-assisted procedure for the preparation of calcium phosphate-based biomaterials. Reprinted with permission from Ref. [45], Copyright 2020, Elsevier.

Power and duration, solvent and pH, precursor concentration and ratio, additives and surfactants, and cooling rate influence the formation of CaP nanoparticles [48]. Higher power and longer durations can lead to increased heating and higher reaction temperatures, affecting the nucleation, growth, and crystallinity of the nano calcium phosphate particles [49]. Different solvents and pH conditions can affect the particle size, morphology, and phase composition of the nano calcium phosphate [17]. Varying the precursor concentrations and ratios can affect the nucleation and growth kinetics, leading to variations in particle size, crystallinity, and surface properties [50]. These additives can act as nucleation promoters, growth modifiers, or surface modifiers, resulting in controlled particle formation, improved dispersibility, and enhanced stability. Rapid cooling can lead to the formation of amorphous or partially crystalline phases, while slower cooling rates may promote the growth of larger crystals [51]. The cooling rate can influence the phase composition, crystallinity, and surface properties of the synthesized nanoparticles. Thus, the structure, morphology, phase, as well as particle size can be regulated via the parameters.

Microwave-assisted synthesis has some advantages, such as high energy efficiency, shorter synthesis time, as well as consuming few samples [39], which make it a promising method for the laboratory. However, the high heat generated can also lead to some disadvantages, such as the deterioration of the sample constituents and the high cost of industry-level equipment maintenance. It is important to consider both the advantages and disadvantages of this method before using it in research or industrial applications.

2.5. Sonochemical Synthesis

As shown in Figure 5, sonochemical synthesis has the potential to offer several advantages over other synthesis methods, such as being safer and more environmentally friendly, as it does not require the use of toxic solvents [52]. This method also has the advantage of the reduction in reaction time, the ability to control particle size, and the production of highly homogeneous materials. The method can also be carried out at relatively low temperatures and does not require high-pressure conditions, which reduces the energy consumption and cost of the process. Additionally, sonochemistry can be used to modify the surface properties of materials, such as increasing their porosity, improving their biocompatibility, and enhancing their drug delivery capabilities. Additionally, the cavitation effect can lead to smaller and more uniform particle size, which can increase the protein absorption of the nanoparticles [53]. Herein, ultrasonic power and frequency, [54] reactant concentration, [55] pH and temperature, the addition of surfactants and additives, and reaction time [56] all influence the formation of calcium phosphate nanoparticles via sonochemical synthesis.

Further research is needed to fully understand the effects of sonochemical synthesis on the properties of calcium phosphate-based nanoparticles, including their crystallinity and morphology [56]. With continued exploration and the refinement of this method, it may prove to be a valuable approach for the synthesis of high-quality calcium phosphate-based materials with a wide range of potential applications. The main disadvantage of sonochemistry is that it is difficult to scale up to industrial-level production due to the limitations of the equipment and the variability in the cavitation effect.

2.6. Enzyme-Assisted Method

There is also research that shows that calcium phosphate-based nanoparticles, obtained in the enzymatic approach, have strong bioactivity in vivo/vitro experiments due to functional enzymes in promoting biomineralization [57]. As shown in Figure 6, Jiang et al. developed bioactive minerals via the enzymatic reaction based on the use of alkaline phosphatase (ALP) to catalyze the hydrolysis of ATP molecules and the release of phosphate ions combined with the unconstrained calcium ions in the precursor solutions. Thereafter, the organic-inorganic composites containing amorphous calcium phosphate, ATP, ADP, and AMP were obtained, and the composites showed superior biocompatibility, enhanced osteogenic differentiation, and reduced repair time for bone regeneration [58]. Additionally, the control of rate of deposition and final coating morphology can be reached by adjusting the value of the pH, the concentration of the enzyme, the ratio of calcium and phosphate ions, and the time of reaction [59].

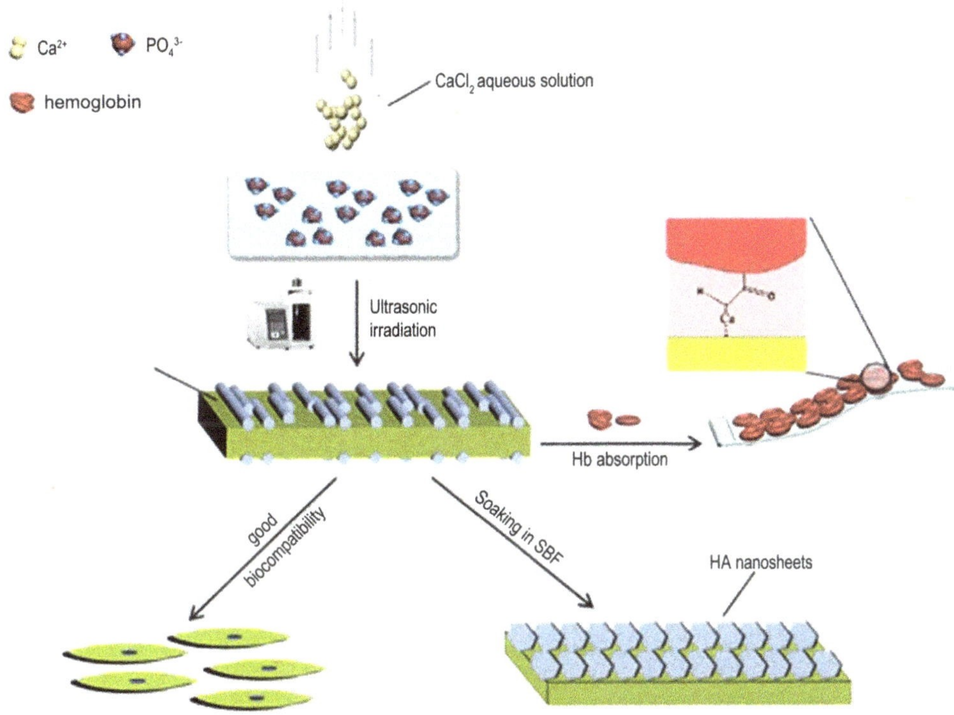

Figure 5. Schematic representation of the sonochemical synthesis for the preparation of calcium phosphate-based biomaterials. Reprinted with permission from Ref. [52], Copyright 2018, Nature Publishing Group (Berlin, Germany).

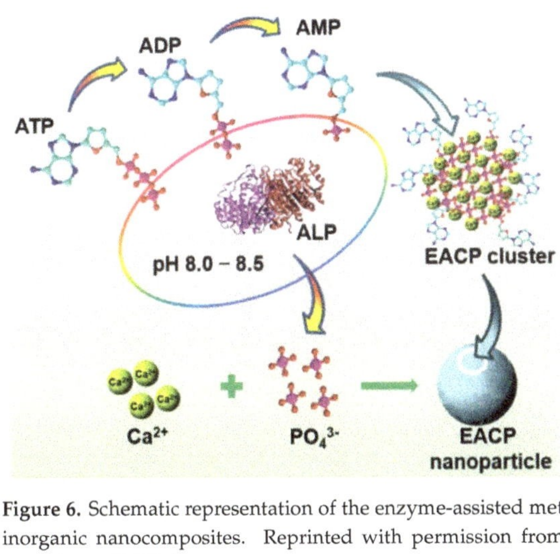

Figure 6. Schematic representation of the enzyme-assisted method for the preparation of organic-inorganic nanocomposites. Reprinted with permission from Ref. [58], Copyright 2018, Wiley (Hoboken, NJ, USA).

Enzymatic methods offer several advantages in the synthesis of calcium phosphate-based biomaterials. Firstly, they are mild and environmentally friendly because the reaction is performed under mild conditions without the use of harsh chemicals or high temperatures [60]. Secondly, the obtained materials are usually of highly purity, which is essential for their biological activity. Thirdly, enzymatic methods have the potential to mimic the biomineralization processes that occur in living organisms, leading to the synthesis of biomaterials with unique properties that are not possible to achieve via other methods [57]. The enzymatic synthesis method also has some drawbacks. The enzymatic reaction is often slow and requires longer reaction times than other methods. Additionally, the enzyme used in the process can be expensive and can affect the final product yield.

2.7. Spray Drying and Electrospinning

Spray drying and electrospinning are two other methods used for the preparation of calcium phosphate nanomaterials. In the spray drying method, a solution containing the calcium and phosphate precursors is sprayed into a hot air stream, resulting in the formation of nanoparticles. In addition, the spray process can also be applied to the preparation of calcium phosphate coating [61]. In the electrospinning method, a polymer solution containing calcium and phosphate precursors is used to form nanofibers, which are then calcined to obtain the desired calcium phosphate nanomaterials.

Additionally, plasma spraying can also be used for the preparation of calcium phosphate coating, which can effectively prevent the corrosion and loosening of metal implants in clinic. Plasma spraying requires a high cost; therefore, the application is limited. Liu et al. developed a double-layer calcium phosphate-sandwiched siloxane composite coating that can decrease the cost by using the chemical conversion method and the sequential mineralization method to promote the loading of Ca and P elements with the coating so that this magnesium alloy with the composite coating can achieve good mineralization ability and biocompatibility in vivo [62]. Moreover, calcium phosphate coatings can also be obtained via sequential mineralization in SBF [63] or electrochemical-assisted deposition [64].

For spray drying and electrospinning, the concentration of the calcium and phosphate precursors in the spray drying and electrospinning solutions affects the viscosity and surface tension of the solution. Higher concentrations typically result in increased particle size and improved crystallinity. Different solvents have varying evaporation rates and compatibility with the precursors, [65] leading to differences in particle size, porosity, and surface characteristics. Higher airflow rates and temperatures generally result in smaller particle sizes and improved crystallinity. Optimal feed rates ensure uniform particle distribution [66]. Different polymers have varying viscosities, conductivity, and compatibility with the precursors, leading to differences in fiber morphology, diameter, and mechanical properties [67]. Post-treatment techniques, such as heat treatment or cross-linking, can influence the crystallinity, porosity, and mechanical strength of the nanoparticles.

As described above, each synthesis method has its own unique advantages and limitations for the preparation of calcium phosphate nanomaterials, and a summary is given in Table 1. Proper synthesis methods can be employed for preparing calcium phosphate nanomaterials with desired properties.

Table 1. A summary of synthesis methods for the preparation of calcium phosphate-based nanomaterials.

Synthesis Methods	Advantages	Disadvantages
Wet chemical precipitation	1. Simple, efficient [68] 2. Easy control of the reaction system environment [19]	1. Needs a long reaction time [19] 2. Difficult to purify composites [69]
Solvothermal synthesis	1. Short reaction time [28] 2. Simple operation process [29]	1. Security risks in the reaction process [70] 2. Hard to control materials' properties [71] 3. More energy consumption [72]

Table 1. *Cont.*

Synthesis Methods	Advantages	Disadvantages
Sol-gel method	1. Simple synthesis process [73] 2. Excellent calcium phosphate crystallization [74]	1. The physicochemical properties of the product are uncontrollable [75] 2. Mixed with impurities [76]
Microwave-assisted method	1. Short reaction time [51] 2. Less raw material consumption [48]	1. Raw materials require full dissolution [45] 2. Limited application range [17] 3. High equipment maintenance costs [77]
Sonochemical synthesis	1. Less cost of the process [55] 2. The cavitation effect [52]	1. Few studies on the preparation of calcium phosphate materials [78] 2. Hard to industrialize [53]
Enzyme-assisted method	1. Environmentally friendly [79] 2. The reaction conditions are controllable [58]	1. Longer reaction time [80] 2. Whole process monitoring [81]
Spray drying and electrospinning	1. Machine parameters control product structure [82]	1. High equipment costs [83] 2. Difficult preparation of precursor solution [84]

3. Multifunctional Properties of Calcium Phosphate-Based Nanomaterials

The various synthesis methods contribute to the diversity of calcium phosphate-based nanoparticles. Herein, calcium phosphate-based nanomaterials have favorable properties, involving biocompatibility, biodegradability, and the fact that calcium is a critical mineral composition of human bones and teeth [85], and calcium phosphate-based nanomaterials can also decompose in an aqueous solution with the pH value in human internal environment [86]. Thus, it can be used as a great carrier to load drugs and can protect them in blood [87], leading to controllable release in the human internal situation.

Moreover, large specific surface areas of calcium phosphate-based nanomaterials lead to loading more therapeutic drugs, increasing the concentration of the drug around the targeted sites to achieve efficient bone healing [88,89]. Based on this reason, Kans et al. developed CaP-based coatings with interconnected pores via ultrasound-assisted microarc oxidation method. The porous structure of the coatings contributes to the improvement of the vancomycin loading capacity to achieve more effective antibacterial properties. Additionally, by taking advantage of the electrostatic interaction between Ca^{2+} ions, on the surface of the CaP, and COO^{-} in bovine serum albumin (BSA), Kanupriya et al. found that anhydrous dicalcium phosphate synthesized via rapid microwave-assisted synthesis had higher porosity (77.8 m^2/g), providing more binding sites for BSA. The porous anhydrous dicalcium phosphate showed about a 59 wt% loading capacity of BSA, which is much higher than that of hydroxyapatite with a lower specific surface area (16.1 m^2/g) [90].

As shown above, calcium phosphates have the ability to incorporate biomolecules, inside or on the surface, to reach the target sites and deliver therapeutic compounds. In addition, some biomolecules can combine with inorganic structures to repair bone defects by suppressing the acute inflammatory response [91,92] or various active ingredients, promoting the formation of new blood vessels, inhibiting the fusion and migration of osteoclasts [93] or directly encouraging osteogenic differentiation [94–96]. As shown in Figure 7a, Kai-Chi et al. developed uniform carbonate-based apatite nanorods, which upregulate cellular attachment and mineralization, by combining ferulic acid through the regulation of heparin [97]. Additionally, many growth factors show various functions to control the evolution, differentiation, and metabolism of stem cells in the process of bone regeneration, including platelet-derived growth factor (PDGF), transforming growth factor beta1 (TGFbeta1), vascular endothelial growth factor (VEGF), basic fibroblast growth factor (bFGF), hepatocyte growth factor (HGF), epidermal growth factor (EGF), insulin-like growth factor-1 (IGF-1), and so on. Bone-morphogenetic proteins (BMP) show especially promising results when used in bone regeneration. As shown in Figure 7b, Seong et al. combined BMP-2 with the crosslinked porous biphasic calcium phosphate, invented by applying a water-in-oil emulsion technique with camphene as a pore generator, to achieve high loading efficiency and constant release [95]. In another study shown in Figure 7c, there is a phenomenon that the calcium pyrophosphate can keep the shape of nanofiber microspheres in the presence of a low pH value (pH~4), consisting of a stomach environment, and can reorganize into fiber and even into mineral plates in the intestinal environment (pH~7), which means that the large specific surface area of 65 m^2/g turns into only 1.5 m^2/g; thus, the loaded protein can keep its high activity when exposed to the stomach environment. Subsequently, the loaded proteins would be released in the intestinal environment, which leads to targeted enteric delivery [98].

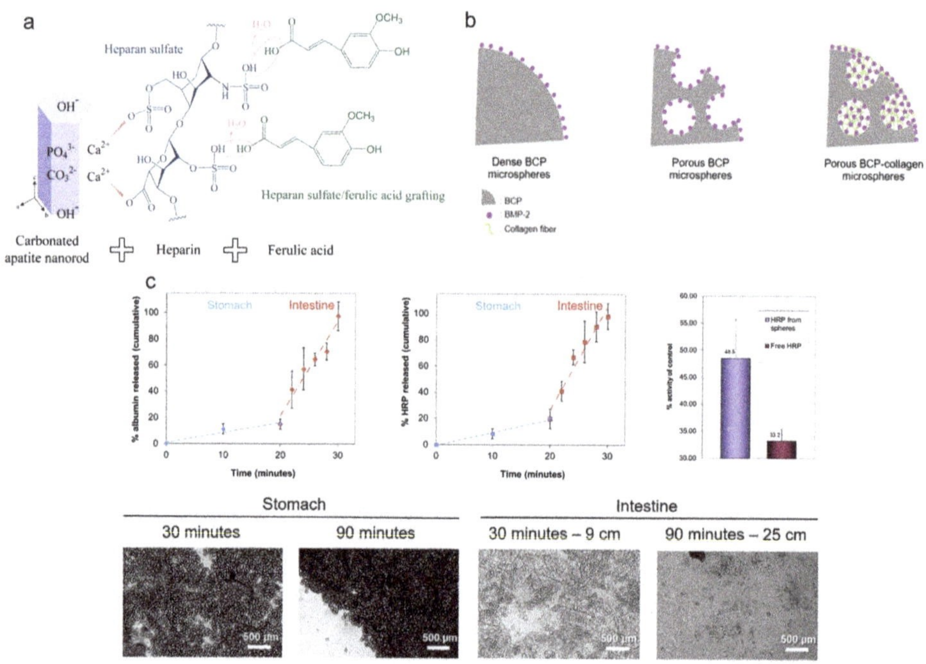

Figure 7. Strategies for the component engineering of nano-calcium phosphate-based biomaterials. (**a**) Calcium phosphate-based biomaterial coated with heparin to crosslink with ferulic acid; reprinted with permission from Ref. [97], Copyright 2021, MDPI (Basel, Switzerland). (**b**) The crosslinked porous biphasic calcium phosphate loading more BMP-2; reprinted with permission from Ref. [95]. (**c**) The structure of the calcium phosphate-based biomaterial influenced by the pH value, leading to the drug release; reprinted with permission from Ref. [98], Copyright 2019, Elsevier.

Stem cells, such as hBMSCs [10], hESC-MSCs [99], and hiPSC-MSCAs [100], play a critical role in the process of bone regeneration. Several studies have investigated that calcium-based materials can load these cells [101], and the interaction between nanostructures and cells contributes to bone healing [102,103]. Calcium phosphate bone cement (CPC) was compounded with bone marrow mesenchymal stem cells (BMSCs) and was condensed in alginate chitosan alginate (ACA) microcapsules. This can protect cells from the negative influence of the CPC setting reaction and effectively form macropores in the composite to help CPC display better bone regeneration functions in the performance of ectopic osteogenesis and high effective degradability in vivo compared to the CPC with the addition of pure microcapsules or cell microcapsules [103]. Calcium phosphates, which are osteoconductive, injectable, and moldable, can provide strong sites for the proliferation and differentiation of cells and can promote bone healing.

Gene therapy is a potential and new approach to achieve highly efficient bone regeneration [104]. Calcium phosphate nanomaterials can be used as carriers for RNA [85,105] or DNA [106,107]. BMP-2 promotes bone regeneration effectively, and a high dosage of it can be loaded on the calcium phosphate nanocarriers to achieve the satisfied release of the growth factor during the stage of bone regeneration. However, there is difficulty in achieving the controlled release of growth factors during bone regeneration. A fast degradation rate leads to the release of BMP-2 at a high level, as well as bone or tooth resorption. To solve this problem, achieving larger, longer, and a more gradual release of BMP-2, as shown in Figure 8a, Tenkumo et al. designed a multi-shell calcium phosphate nanoparticle as a carrier with BMP-2-encoding-plasmid DNA. Thereafter, the drug delivery system was incorporated with a nanohydroxyapatite-collagen scaffold to promote gene transfection successfully [96]. The efficient cellular uptake of nanoparticle-loaded nucleic acid molecules has a huge influence on the efficiency of bone regeneration. In Figure 8b, it is shown that Bogyu Choi et al. found that nucleic acid-loaded CaP nanoparticles with a Gln-Ochi chitosan coating can protect these particles from forming large aggregates due to electrostatic repulsion and can achieve higher cellular uptake to promote bone tissue regeneration.

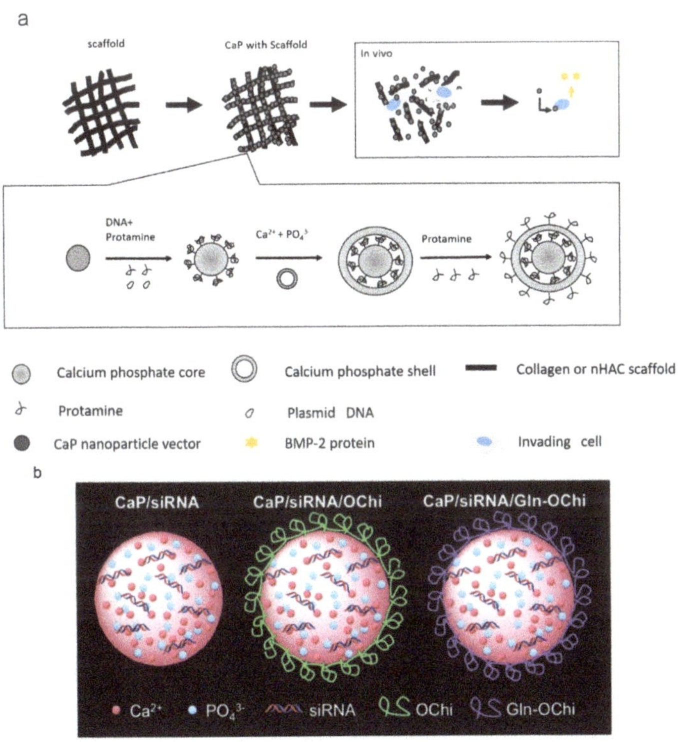

Figure 8. Strategies for calcium phosphate-based material loading genes. (**a**) Calcium phosphate-loading DNA fixed in a scaffold to promote BMP-2 protein; reprinted with permission from Ref. [96], Copyright 2018, Elsevier. (**b**) The nucleic acid-loaded nanoparticles, combining nucleic acid molecule-loaded CaP nanoparticles with a Gln-Ochi chitosan coating to avoid aggregating; reprinted with permission from Ref. [108], Copyright 2015, Royal Society of Chemistry.

Metal ions can also be integrated within calcium phosphate-based nanomaterials, regulating gene expression and promoting bone repair [109–113]. As shown in Figure 9, Wu et al. introduced strontium ions, which came from $SrCO_3$, into the modified calcium phosphate cement, composed of 20 wt% pregelatinized starch and 10 wt% $BaSO_4$, to improve the flexibility, uniformity, and radiopacity performance of the cement. A total of 0.25 M of the Na_2HPO_4 solution acted as the setting liquid. This mixture performed well in a calvarial defect model of a rat and showed suitable mechanical strength [114].

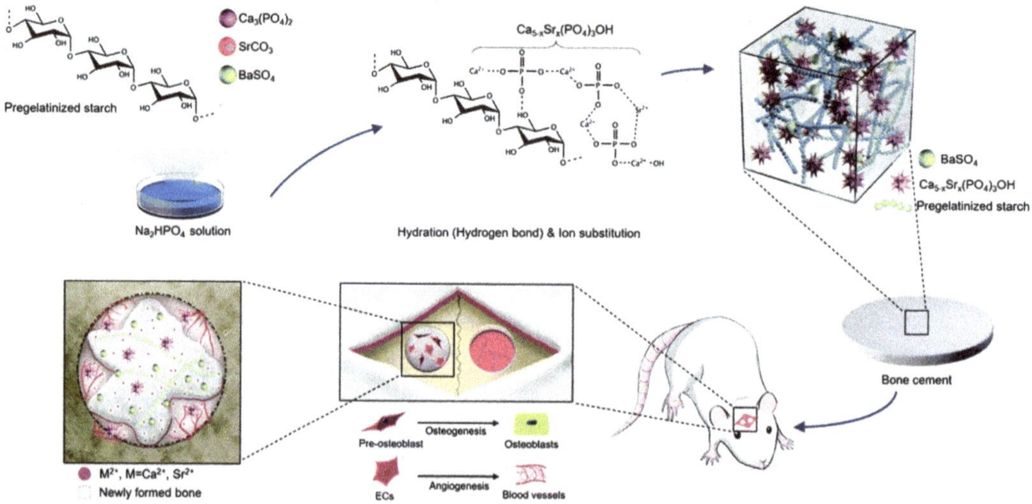

Figure 9. Strategies for mixing metal ions with calcium phosphate. Calcium phosphate cement mixed with Ba/Sr ions to achieve bone regeneration. Reprinted with permission from Ref. [114], Copyright 2021, Royal Society of Chemistry.

4. Applications of Calcium Phosphate-Based Nanomaterials in Bone Tissue Engineering

Calcium phosphate-based nanomaterials show superior biocompatibility, show osteoinductivity, and have high surface area and porosity. Thus, they have been widely used for bone regeneration [115]. Additionally, calcium phosphate-based nanomaterials can be doped with special compounds to promote bone repair directly. Susmita et al. designed 3D calcium phosphate scaffolds, resembling the structure of cortical and cancellous bones, to provide a stronger, denser structure to develop compressive strengths of the scaffold and maintain the central interconnected porosity for cell proliferation and vascularization. The scaffold was incorporated with natural compounds from ginger root and garlic powder, which can enhance bone healing when used in vivo, and improved the bioavailability of these medicinal compounds [116] (Figure 10a). Furthermore, many metal elements also have various influences on the process of bone regeneration, such as silicon, magnesium, cerium, and so on. Based on this theory, Fe and Zn were combined with tricalcium phosphate (TCP) via co-deposition because these two elements can improve new blood vessel formation, which can significantly promote bone regeneration; then, the Fe/Zn-modified TCP powders were turned into a solid, and micropores were formed inside at room temperature. The composites achieved the sustained release of metal (Ca^{2+}, Zn^{2+} and Fe^{3+}) ions, which can promote the process of bone repair [117] (Figure 10b). Additionally, because of the low mechanical strength, brittleness, and quick resorption rate, CaP-based scaffolds need to be reinforced with mechanical strength and be improved regarding bioactivity. It is reported that bioceramic powders (hydroxyapatite and β-tricalcium phosphate) have been embedded in mixed solutions of chitosan and silk fibroin to improve both the mechanical properties and the differentiation of mesenchymal stem cells since chitosan and silk fibroin have shown better bioactivity in supporting the growth and differentiation of BMSCs.

Additionally, the polymer solution can be used as the bioink of robocasting equipment to print 3D scaffolds with fixed system parameters at room temperature, and this scaffold achieved great performance regarding mechanical properties and biocompatibility [118]. Calcium phosphate-based materials can also be used as carriers to load cells or growth factors, which can improve effective therapeutic ingredients in bone defect areas, can keep the sustained release of these factors, and can provide enough room for osteoblasts and new blood vessels [119]. Li et al. reported that bone marrow mesenchymal stem cells and platelet-rich plasma combined with a calcium phosphate cement scaffold achieved more newly formed bone areas than normal calcium phosphate cement scaffolds in an in vivo experiment [120].

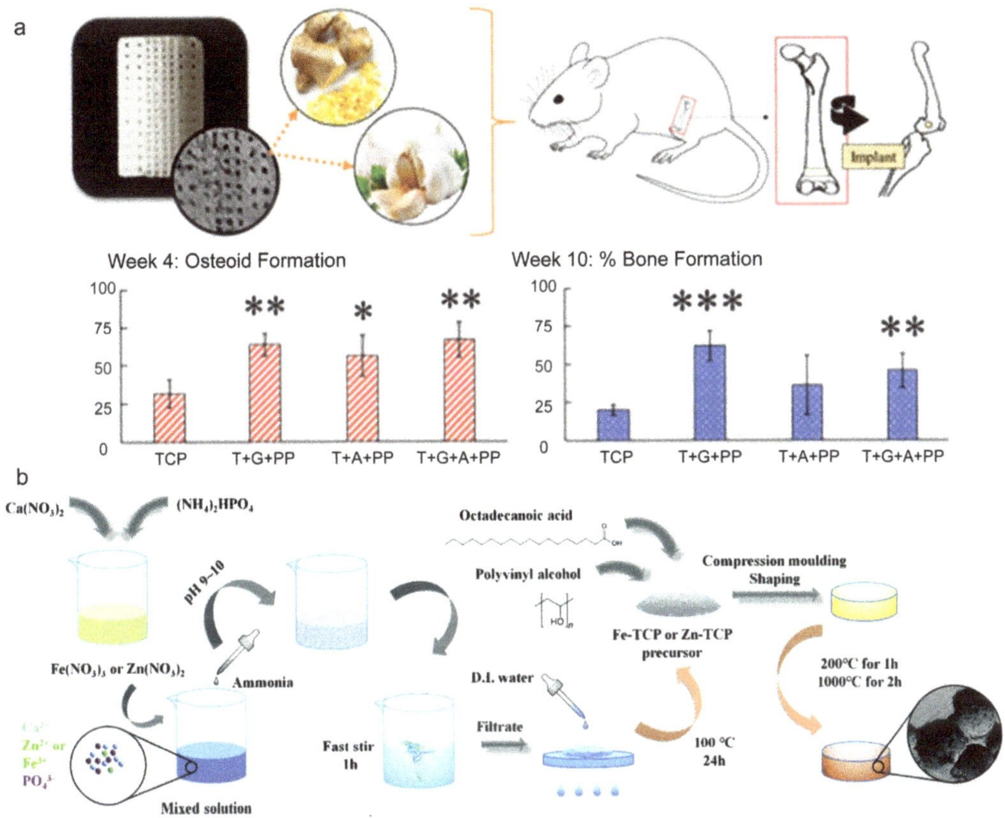

Figure 10. Calcium phosphate composite materials with different properties for bone repair. (**a**) Calcium phosphate scaffolds loaded with ginger and garlic extracts can improve bone regeneration and osteogenic differentiation (* $p < 0.05$; ** $0.05 < p < 0.01$; and *** $p < 0.01$); reprinted with permission from Ref. [116], Copyright 2022, American Chemical Society. (**b**) Calcium phosphate materials were combined with Zn/Fe ions to turn micropores into a dispersed solid; reprinted with permission from Ref. [117], Copyright 2019, Royal Society of Chemistry.

Recently, near-infrared-emitting persistent luminescence nanoparticles have been used as an optical probe for bioimaging and biosensing [121,122]. Though they show low absorptivity in deep-tissue imaging, achieving stable in vivo luminescence is still a great challenge [123]. Chen et al. developed Eu^{3+}/Gd^{3+} ion-dual-doped CaP nanoparticles via co-precipitation using block copolymer polylactide-block-monomethoxy as a template. The nanoparticles showed prolonged stability (more than 80 days), improved the T1-weighted

MRI signal intensity, and decreased T2-weighted MRI signal intensity, which resulted in darker images for the better observation of changes in local areas in vivo [124] (Figure 11a). Additionally, to monitor the in vivo performance of calcium phosphate cements, which show a high structural similarity to bone [125], calcium phosphate cements linked with gadolinium (III) by bisphosphonates were developed, and they showed shortened T1 relaxation times of the water in tissues and achieved signal enhancement in a T1-weighted MRI. In this way, the highly accurate evaluation of the implant shape both in MRI and CT for a prolonged time period (about 8 weeks) was achieved [126] (Figure 11b).

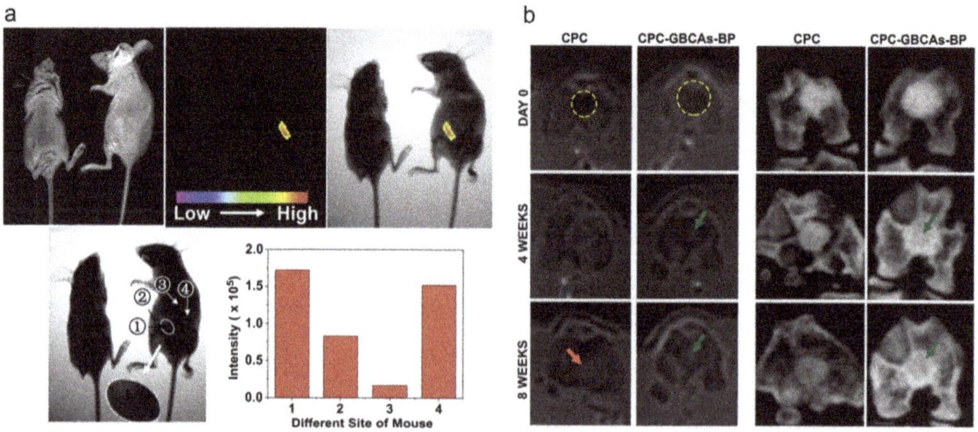

Figure 11. Multi-application in the imaging area. (**a**) Calcium phosphate-based materials used in bioimaging; reprinted with permission from Ref. [124], Copyright 2012, Elsevier. (**b**) Simple flow chart of calcium phosphate composite gadolinium and for CT and MRI bone defect repair evaluation. Green arrows indicate the bright area which appears in the middle of the implant on the MRI acquisitions after 4 weeks from the surgery. Red arrow displays the calcium phosphate cements that become indistinguishable from the surrounding bone after 8 weeks from implantation in vivo; reprinted with permission from Ref. [126], Copyright 2018, Wiley.

Calcium phosphate-based nanoparticles are also desirable materials for drug delivery [127]. Doxorubicin could activate the immunogenic cell death of tumor cells through an apoptosis pathway, including reactive oxygen species, which could lead to DNA cleavage and mitochondrial dysfunction [128], while the multidrug resistance of cancers may result in poor prognosis [129]. To address this issue, a selenium-doped CaP, serving as the doxorubicin carrier, was designed for reversing the multidrug resistance of tumors. Se-doped CaP is pH-sensitive and dox can be released specifically in the tumor sites due to the acid microenvironment. Thus, the uptake of anticancer drugs of tumor cells was raised, and Se ions released could decrease reactive oxygen species of tumor cells and the expression of ATP-binding cassette transporters, which reverse multidrug resistance [130] (Figure 12a). The surgery of bone tumors causes large bone defects, and calcium phosphate bone pastes have been widely used as bone substitutes in clinics to replace allogenous bone, providing strong and stable support for the defect sites without internal fixation [131,132], for many years, and the result of anticancer is also well described in the long run [133,134]. Furthermore, there is the theory that calcium ions play a vital role in tumor necrosis by regulating the stability of the intracellular concentration of calcium ions [135–137], and a high concentration of calcium in the microenvironment of the tumor can encourage tumor calcification [138,139]. Based on this phenomenon, calcium phosphate can combine with some special materials, such as ferritin, which is a promising load for targeted delivery, to protect ferritin from interception to achieve the function of targeted delivery to the tumor effectively, and the shell of calcium phosphate not only counterbalances the acidic microenvironment around tumors but also accelerates the immunomodulation and calcification of cancers [140,141]. CaP nanoparticles can also be coated to camouflage, which may result in intracellular calcium overload and induce apoptosis. For example, TiO_2-coated CaP can elevate the generation of reactive oxygen species, due to the demonstrative property of inorganic sonosensitizers, and can provide calcium ions due to the acidic microenvironment of the tumor (Figure 12b) [142–144].

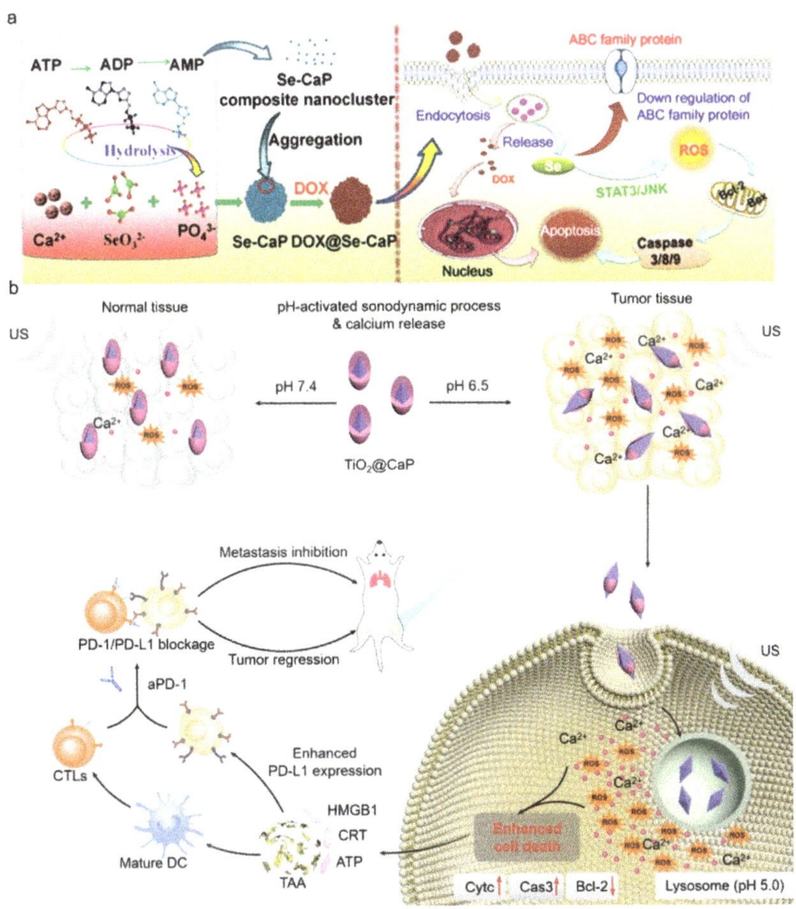

Figure 12. Strategies for calcium phosphate-based materials to kill cancer cells. (**a**) Reversal of the multidrug resistance of tumors by combining calcium phosphate with Se element; reprinted with permission from Ref. [130], Copyright 2020, Elsevier. (**b**) Construction of calcium phosphate and TiO_2 to promote cancer therapy; reprinted with permission from Ref. [142], Copyright 2021, Wiley.

5. Conclusions and Perspectives

Nano-calcium phosphate-based biomaterials have shown great potential in bone tissue engineering due to their unique properties, including their small size, high surface area to volume ratio, and multifunctionality. Various preparation methods, including sol-gel, hydrothermal synthesis, spray drying, and electrospinning, have been used to obtain these biomaterials with controlled size, morphology, and composition.

The multifunctionality of nano-calcium phosphate-based biomaterials is attributed to their abilities to enhance the osteogenic differentiation and mineralization of mesenchymal stem cells, to promote angiogenesis, and to exhibit antimicrobial properties. These properties make them attractive for various applications in bone tissue engineering, including bone defect repair, bioimaging, and anticancer applications.

The preparation, multifunctionality, and application of nano-calcium phosphate-based biomaterials for bone tissue engineering have been extensively studied and reviewed in the literature. These biomaterials have shown great potential in the regeneration and repair of bone tissues and can provide a scaffold for the adhesion, proliferation, and differentiation of stem cells. Further research is needed to optimize the preparation methods, functionalization, and characterization of these biomaterials to improve their performance and clinical outcomes. Nonetheless, these biomaterials represent a promising avenue for the development of effective and safe bone tissue engineering therapies.

The future exploration of calcium phosphate-based nanomaterials could be based on the following points: more effective binding of active substances; more effective targeting methods to achieve more effective treatment goals in local areas; and the interaction mechanism between calcium phosphate and substances. Calcium phosphate binds to the active ingredient and can protect the bioactivity of the component from being affected to maximize the function of the ingredient, such as promoting bone regeneration and anticancer properties. In addition, effective targeting strategies can deliver calcium phosphate-loaded components to the relevant areas so that the local area has a high concentration of therapeutic components, which minimizes the harm caused by therapeutic components. In order to achieve the above objectives, it is necessary to further explore the interaction mechanism between calcium phosphate and various substances to achieve the stable synthesis of calcium phosphate materials with related functions and even commercial production into clinical applications. Thus, it is conducive to the stable output of bioactive calcium phosphate material for large-scale production and application in practice.

Thus far, based on the consideration of biosafety, only a few calcium phosphate-based nanoparticles have been applied in clinics. Therefore, we hope that this review inspires readers to obtain more ideas for the design of bone repair materials.

Author Contributions: X.C. and H.L. gave the conceptualization, conducted the investigation, and wrote the original draft; Y.M. and Y.J. revised the manuscript; Y.J. contributed to the funding acquisition. All authors have read and agreed to the published version of the manuscript.

Funding: The authors acknowledge the grants by support from National Natural Science Foundation of China (No. 82102217), Science and Technology Commission of Shanghai Municipality (No. 21YF1413100).

Institutional Review Board Statement: Not applicable.

Informed Consent Statement: Not applicable.

Data Availability Statement: Not applicable.

Conflicts of Interest: The authors declare no conflict of interest.

Sample Availability: Not applicable.

References

1. Kahar, N.N.F.; Ahmad, N.; Jaafar, M.; Yahaya, B.H.; Sulaiman, A.R.; Hamid, Z.A.A. A review of bioceramics scaffolds for bone defects in different types of animal models: HA andbeta-TCP. *Biomed. Phys. Eng. Express* **2022**, *8*, 21. [CrossRef]
2. Greenwald, A.S.; Boden, S.D.; Goldberg, V.M.; Khan, Y.; Laurencin, C.T.; Rosier, R.N. Bone-graft substitutes: Facts, fictions, and applications. *J. Bone Joint Surg. Am.* **2001**, *83* (Suppl. 2), S98–S103. [CrossRef] [PubMed]
3. Wang, J.; Li, W.; He, X.; Li, S.; Pan, H.; Yin, L. Injectable platelet-rich fibrin positively regulates osteogenic differentiation of stem cells from implant hole via the ERK1/2 pathway. *Platelets* **2023**, *34*, 2159020. [CrossRef] [PubMed]
4. Ng, J.; Spiller, K.; Bernhard, J.; Vunjak-Novakovic, G. Biomimetic Approaches for Bone Tissue Engineering. *Tissue Eng. Part B Rev.* **2017**, *23*, 480–493. [CrossRef] [PubMed]
5. Fu, Q.; Saiz, E.; Rahaman, M.N.; Tomsia, A.P. Toward Strong and Tough Glass and Ceramic Scaffolds for Bone Repair. *Adv. Funct. Mater.* **2013**, *23*, 5461–5476. [CrossRef] [PubMed]
6. Tomasi, C.; Regidor, E.; Ortiz-Vigón, A.; Derks, J. Efficacy of reconstructive surgical therapy at peri-implantitis-related bone defects. A systematic review and meta-analysis. *J. Clin. Periodontol.* **2019**, *46* (Suppl. 21), 340–356. [CrossRef]

7. Amini, Z.; Lari, R. A systematic review of decellularized allograft and xenograft-derived scaffolds in bone tissue regeneration. *Tissue Cell* **2021**, *69*, 101494. [CrossRef]
8. Fillingham, Y.; Jacobs, J. Bone grafts and their substitutes. *Bone Joint J.* **2016**, *98-B*, 6–9. [CrossRef]
9. Zhao, R.; Yang, R.; Cooper, P.R.; Khurshid, Z.; Shavandi, A.; Ratnayake, J. Bone Grafts and Substitutes in Dentistry: A Review of Current Trends and Developments. *Molecules* **2021**, *26*, 3007. [CrossRef]
10. Xu, H.H.; Wang, P.; Wang, L.; Bao, C.; Chen, Q.; Weir, M.D.; Chow, L.C.; Zhao, L.; Zhou, X.; Reynolds, M.A. Calcium phosphate cements for bone engineering and their biological properties. *Bone Res.* **2017**, *5*, 17056. [CrossRef]
11. Yang, Y.; Su, S.; Liu, S.; Liu, W.; Yang, Q.; Tian, L.; Tan, Z.; Fan, L.; Yu, B.; Wang, J.; et al. Triple-functional bone adhesive with enhanced internal fixation, bacteriostasis and osteoinductive properties for open fracture repair. *Bioact. Mater.* **2023**, *25*, 273–290. [CrossRef] [PubMed]
12. Idaszek, J.; Jaroszewicz, J.; Choinska, E.; Gorecka, Z.; Hyc, A.; Osiecka-Iwan, A.; Wielunska-Kus, B.; Swieszkowski, W.; Moskalewski, S. Toward osteomimetic formation of calcium phosphate coatings with carbonated hydroxyapatite. *Biomater. Adv.* **2023**, *149*, 213403. [CrossRef] [PubMed]
13. Tabaković, A.; Kester, M.; Adair, J.H. Calcium phosphate-based composite nanoparticles in bioimaging and therapeutic delivery applications. *Wiley Interdiscip. Rev.—Nanomed. Nanobiotechnol.* **2012**, *4*, 96–112. [CrossRef] [PubMed]
14. Zhu, Q.; Chen, Z.; Paul, P.K.; Lu, Y.; Wu, W.; Qi, J. Oral delivery of proteins and peptides: Challenges, status quo and future perspectives. *Acta Pharm. Sin. B* **2021**, *11*, 2416–2448. [CrossRef] [PubMed]
15. Szurkowska, K.; Szeleszczuk, Ł.; Kolmas, J. Effects of Synthesis Conditions on the Formation of Si-Substituted Alpha Tricalcium Phosphates. *Int. J. Mol. Sci.* **2020**, *21*, 9164. [CrossRef]
16. Kim, H.-W.; Kim, Y.-J. Effect of silicon or cerium doping on the anti-inflammatory activity of biphasic calcium phosphate scaffolds for bone regeneration. *Prog. Biomater.* **2022**, *11*, 421–430. [CrossRef]
17. Sanchez-Campos, D.; Valderrama, M.I.R.; Lopez-Ortiz, S.; Salado-Leza, D.; Fernandez-Garcia, M.E.; Mendoza-Anaya, D.; Salinas-Rodriguez, E.; Rodriguez-Lugo, V. Modulated Monoclinic Hydroxyapatite: The Effect of pH in the Microwave Assisted Method. *Minerals* **2021**, *11*, 13. [CrossRef]
18. Latocha, J.; Wojasinski, M.; Sobieszuk, P.; Gierlotka, S.; Ciach, T. Impact of morphology-influencing factors in lecithin-based hydroxyapatite precipitation. *Ceram. Int.* **2019**, *45*, 21220–21227. [CrossRef]
19. Esposti, L.D.; Dotti, A.; Adamiano, A.; Fabbi, C.; Quarta, E.; Colombo, P.; Catalucci, D.; De Luca, C.E.; Iafisco, M. Calcium Phosphate Nanoparticle Precipitation by a Continuous Flow Process: A Design of an Experiment Approach. *Crystals* **2020**, *10*, 17. [CrossRef]
20. Khayrutdinova, D.R.; Goldberg, M.A.; Antonova, O.S.; Krokhicheva, P.A.; Fomin, A.S.; Obolkina, T.O.; Konovalov, A.A.; Akhmedova, S.A.; Sviridova, I.K.; Kirsanova, V.A.; et al. Effects of Heat Treatment on Phase Formation in Cytocompatible Sulphate-Containing Tricalcium Phosphate Materials. *Minerals* **2023**, *13*, 147. [CrossRef]
21. Goh, K.W.; Wong, Y.H.; Ramesh, S.; Chandran, H.; Krishnasamy, S.; Ramesh, S.; Sidhu, A.; Teng, W.D. Effect of pH on the properties of eggshell-derived hydroxyapatite bioceramic synthesized by wet chemical method assisted by microwave irradiation. *Ceram. Int.* **2021**, *47*, 8879–8887. [CrossRef]
22. Latocha, J.; Wojasinski, M.; Janowska, O.; Chojnacka, U.; Gierlotka, S.; Ciach, T.; Sobieszuk, P. Morphology-controlled precipitation/remodeling of plate and rod-shaped hydroxyapatite nanoparticles. *Aiche J.* **2022**, *68*, 12. [CrossRef]
23. Lv, L.; Liao, H.; Zhang, T.; Tang, S.W.; Liu, W.Z. Separation of calcium chloride from waste acidic raffinate in HCl wet process for phosphoric acid manufacture: Simulated and experimental study. *J. Environ. Chem. Eng.* **2022**, *10*, 108076. [CrossRef]
24. Cai, F.; Yang, L.; Shan, S.; Mott, D.; Chen, B.H.; Luo, J.; Zhong, C.-J. Preparation of PdCu Alloy Nanocatalysts for Nitrate Hydrogenation and Carbon Monoxide Oxidation. *Catalysts* **2016**, *6*, 96. [CrossRef]
25. Zhong, H.; Mirkovic, T.; Scholes, G.D. 5.06—Nanocrystal Synthesis. In *Comprehensive Nanoscience and Technology*; Andrews, D.L., Scholes, G.D., Wiederrecht, G.P., Eds.; Academic Press: Amsterdam, The Netherlands, 2011; pp. 153–201. [CrossRef]
26. Mutalib, A.A.A.; Jaafar, N.F. Potential of deep eutectic solvent in photocatalyst fabrication methods for water pollutant degradation: A review. *J. Environ. Chem. Eng.* **2022**, *10*, 107422. [CrossRef]
27. Verma, S.; Murugavel, R. Alkali Metal Di-tert-butyl Phosphates: Single-Source Precursors for Homo- and Heterometallic Inorganic Phosphate Materials. *Inorg. Chem.* **2022**, *61*, 6807–6818. [CrossRef]
28. Qi, C.; Zhu, Y.-J.; Ding, G.-J.; Wu, J.; Chen, F. Solvothermal synthesis of hydroxyapatite nanostructures with various morphologies using adenosine 5′-monophosphate sodium salt as an organic phosphorus source. *RSC Adv.* **2015**, *5*, 3792–3798. [CrossRef]
29. Hao, H.; Wang, Y.; Shi, B. NaLa$(CO_3)(2)$ hybridized with Fe_3O_4 for efficient phosphate removal: Synthesis and adsorption mechanistic study. *Water Res.* **2019**, *155*, 1–11. [CrossRef]
30. Nur, A.; Jumari, A.; Budiman, A.W.; Ruzicka, O.; Fajri, M.A.; Nazriati, N.; Fajaroh, F. Electrosynthesis of Cobalt—Hydroxyapatite Nanoparticles. In Proceedings of the 4th International Conference on Industrial, Mechanical, Electrical, and Chemical Engineering (ICIMECE), Surakarta, Indonesia, 9–11 October 2018.
31. Bharath, G.; Latha, S.B.; Alsharaeh, E.H.; Prakash, P.; Ponpandian, N. Enhanced hydroxyapatite nanorods formation on graphene oxide nanocomposite as a potential candidate for protein adsorption, pH controlled release and an effective drug delivery platform for cancer therapy. *Anal. Methods* **2016**, *9*, 240–252. [CrossRef]
32. Verma, S.; Murugavel, R. Di-tert-butylphosphate Derived Thermolabile Calcium Organophosphates: Precursors for $Ca(H_2PO_4)_2$, $Ca(HPO_4)$, α-/β-$Ca(PO_3)_2$, and Nanocrystalline $Ca_{10}(PO_4)_6(OH)_2$. *Inorg. Chem.* **2020**, *59*, 13233–13244. [CrossRef]

33. Zhang, Y.-G.; Zhu, Y.-J.; Chen, F.; Sun, T.-W.; Jiang, Y.-Y. Ultralong hydroxyapatite microtubes: Solvothermal synthesis and application in drug loading and sustained drug release. *Crystengcomm* **2017**, *19*, 1965–1973. [CrossRef]
34. Yang, M.S.; Xu, P.F.; Zhao, X.Y.; Tian, C.; Han, C.R.; Song, J. Systematic studies of hydroxyapatite/terpene hybrid microspheres: Natural rosin-based phosphorus sources and chemical structures of coordination compounds. *Mater. Res. Express* **2019**, *6*, 8. [CrossRef]
35. Bueno, O.M.V.M.; Herrera, C.L.; Bertran, C.A.; San-Miguel, M.A.; Lopes, J.H. An experimental and theoretical approach on stability towards hydrolysis of triethyl phosphate and its effects on the microstructure of sol-gel-derived bioactive silicate glass. *Mater. Sci. Eng. C Mater. Biol. Appl.* **2021**, *120*, 111759. [CrossRef]
36. Coelho, S.A.R.; Almeida, J.C.; Unalan, I.; Detsch, R.; Miranda Salvado, I.M.; Boccaccini, A.R.; Fernandes, M.H.V. Cellular Response to Sol-Gel Hybrid Materials Releasing Boron and Calcium Ions. *ACS Biomater. Sci. Eng.* **2021**, *7*, 491–506. [CrossRef] [PubMed]
37. Snyder, K.L.; Holmes, H.R.; McCarthy, C.; Rajachar, R.M. Bioactive vapor deposited calcium-phosphate silica sol-gel particles for directing osteoblast behavior. *J. Biomed. Mater. Res. A* **2016**, *104*, 2135–2148. [CrossRef] [PubMed]
38. Akbarzade, T.; Farmany, A.; Farhadian, M.; Khamverdi, Z.; Dastgir, R. Synthesis and characterization of nano bioactive glass for improving enamel remineralization ability of casein phosphopeptide-amorphous calcium phosphate (CPP-ACP). *BMC Oral. Health* **2022**, *22*, 9. [CrossRef]
39. Christ, B.; Glaubitt, W.; Berberich, K.; Weigel, T.; Probst, J.; Sextl, G.; Dembski, S. Sol-Gel-Derived Fibers Based on Amorphous alpha-Hydroxy-Carboxylate-Modified Titanium(IV) Oxide as a 3-Dimensional Scaffold. *Materials* **2022**, *15*, 12. [CrossRef] [PubMed]
40. Yilmaz, E.; Soylak, M. 15—Functionalized Nanomaterials for Sample Preparation Methods. In *Handbook of Nanomaterials in Analytical Chemistry*; Mustansar Hussain, C., Ed.; Elsevier: Amsterdam, The Netherlands, 2020; pp. 375–413. [CrossRef]
41. Singh, L.P.; Bhattacharyya, S.K.; Kumar, R.; Mishra, G.; Sharma, U.; Singh, G.; Ahalawat, S. Sol-Gel processing of silica nanoparticles and their applications. *Adv. Colloid. Interface Sci.* **2014**, *214*, 17–37. [CrossRef] [PubMed]
42. Joughehdoust, S.; Behnamghader, A.; Jahandideh, R.; Manafi, S. Effect of aging temperature on formation of sol-gel derived fluor-hydroxyapatite nanoparticles. *J. Nanosci. Nanotechnol.* **2010**, *10*, 2892–2896. [CrossRef]
43. Jmal, N.; Bouaziz, J. Synthesis, characterization and bioactivity of a calcium-phosphate glass-ceramics obtained by the sol-gel processing method. *Mater. Sci. Eng. C Mater. Biol. Appl.* **2017**, *71*, 279–288. [CrossRef]
44. Morsali, A.; Hashemi, L. Chapter Two—Nanoscale coordination polymers: Preparation, function and application. In *Advances in Inorganic Chemistry*; Ruiz-Molina, D., van Eldik, R., Eds.; Academic Press: Cambridge, MA, USA, 2020; Volume 76, pp. 33–72.
45. Sikder, P.; Ren, Y.; Bhaduri, S.B. Microwave processing of calcium phosphate and magnesium phosphate based orthopedic bioceramics: A state-of-the-art review. *Acta Biomater.* **2020**, *111*, 29–53. [CrossRef] [PubMed]
46. Zhao, J.; Zhu, Y.-J.; Cheng, G.-F.; Ruan, Y.-J.; Sun, T.-W.; Chen, F.; Wu, J.; Zhao, X.-Y.; Ding, G.-J. Microwave-assisted hydrothermal rapid synthesis of amorphous calcium phosphate nanoparticles and hydroxyapatite microspheres using cytidine 5′-triphosphate disodium salt as a phosphate source. *Mater. Lett.* **2014**, *124*, 208–211. [CrossRef]
47. Dharmalingam, K.; Padmavathi, G.; Kunnumakkara, A.B.; Anandalakshmi, R. Microwave-assisted synthesis of cellulose/zinc-sulfate-calcium-phosphate (ZSCAP) nanocomposites for biomedical applications. *Mater. Sci. Eng. C Mater. Biol. Appl.* **2019**, *100*, 535–543. [CrossRef]
48. Jodati, H.; Tezcaner, A.; Alshemary, A.Z.; Sahin, V.; Evis, Z. Effects of the doping concentration of boron on physicochemical, mechanical, and biological properties of hydroxyapatite. *Ceram. Int.* **2022**, *48*, 22743–22758. [CrossRef]
49. Srinivasan, B.; Kolanthai, E.; Nivethaa, E.A.K.; Pandian, M.S.; Ramasamy, P.; Catalani, L.H.; Kalkura, S.N. Enhanced in vitro inhibition of MCF-7 and magnetic properties of cobalt incorporated calcium phosphate (HAp and ss-TCP) nanoparticles. *Ceram. Int.* **2023**, *49*, 855–861. [CrossRef]
50. Matamoros-Veloza, Z.; Rendon-Angeles, J.C.; Yanagisawa, K.; Ueda, T.; Zhu, K.J.; Moreno-Perez, B. Preparation of Silicon Hydroxyapatite Nanopowders under Microwave-Assisted Hydrothermal Method. *Nanomaterials* **2021**, *11*, 16. [CrossRef]
51. Sozugecer, S.; Bayramgil, N.P. Preparation and characterization of polyacrylic acid-hydroxyapatite nanocomposite by microwave-assisted synthesis method. *Heliyon* **2021**, *7*, 8. [CrossRef] [PubMed]
52. Fu, L.-H.; Qi, C.; Liu, Y.-J.; Cao, W.-T.; Ma, M.-G. Sonochemical synthesis of cellulose/hydroxyapatite nanocomposites and their application in protein adsorption. *Sci. Rep.* **2018**, *8*, 8292. [CrossRef]
53. Gausterer, J.C.; Schüßler, C.; Gabor, F. The impact of calcium phosphate on FITC-BSA loading of sonochemically prepared PLGA nanoparticles for inner ear drug delivery elucidated by two different fluorimetric quantification methods. *Ultrason. Sonochemistry* **2021**, *79*, 105783. [CrossRef]
54. Muthumariyappan, A.; Rajaji, U.; Chen, S.-M.; Baskaran, N.; Chen, T.-W.; Ramalingam, R.J. Sonochemical synthesis of perovskite-type barium titanate nanoparticles decorated on reduced graphene oxide nanosheets as an effective electrode material for the rapid determination of ractopamine in meat samples. *Ultrason. Sonochemistry* **2019**, *56*, 318–326. [CrossRef] [PubMed]
55. Liu, X.; Wu, Z.; Cavalli, R.; Cravotto, G. Sonochemical Preparation of Inorganic Nanoparticles and Nanocomposites for Drug Release-A Review. *Ind. Eng. Chem. Res.* **2021**, *60*, 10011–10032. [CrossRef]
56. Qi, C.; Zhou, D.; Zhu, Y.J.; Sun, T.W.; Chen, F.; Zhang, C.Q. Sonochemical synthesis of fructose 1,6-bisphosphate dicalcium porous microspheres and their application in promotion of osteogenic differentiation. *Mater. Sci. Eng. C-Mater. Biol. Appl.* **2017**, *77*, 846–856. [CrossRef]

57. Guibert, C.; Landoulsi, J. Enzymatic Approach in Calcium Phosphate Biomineralization: A Contribution to Reconcile the Physicochemical with the Physiological View. *Int. J. Mol. Sci.* **2021**, *22*, 24. [CrossRef]
58. Jiang, Y.-Y.; Zhou, Z.-F.; Zhu, Y.-J.; Chen, F.-F.; Lu, B.-Q.; Cao, W.-T.; Zhang, Y.-G.; Cai, Z.-D.; Chen, F. Enzymatic Reaction Generates Biomimic Nanominerals with Superior Bioactivity. *Small* **2018**, *14*, e1804321. [CrossRef]
59. Nijhuis, A.W.G.; Nejadnik, M.R.; Nudelman, F.; Walboomers, X.F.; te Riet, J.; Habibovic, P.; Tahmasebi Birgani, Z.; Li, Y.; Bomans, P.H.H.; Jansen, J.A.; et al. Enzymatic pH control for biomimetic deposition of calcium phosphate coatings. *Acta Biomater.* **2014**, *10*, 931–939. [CrossRef] [PubMed]
60. Medvecky, L.; Stulajterova, R.; Giretova, M.; Luptakova, L.; Sopcak, T. Injectable Enzymatically Hardened Calcium Phosphate Biocement. *J. Funct. Biomater.* **2020**, *11*, 74. [CrossRef] [PubMed]
61. Chahal, H.K.; Matthews, S.; Jones, M.I. Effect of process conditions on spray dried calcium carbonate powders for thermal spraying. *Ceram. Int.* **2021**, *47*, 351–360. [CrossRef]
62. Liu, Z.; Wang, T.; Xu, Y.; Liang, C.; Li, G.; Guo, Y.; Zhang, Z.; Lian, J.; Ren, L. Double-layer calcium phosphate sandwiched siloxane composite coating to enhance corrosion resistance and biocompatibility of magnesium alloys for bone tissue engineering. *Prog. Org. Coat.* **2023**, *177*, 107417. [CrossRef]
63. Chen, S.J.; Wang, Q.; Eltit, F.; Guo, Y.B.; Cox, M.; Wang, R.Z. An Ammonia-Induced Calcium Phosphate Nanostructure: A Potential Assay for Studying Osteoporosis and Bone Metastasis. *Acs Appl. Mater. Interfaces* **2021**, *13*, 17207–17219. [CrossRef] [PubMed]
64. Zai, W.; Sun, S.; Man, H.; Lian, J.S.; Zhang, Y.S. Preparation and anticorrosion properties of electrodeposited calcium phosphate (CaP) coatings on Mg-Zn-Ca metallic glass. *Mater. Chem. Phys.* **2022**, *290*, 15. [CrossRef]
65. Le Grill, S.; Soulie, J.; Coppel, Y.; Roblin, P.; Lecante, P.; Marsan, O.; Charvillat, C.; Bertrand, G.; Rey, C.; Brouillet, F. Spray-drying-derived amorphous calcium phosphate: A multi-scale characterization. *J. Mater. Sci.* **2021**, *56*, 1189–1202. [CrossRef]
66. Ye, H.; Zhu, J.; Deng, D.; Jin, S.; Li, J.; Man, Y. Enhanced osteogenesis and angiogenesis by PCL/chitosan/Sr-doped calcium phosphate electrospun nanocomposite membrane for guided bone regeneration. *J. Biomater. Sci. -Polym. Ed.* **2019**, *30*, 1505–1522. [CrossRef] [PubMed]
67. Singh, Y.P.; Mishra, B.; Gupta, M.K.; Bhaskar, R.; Han, S.S.; Mishra, N.C.; Dasgupta, S. Gelatin/monetite electrospun scaffolds to regenerate bone tissue: Fabrication, characterization, and in-vitro evaluation. *J. Mech. Behav. Biomed. Mater.* **2023**, *137*, 11. [CrossRef]
68. Sadiq, T.O.; Sudin, I.; Idris, J.; Fadil, N.A. Synthesis Techniques of Bioceramic Hydroxyapatite for Biomedical. *J. Biomim. Biomater. Biomed. Eng.* **2023**, *59*, 59–80. [CrossRef]
69. Chou, Y.J.; Ningsih, H.S.; Shih, S.J. Preparation, characterization and investigation of antibacterial silver-zinc co-doped beta-tricalcium phosphate by spray pyrolysis. *Ceram. Int.* **2020**, *46*, 16708–16715. [CrossRef]
70. Nosrati, H.; Sarraf-Mamoory, R.; Kazemi, M.H.; Perez, M.C.; Shokrollahi, M.; Emameh, R.Z.; Falak, R. Characterization of hydroxyapatite-reduced graphene oxide nanocomposites consolidated via high frequency induction heat sintering method. *J. Asian Ceram. Soc.* **2020**, *8*, 1296–1309. [CrossRef]
71. Karalkeviciene, R.; Raudonyte-Svirbutaviciene, E.; Zarkov, A.; Yang, J.C.; Popov, A.I.; Kareiva, A. Solvothermal Synthesis of Calcium Hydroxyapatite via Hydrolysis of Alpha-Tricalcium Phosphate in the Presence of Different Organic Additives. *Crystals* **2023**, *13*, 265. [CrossRef]
72. Farahani, S.D.; Zolgharnein, J. Removal of Alizarin red S by calcium-terephthalate MOF synthesized from recycled PET-waste using Box-Behnken and Taguchi designs optimization approaches. *J. Solid State Chem.* **2022**, *316*, 123560. [CrossRef]
73. Ray, S.; Yadav, J.; Mishra, A.; Dasgupta, S. In-Vitro antimicrobial & biocompatibility study of Spherical 52S4.6 Submicron-Bioactive glass synthesized by Stober Method: Effect of Ag Doping. *J. Sol-Gel Sci. Technol.* **2023**, *106*, 67–84. [CrossRef]
74. Novak, S.; Orives, J.R.; Nalin, M.; Unalan, I.; Boccaccini, A.R.; de Camargo, E.R. Quaternary bioactive glass-derived powders presenting submicrometric particles and antimicrobial activity. *Ceram. Int.* **2022**, *48*, 29982–29990. [CrossRef]
75. Kazeli, K.; Tsamesidis, I.; Theocharidou, A.; Malletzidou, L.; Rhoades, J.; Pouroutzidou, G.K.; Likotrafiti, E.; Chrissafis, K.; Lialiaris, T.; Papadopoulou, L.; et al. Synthesis and Characterization of Novel Calcium-Silicate Nanobioceramics with Magnesium: Effect of Heat Treatment on Biological, Physical and Chemical Properties. *Ceramics* **2021**, *4*, 628–651. [CrossRef]
76. Guo, X.; Hu, Y.P.; Yuan, K.Z.; Qiao, Y. Review of the Effect of Surface Coating Modification on Magnesium Alloy Biocompatibility. *Materials* **2022**, *15*, 3291. [CrossRef] [PubMed]
77. Citradewi, P.W.; Hidayat, H.; Purwiandono, G.; Fatimah, I.; Sagadevan, S. Clitorea ternatea-mediated silver nanoparticle-doped hydroxyapatite derived from cockle shell as antibacterial material. *Chem. Phys. Lett.* **2021**, *769*, 8. [CrossRef]
78. Akhtar, K.; Pervez, C. Evaluation of the experimental parameters for the morphological tunning of monodispersed calcium hydroxyapatite. *J. Dispers. Sci. Technol.* **2021**, *42*, 984–997. [CrossRef]
79. Colaco, E.; Guibert, C.; Lee, J.; Maisonhaute, E.; Brouri, D.; Dupont-Gillain, C.; El Kirat, K.; Demoustier-Champagne, S.; Landoulsi, J. Embedding Collagen in Multilayers for Enzyme-Assisted Mineralization: A Promising Way to Direct Crystallization in Confinement. *Biomacromolecules* **2021**, *22*, 3460–3473. [CrossRef]
80. Kordesedehi, R.; Asadollahi, M.A.; Shahpiri, A.; Biria, D.; Nikel, P.I. Optimized enantioselective (S)-2-hydroxypropiophenone synthesis by free- and encapsulated-resting cells of Pseudomonas putida. *Microb. Cell Factories* **2023**, *22*, 11. [CrossRef] [PubMed]

81. Colaco, E.; Lefevre, D.; Maisonhaute, E.; Brouri, D.; Guibert, C.; Dupont-Gillain, C.; El Kirat, K.; Demoustier-Champagne, S.; Landoulsi, J. Enzyme-assisted mineralization of calcium phosphate: Exploring confinement for the design of highly crystalline nano-objects. *Nanoscale* **2020**, *12*, 10051–10064. [CrossRef]
82. Nakhaei, M.; Jirofti, N.; Ebrahimzadeh, M.H.; Moradi, A. Different methods of hydroxyapatite-based coatings on external fixator pin with high adhesion approach. *Plasma Process. Polym.* **2023**, e2200219. [CrossRef]
83. Akhtar, M.; Uzair, S.A.; Rizwan, M.; Rehman, M.A.U. The Improvement in Surface Properties of Metallic Implant via Magnetron Sputtering: Recent Progress and Remaining Challenges. *Front. Mater.* **2022**, *8*, 18. [CrossRef]
84. Miller, F.; Wenderoth, S.; Wintzheimer, S.; Mandel, K. Rising Like a Phoenix from the Ashes: Fire-Proof Magnetically Retrievable Supraparticles with an Optical Fingerprint for Postmortem Identification of Products. *Adv. Opt. Mater.* **2022**, *10*, 11. [CrossRef]
85. Levingstone, T.J.; Herbaj, S.; Redmond, J.; McCarthy, H.O.; Dunne, N.J. Calcium Phosphate Nanoparticles-Based Systems for RNAi Delivery: Applications in Bone Tissue Regeneration. *Nanomaterials* **2020**, *10*, 146. [CrossRef] [PubMed]
86. Qi, C.; Zhu, Y.-J.; Zhang, Y.-G.; Jiang, Y.-Y.; Wu, J.; Chen, F. Vesicle-like nanospheres of amorphous calcium phosphate: Sonochemical synthesis using the adenosine 5′-triphosphate disodium salt and their application in pH-responsive drug delivery. *J. Mater. Chem. B* **2015**, *3*, 7347–7354. [CrossRef] [PubMed]
87. Yang, J.; Wang, X.; Wang, B.; Park, K.; Wooley, K.; Zhang, S. Challenging the fundamental conjectures in nanoparticle drug delivery for chemotherapy treatment of solid cancers. *Adv. Drug. Deliv. Rev.* **2022**, *190*, 114525. [CrossRef] [PubMed]
88. Ding, G.-J.; Zhu, Y.-J.; Qi, C.; Lu, B.-Q.; Chen, F.; Wu, J. Porous hollow microspheres of amorphous calcium phosphate: Soybean lecithin templated microwave-assisted hydrothermal synthesis and application in drug delivery. *J. Mater. Chem. B* **2015**, *3*, 1823–1830. [CrossRef] [PubMed]
89. Sun, R.; Ahlen, M.; Tai, C.W.; Bajnoczi, E.G.; de Kleijne, F.; Ferraz, N.; Persson, I.; Stromme, M.; Cheung, O. Highly Porous Amorphous Calcium Phosphate for Drug Delivery and Bio-Medical Applications. *Nanomaterials* **2020**, *10*, 18. [CrossRef]
90. Ching Lau, C.; Reardon, P.J.T.; Campbell Knowles, J.; Tang, J. Phase-Tunable Calcium Phosphate Biomaterials Synthesis and Application in Protein Delivery. *ACS Biomater. Sci. Eng.* **2015**, *1*, 947–954. [CrossRef]
91. Ge, Y.-W.; Chu, M.; Zhu, Z.-Y.; Ke, Q.-F.; Guo, Y.-P.; Zhang, C.-Q.; Jia, W.-T. Nacre-inspired magnetically oriented micro-cellulose fibres/nano-hydroxyapatite/chitosan layered scaffold enhances pro-osteogenesis and angiogenesis. *Mater. Today Bio* **2022**, *16*, 100439. [CrossRef]
92. Ge, Y.-W.; Fan, Z.-H.; Ke, Q.-F.; Guo, Y.-P.; Zhang, C.-Q.; Jia, W.-T. $SrFe_{12}O_{19}$-doped nano-layered double hydroxide/chitosan layered scaffolds with a nacre-mimetic architecture guide in situ bone ingrowth and regulate bone homeostasis. *Mater. Today Bio* **2022**, *16*, 100362. [CrossRef]
93. Zhou, F.; Shen, Y.; Liu, B.; Chen, X.; Wan, L.; Peng, D. Gastrodin inhibits osteoclastogenesis via down-regulating the NFATc1 signaling pathway and stimulates osseointegration in vitro. *Biochem. Biophys. Res. Commun.* **2017**, *484*, 820–826. [CrossRef]
94. Kuro-O, M. Klotho and calciprotein particles as therapeutic targets against accelerated ageing. *Clin. Sci.* **2021**, *135*, 1915–1927. [CrossRef]
95. Seong, Y.-J.; Song, E.-H.; Park, C.; Lee, H.; Kang, I.-G.; Kim, H.-E.; Jeong, S.-H. Porous calcium phosphate-collagen composite microspheres for effective growth factor delivery and bone tissue regeneration. *Mater. Sci. Engineerin. C Mater. Biol. Appl.* **2020**, *109*, 110480. [CrossRef]
96. Tenkumo, T.; Vanegas Sáenz, J.R.; Nakamura, K.; Shimizu, Y.; Sokolova, V.; Epple, M.; Kamano, Y.; Egusa, H.; Sugaya, T.; Sasaki, K. Prolonged release of bone morphogenetic protein-2 in vivo by gene transfection with DNA-functionalized calcium phosphate nanoparticle-loaded collagen scaffolds. *Mater. Sci. Eng. C Mater. Biol. Appl.* **2018**, *92*, 172–183. [CrossRef]
97. Chang, K.C.; Chen, J.C.; Cheng, I.T.; Haung, S.M.; Liu, S.M.; Ko, C.L.; Sun, Y.S.; Shih, C.J.; Chen, W.C. Strength and Biocompatibility of Heparin-Based Calcium Phosphate Cement Grafted with Ferulic Acid. *Polymers* **2021**, *13*, 19. [CrossRef] [PubMed]
98. Bassett, D.C.; Robinson, T.E.; Hill, R.J.; Grover, L.M.; Barralet, J.E. Self-assembled calcium pyrophosphate nanostructures for targeted molecular delivery. *Biomater. Adv.* **2022**, *140*, 213086. [CrossRef] [PubMed]
99. Zhao, L.; Weir, M.D.; Xu, H.H.K. Human umbilical cord stem cell encapsulation in calcium phosphate scaffolds for bone engineering. *Biomaterials* **2010**, *31*, 3848–3857. [CrossRef] [PubMed]
100. Wang, P.; Zhao, L.; Liu, J.; Weir, M.D.; Zhou, X.; Xu, H.H.K. Bone tissue engineering via nanostructured calcium phosphate biomaterials and stem cells. *Bone Res.* **2014**, *2*, 14017. [CrossRef] [PubMed]
101. Kim, H.D.; Amirthalingam, S.; Kim, S.L.; Lee, S.S.; Rangasamy, J.; Hwang, N.S. Biomimetic Materials and Fabrication Approaches for Bone Tissue Engineering. *Adv. Healthc. Mater.* **2017**, *6*, 18. [CrossRef]
102. Hou, X.D.; Zhang, L.; Zhou, Z.F.; Luo, X.; Wang, T.L.; Zhao, X.Y.; Lu, B.Q.; Chen, F.; Zheng, L.P. Calcium Phosphate-Based Biomaterials for Bone Repair. *J. Funct. Biomater.* **2022**, *13*, 39. [CrossRef]
103. Yuan, Y.; Shen, L.; Liu, T.; He, L.; Meng, D.; Jiang, Q. Physicochemical properties of bone marrow mesenchymal stem cells encapsulated in microcapsules combined with calcium phosphate cement and their ectopic bone formation. *Front. Bioeng. Biotechnol.* **2022**, *10*, 1005954. [CrossRef]
104. Evans, C.H.; Huard, J. Gene therapy approaches to regenerating the musculoskeletal system. *Nat. Rev. Rheumatol.* **2015**, *11*, 234–242. [CrossRef]
105. Dorozhkin, S.V. Bioceramics of calcium orthophosphates. *Biomaterials* **2010**, *31*, 1465–1485. [CrossRef]

106. Zhu, C.; Chang, Q.; Zou, D.; Zhang, W.; Wang, S.; Zhao, J.; Yu, W.; Zhang, X.; Zhang, Z.; Jiang, X. LvBMP-2 gene-modified BMSCs combined with calcium phosphate cement scaffolds for the repair of calvarial defects in rats. *J. Mater. Sci. Mater. Med.* **2011**, *22*, 1965–1973. [CrossRef] [PubMed]
107. Tenkumo, T.; Vanegas Sáenz, J.R.; Takada, Y.; Takahashi, M.; Rotan, O.; Sokolova, V.; Epple, M.; Sasaki, K. Gene transfection of human mesenchymal stem cells with a nano-hydroxyapatite-collagen scaffold containing DNA-functionalized calcium phosphate nanoparticles. *Genes Cells* **2016**, *21*, 682–695. [CrossRef] [PubMed]
108. Choi, B.; Cui, Z.-K.; Kim, S.; Fan, J.; Wu, B.M.; Lee, M. Glutamine-chitosan modified calcium phosphate nanoparticles for efficient siRNA delivery and osteogenic differentiation. *J. Mater. Chem. B* **2015**, *3*, 6448–6455. [CrossRef]
109. Chowdhury, E.H.; Kunou, M.; Nagaoka, M.; Kundu, A.K.; Hoshiba, T.; Akaike, T. High-efficiency gene delivery for expression in mammalian cells by nanoprecipitates of Ca-Mg phosphate. *Gene* **2004**, *341*, 77–82. [CrossRef] [PubMed]
110. Khalifehzadeh, R.; Arami, H. DNA-Templated Strontium-Doped Calcium Phosphate Nanoparticles for Gene Delivery in Bone Cells. *ACS Biomater. Sci. Eng.* **2019**, *5*, 3201–3211. [CrossRef] [PubMed]
111. Mao, L.; Xia, L.; Chang, J.; Liu, J.; Jiang, L.; Wu, C.; Fang, B. The synergistic effects of Sr and Si bioactive ions on osteogenesis, osteoclastogenesis and angiogenesis for osteoporotic bone regeneration. *Acta Biomater.* **2017**, *61*, 217–232. [CrossRef]
112. Zhang, M.; Wu, C.; Lin, K.; Fan, W.; Chen, L.; Xiao, Y.; Chang, J. Biological responses of human bone marrow mesenchymal stem cells to Sr-M-Si (M = Zn, Mg) silicate bioceramics. *J. Biomed. Mater. Res. A* **2012**, *100*, 2979–2990. [CrossRef]
113. Rentsch, B.; Bernhardt, A.; Henß, A.; Ray, S.; Rentsch, C.; Schamel, M.; Gbureck, U.; Gelinsky, M.; Rammelt, S.; Lode, A. Trivalent chromium incorporated in a crystalline calcium phosphate matrix accelerates materials degradation and bone formation in vivo. *Acta Biomater.* **2018**, *69*, 332–341. [CrossRef]
114. Wu, X.; Tang, Z.; Wu, K.; Bai, Y.; Lin, X.; Yang, H.; Yang, Q.; Wang, Z.; Ni, X.; Liu, H.; et al. Strontium-calcium phosphate hybrid cement with enhanced osteogenic and angiogenic properties for vascularised bone regeneration. *J. Mater. Chem. B* **2021**, *9*, 5982–5997. [CrossRef]
115. Duraisamy, K.; Gangadharan, A.; Martirosyan, K.S.; Sahu, N.K.; Manogaran, P.; Easwaradas Kreedapathy, G. Fabrication of Multifunctional Drug Loaded Magnetic Phase Supported Calcium Phosphate Nanoparticle for Local Hyperthermia Combined Drug Delivery and Antibacterial Activity. *ACS Appl. Bio Mater.* **2023**, *6*, 104–116. [CrossRef] [PubMed]
116. Bose, S.; Banerjee, D.; Vu, A.A. Ginger and Garlic Extracts Enhance Osteogenesis in 3D Printed Calcium Phosphate Bone Scaffolds with Bimodal Pore Distribution. *ACS Appl. Mater. Interfaces* **2022**, *14*, 12964–12975. [CrossRef] [PubMed]
117. Xie, L.; Yang, Y.; Fu, Z.; Li, Y.; Shi, J.; Ma, D.; Liu, S.; Luo, D. Fe/Zn-modified tricalcium phosphate (TCP) biomaterials: Preparation and biological properties. *RSC Adv.* **2019**, *9*, 781–789. [CrossRef] [PubMed]
118. Torres, P.M.C.; Ribeiro, N.; Nunes, C.M.M.; Rodrigues, A.F.M.; Sousa, A.; Olhero, S.M. Toughening robocast chitosan/biphasic calcium phosphate composite scaffolds with silk fibroin: Tuning printable inks and scaffold structure for bone regeneration. *Biomater. Adv.* **2022**, *134*, 112690. [CrossRef]
119. Shakoor, S.; Kibble, E.; El-Jawhari, J.J. Bioengineering Approaches for Delivering Growth Factors: A Focus on Bone and Cartilage Regeneration. *Bioengineering* **2022**, *9*, 15. [CrossRef]
120. Li, G.; Shen, W.; Tang, X.; Mo, G.; Yao, L.; Wang, J. Combined use of calcium phosphate cement, mesenchymal stem cells and platelet-rich plasma for bone regeneration in critical-size defect of the femoral condyle in mini-pigs. *Regen. Med.* **2021**, *16*, 451–464. [CrossRef]
121. Xie, W.; Jiang, W.; Zhou, R.; Li, J.; Ding, J.; Ni, H.; Zhang, Q.; Tang, Q.; Meng, J.-X.; Lin, L. Disorder-Induced Broadband Near-Infrared Persistent and Photostimulated Luminescence in Mg_2SnO_4:Cr_3. *Inorg. Chem.* **2021**, *60*, 2219–2227. [CrossRef]
122. Xue, Z.; Li, X.; Li, Y.; Jiang, M.; Liu, H.; Zeng, S.; Hao, J. X-ray-Activated Near-Infrared Persistent Luminescent Probe for Deep-Tissue and Renewable In Vivo Bioimaging. *ACS Appl. Mater. Interfaces* **2017**, *9*, 22132–22142. [CrossRef]
123. Shiu, W.-T.; Chang, L.-Y.; Jiang, Y.; Shakouri, M.; Wu, Y.-H.; Lin, B.-H.; Liu, L. Synthesis and characterization of a near-infrared persistent luminescent Cr-doped zinc gallate-calcium phosphate composite. *Phys. Chem. Chem. Phys.* **2022**, *24*, 21131–21140. [CrossRef]
124. Chen, F.; Huang, P.; Zhu, Y.-J.; Wu, J.; Cui, D.-X. Multifunctional Eu^{3+}/Gd^{3+} dual-doped calcium phosphate vesicle-like nanospheres for sustained drug release and imaging. *Biomaterials* **2012**, *33*, 6447–6455. [CrossRef]
125. Zhang, J.; Liu, W.; Schnitzler, V.; Tancret, F.; Bouler, J.-M. Calcium phosphate cements for bone substitution: Chemistry, handling and mechanical properties. *Acta Biomater.* **2014**, *10*, 1035–1049. [CrossRef] [PubMed]
126. Mastrogiacomo, S.; Kownacka, A.E.; Dou, W.; Burke, B.P.; de Rosales, R.T.M.; Heerschap, A.; Jansen, J.A.; Archibald, S.J.; Walboomers, X.F. Bisphosphonate Functionalized Gadolinium Oxide Nanoparticles Allow Long-Term MRI/CT Multimodal Imaging of Calcium Phosphate Bone Cement. *Adv. Healthc. Mater.* **2018**, *7*, e1800202. [CrossRef] [PubMed]
127. Rong, Z.-J.; Yang, L.-J.; Cai, B.-T.; Zhu, L.-X.; Cao, Y.-L.; Wu, G.-F.; Zhang, Z.-J. Porous nano-hydroxyapatite/collagen scaffold containing drug-loaded ADM-PLGA microspheres for bone cancer treatment. *J. Mater. Sci. Mater. Med.* **2016**, *27*, 89. [CrossRef]
128. Xie, L.; Wang, G.; Sang, W.; Li, J.; Zhang, Z.; Li, W.; Yan, J.; Zhao, Q.; Dai, Y. Phenolic immunogenic cell death nanoinducer for sensitizing tumor to PD-1 checkpoint blockade immunotherapy. *Biomaterials* **2021**, *269*, 120638. [CrossRef] [PubMed]
129. Schwartz, C.L.; Gorlick, R.; Teot, L.; Krailo, M.; Chen, Z.; Goorin, A.; Grier, H.E.; Bernstein, M.L.; Meyers, P. Multiple drug resistance in osteogenic sarcoma: INT0133 from the Children's Oncology Group. *J. Clin. Oncol.* **2007**, *25*, 2057–2062. [CrossRef]
130. Hu, J.; Jiang, Y.; Tan, S.; Zhu, K.; Cai, T.; Zhan, T.; He, S.; Chen, F.; Zhang, C. Selenium-doped calcium phosphate biomineral reverses multidrug resistance to enhance bone tumor chemotherapy. *Nanomedicine* **2021**, *32*, 102322. [CrossRef] [PubMed]

131. Takeuchi, A.; Suwanpramote, P.; Yamamoto, N.; Shirai, T.; Hayashi, K.; Kimura, H.; Miwa, S.; Higuchi, T.; Abe, K.; Tsuchiya, H. Mid- to long-term clinical outcome of giant cell tumor of bone treated with calcium phosphate cement following thorough curettage and phenolization. *J. Surg. Oncol.* **2018**, *117*, 1232–1238. [CrossRef]
132. Wang, Y.; Li, X.; Luo, Y.; Zhang, L.; Chen, H.; Min, L.; Chang, Q.; Zhou, Y.; Tu, C.; Zhu, X.; et al. Application of osteoinductive calcium phosphate ceramics in giant cell tumor of the sacrum: Report of six cases. *Regen. Biomater.* **2022**, *9*, rbac017. [CrossRef]
133. Higuchi, T.; Yamamoto, N.; Hayashi, K.; Takeuchi, A.; Kimura, H.; Miwa, S.; Igarashi, K.; Abe, K.; Taniguchi, Y.; Aiba, H.; et al. Calcium Phosphate Cement in the Surgical Management of Benign Bone Tumors. *Anticancer. Res.* **2018**, *38*, 3031–3035.
134. Verlaan, J.J.; van Helden, W.H.; Oner, F.C.; Verbout, A.J.; Dhert, W.J.A. Balloon vertebroplasty with calcium phosphate cement augmentation for direct restoration of traumatic thoracolumbar vertebral fractures. *Spine* **2002**, *27*, 543–548. [CrossRef]
135. Blumenthal, D.T.; Aisenstein, O.; Ben-Horin, I.; Ben Bashat, D.; Artzi, M.; Corn, B.W.; Kanner, A.A.; Ram, Z.; Bokstein, F. Calcification in high grade gliomas treated with bevacizumab. *J. Neurooncol.* **2015**, *123*, 283–288. [CrossRef] [PubMed]
136. Kozai, D.; Ogawa, N.; Mori, Y. Redox regulation of transient receptor potential channels. *Antioxid. Redox Signal.* **2014**, *21*, 971–986. [CrossRef] [PubMed]
137. Sun, Q.; Liu, B.; Zhao, R.; Feng, L.; Wang, Z.; Dong, S.; Dong, Y.; Gai, S.; Ding, H.; Yang, P. Calcium Peroxide-Based Nanosystem with Cancer Microenvironment-Activated Capabilities for Imaging Guided Combination Therapy via Mitochondrial Ca^{2+} Overload and Chemotherapy. *ACS Appl. Mater. Interfaces* **2021**, *13*, 44096–44107. [CrossRef] [PubMed]
138. Yao, S.S.; Jin, B.A.; Liu, Z.M.; Shao, C.Y.; Zhao, R.B.; Wang, X.Y.; Tang, R.K. Biomineralization: From Material Tactics to Biological Strategy. *Adv. Mater.* **2017**, *29*, 19. [CrossRef] [PubMed]
139. Zhou, Y.; Zhang, J.; Dan, P.; Bi, F.; Chen, Y.; Liu, J.; Li, Q.; Gou, H.; Wu, B.; Qiu, M. Tumor calcification as a prognostic factor in cetuximab plus chemotherapy-treated patients with metastatic colorectal cancer. *Anticancer. Drugs* **2019**, *30*, 195–200. [CrossRef] [PubMed]
140. Wang, C.; Wang, X.; Zhang, W.; Ma, D.; Li, F.; Jia, R.; Shi, M.; Wang, Y.; Ma, G.; Wei, W. Shielding Ferritin with a Biomineralized Shell Enables Efficient Modulation of Tumor Microenvironment and Targeted Delivery of Diverse Therapeutic Agents. *Adv. Mater.* **2022**, *34*, e2107150. [CrossRef]
141. Zhao, R.; Wang, B.; Yang, X.; Xiao, Y.; Wang, X.; Shao, C.; Tang, R. A Drug-Free Tumor Therapy Strategy: Cancer-Cell-Targeting Calcification. *Angew. Chem. Int. Ed. Engl.* **2016**, *55*, 5225–5229. [CrossRef] [PubMed]
142. Tan, X.; Huang, J.; Wang, Y.; He, S.; Jia, L.; Zhu, Y.; Pu, K.; Zhang, Y.; Yang, X. Transformable Nanosensitizer with Tumor Microenvironment-Activated Sonodynamic Process and Calcium Release for Enhanced Cancer Immunotherapy. *Angew. Chem. Int. Ed. Engl.* **2021**, *60*, 14051–14059. [CrossRef] [PubMed]
143. Hu, H.; Xu, Q.; Mo, Z.; Hu, X.; He, Q.; Zhang, Z.; Xu, Z. New anti-cancer explorations based on metal ions. *J. Nanobiotechnology* **2022**, *20*, 457. [CrossRef] [PubMed]
144. Zhao, H.; Wang, L.; Zeng, K.; Li, J.; Chen, W.; Liu, Y.-N. Nanomessenger-Mediated Signaling Cascade for Antitumor Immunotherapy. *ACS Nano* **2021**, *15*, 13188–13199. [CrossRef]

molecules

MDPI

Review

Cell Membrane Biomimetic Nanoparticles with Potential in Treatment of Alzheimer's Disease

Xinyu Zhong [1], Yue Na [1], Shun Yin [1], Chang Yan [1], Jinlian Gu [1], Ning Zhang [2,3,*] and Fang Geng [1,4,*]

1 School of Chemistry & Chemical Engineering, College of Chemistry & Chemical Engineering, Harbin Normal University, Harbin 150025, China
2 College of Jiamusi, Heilongjiang University of Chinese Medicine, Harbin 150004, China
3 Wuxi Traditional Chinese Medicine Hospital, Wuxi 214071, China
4 Wuxi School of Medicine, Jiangnan University, Wuxi 214122, China
* Correspondence: zhangning0454@163.com (N.Z.); f.geng@hrbnu.edu.cn (F.G.);

Abstract: Alzheimer's disease (AD) is to blame for about 60% of dementia cases worldwide. The blood–brain barrier (BBB) prevents many medications for AD from having clinical therapeutic effects that can be used to treat the affected area. Many researchers have turned their attention to cell membrane biomimetic nanoparticles (NPs) to solve this situation. Among them, NPs can extend the half-life of drugs in the body as the "core" of the wrapped drug, and the cell membrane acts as the "shell" of the wrapped NPs to functionalize the NPs, which can further improve the delivery efficiency of nano-drug delivery systems. Researchers are learning that cell membrane biomimetic NPs can circumvent the BBB's restriction, prevent harm to the body's immune system, extend the period that NPs spend in circulation, and have good biocompatibility and cytotoxicity, which increases efficacy of drug release. This review summarized the detailed production process and features of core NPs and further introduced the extraction methods of cell membrane and fusion methods of cell membrane biomimetic NPs. In addition, the targeting peptides for modifying biomimetic NPs to target the BBB to demonstrate the broad prospects of cell membrane biomimetic NPs drug delivery systems were summarized.

Keywords: Alzheimer's disease; blood–brain barrier; cell membrane biomimetic nanoparticles; targeting peptides

1. Introduction

The most prevalent type of dementia in the world is Alzheimer's disease (AD), which is a progressive and irreversible neurodegenerative disease [1]. The possible predisposing factor of dementia in elder citizens is neuronal loss and cognitive impairment brought on by buildup of aggregation of amyloid-β (Aβ) and intracellular neurofibrillary tangles with aging [2]. According to World Health Organization projections, more than 55 million people worldwide already suffer from dementia, and that number is projected to increase to 78 million in 2030 and even more than 139 million in 2050 [3]. The researchers also found that the median survival time of AD diagnosis age was 3.2 to 6.6 years [4], and the probability of heritability was about 70%. As the number of AD patients increases, the situation facing patients and their families is dire [5]. A number of drugs for AD have also advanced to the clinical research stage, costing billions of dollars [6]. However, 98% of drugs currently available on the market are blocked by the blood–brain barrier (BBB) in treating AD [7], which prevents pathogens and drugs from entering the brain from the circulatory system [8]. Drug delivery that targets the central nervous system for diagnosis and treatment of neurodegenerative diseases such as AD is restricted.

To solve this problem, many researchers have designed a class of cell membrane biomimetic nanoparticles (NPs) that can cross the BBB to the affected area in the brain. Cell membrane biomimetic NPs typically consist of a thin cytoplasmic membrane and encapsulated therapeutic NPs, resulting in a "core–shell" structure in which drug-encapsulated NPs (polymeric NPs, lipid-based NPs, inorganic NPs) are the "core" [9] and the outer layer of the cell membrane that wraps the NPs is the "shell" (Figure 1).

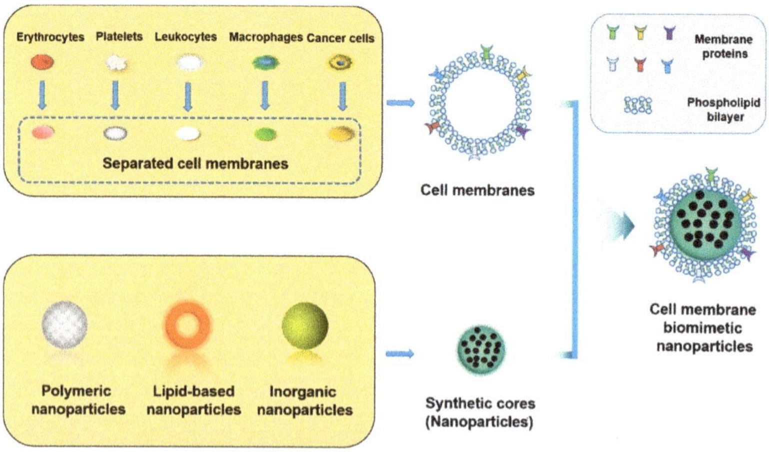

Figure 1. Schematic diagram of the preparation method of cell-membrane-coated NPs.

The "core" of drug-carrying cell membrane biomimetic NPs is prepared from nanomaterials and drugs, which can prolong the drug's half-life and increase biocompatibility in nerve tissues to enhance the therapeutic effect [10]. To further improve delivery efficiency, the NPs are wrapped with appreciable amounts of natural cell membranes that could be easily resized to form the "shell" of NPs [11]. Cell membrane biomimetic NPs, as a new type of nanomedicine, can target disease sites through the homing tendency of membrane proteins while also evading immune elimination, extending circulation time, and other biological functions of the parent cell [12]. In contrast, "core–shell" cell membrane biomimetic NPs are more complex but more flexible and less repulsive than simple NPs without biomimetic membranes [13]. Core NPs can also be formulated to be loaded with drugs to enhance stability of NPs in blood. Cell membrane biomimetic NPs can also be modified with specific peptides targeting the BBB or diseased sites. Taking advantage of the high transmembrane transport efficiency of targeting peptides, targeting peptides are used as carriers to couple with cell membrane biomimetic NPs to "carry" the cell membrane biomimetic NPs to penetrate the BBB, thereby significantly increasing the efficiency of cell membrane biomimetic NPs and enhancing active targeted delivery of NPs. Biomimetic nanotechnology provides a new idea for designing nanomaterials that cross the BBB, which is expected to be used in treatment of AD [14].

In the following review, we focused on the influence of BBB and application of cell membrane biomimetic NPs in treatment of AD. In addition, NPs synthesis methods, cell membrane extraction methods, and cell membrane biomimetic NPs fusion methods were reviewed in this paper. Finally, targeting peptides commonly used to enhance BBB targeting of biomimetic NPs were summarized, aiming to achieve drug delivery to AD lesion areas.

2. BBB Hinders AD Treatment

2.1. Current Therapy Strategy

Less successful treatment drugs have been developed to treat AD [15], and most of them can only temporarily relieve symptoms and improve cognitive function. For symptomatic alleviation of AD, the European Medicines Agency (EMA) suggested cholinesterase inhibitors (ChEIs) and *N*-methyl-D-aspartate (NMDA) receptor antagonists [16]. ChEIs, including donepezil, galantamine, tacrine, and rivastigmine, increase acetylcholine levels in the synaptic cleft by inhibiting acetylcholinesterase, cause temporary cognitive enhancement, and are licensed for mild to moderate AD. NMDA receptor antagonists, such as memantine, reduce neurotoxicity of glutamate for symptomatic relief of moderate to severe AD phases [17]. In addition, the Food and Drug Administration (FDA) also approved marketing of a combination therapy (a fixed-dose mixture of donepezil and memantine) [18] and aducanumab besides ChEIs and NMDA receptor antagonists. The fixed-dose mixture of donepezil and memantine showed more significant effectiveness than donepezil alone [19]. Aducanumab is a monoclonal antibody that treats early-stage AD by reducing amyloid deposition and is the first approved therapy targeting amyloid [20]. However, the EMA rejected marketing of aducanumab after finding abnormal swelling or bleeding in brain of minor patients. Although clinical trials of aducanumab are controversial, treatment with aducanumab still offers advantages over existing treatments [21].

2.2. The Impact of BBB on Treatment of AD

Drug efficiency is enormously limited due to the existence of BBB [22]. BBB is assembled by the blood–brain, cerebrospinal fluid–brain, and blood–cerebrospinal fluid barriers. BBB is composed of brain capillary endothelial cells (BCECs), astrocytes (AS), basement membrane, microglia, tight junctions, neurons, and pericyte, showing high selectivity [23] (Figure 2).

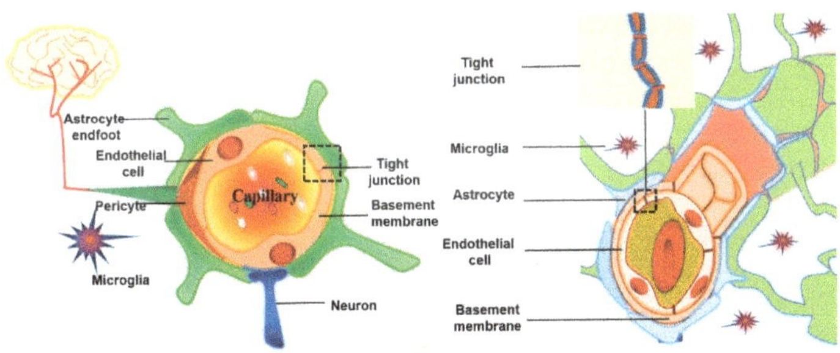

Figure 2. Schematic diagram of the structure of the BBB. The basement membrane surrounds the BCECs and embeds pericytes that span several BCECs. AS end-feet are in contact with the BCECs.

The BBB's BCECs are surrounded by AS, whose feet processes form connections to neurons. Pericytes are sporadically scattered along the brain capillaries and work with the basement membrane to stabilize the BBB. Microglia are sorts of immune cells exiting the central nervous system. Tight junctions are created by a complex network of parallel, linked transmembrane, and cytoplasmic proteins and are found in the apical/luminal area of BMECs. Only particles smaller than 1 nm are permitted to cross the passage of tight junctions. Thus, the BBB provides a protective mechanism for maintaining brain homeostasis and protecting the central nervous system from harmful hematogenous, endogenous, and exogenous substances. Although drugs or endogenous components cross the BBB into the brain via transcellular pathways [24] (passive transcellular diffusion pathway, paracellular pathway, adsorption mediated endocytosis, carrier mediated transport, receptor mediated transcytosis, and efflux pumps that expel materials from the brain [25], as shown in Figure 3, the transcellular pathways still require certain conditions for molecules to enter the brain, including molecular weight (less than 400 Da), shape (spherical), size (nano range), ionization (physiological pH value), lipophilicity, etc. As a result, all macromolecular drugs and more than 98% of small-molecule drugs are excluded from the brain [26]. Even though many drugs show satisfactory therapeutic effects in vitro, most of the activities are blocked by the BBB in vivo. According to the study of Zhao et al., the bioavailability of donepezil administrated orally in the brain is only 0.024–0.05% [27]. The research of Karasova also revealed that the oral bioavailability of tacrine in the brain is only 0.0014–0.0018% [28].

Presence of BBB has a significant impact on bioavailability of drugs into the brain, which is a great challenge for treatment of AD [29].

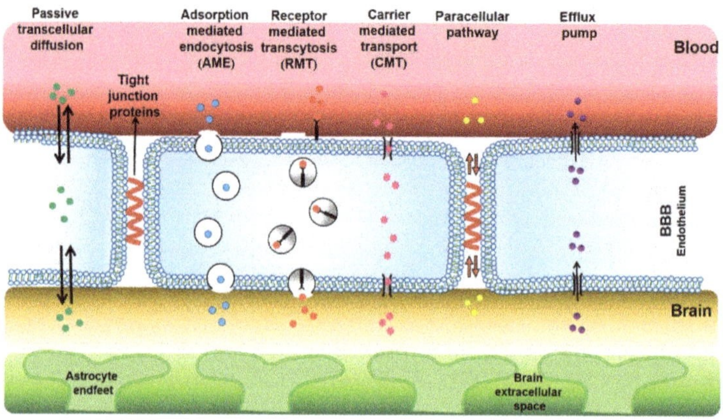

Figure 3. Schematic diagram of the physiological mechanisms by which drugs cross the BBB.

2.3. *New Strategies for Treating AD through BBB*

2.3.1. Route of Administration for Treating AD

Faced with the difficulty of delivering drugs into the brain for diagnosis and treatment, there are currently three main approaches to solving this problem: (A) local sustained release, a highly invasive procedure in which a drug is injected directly into the brain through the meninges. However, it is clinically prone to bleeding and central nervous system infection and should be used in very severe cases or only when a patient is hospitalized. (B) Intranasal administration: the brain receives medication directly by bypassing the BBB via the olfactory and trigeminal pathways. However, there are problems, such as insufficient absorption of drugs from the nasal mucosa, small nasal volume, large variability, and poor stability [30]. (C) Systemically administered, where a drug can cross the BBB and arrive in brain when administered orally or intravenously [31]. To date, the systemic delivery route is the most interesting and receptive strategy for AD treatment.

2.3.2. Potential Agents for AD Treatment

In addition to medicines already in use mentioned in Section 2.1, some natural products have shown great potential in treatment of AD, such as curcumin (Cur), quercetin [32], thymoquinone [33], huperzine A [34], and rhynchophylline [35]. At the same time, many potential natural products, such as fucosterol, lectin, fucoxanthin, and astaxanthin, have been isolated from marine algae [36]. Marine actinomyces produce a variety of halogenated compounds and can also be a rich source of natural medicines to treat AD [37]. However, most natural products are poorly water-soluble, resulting in difficulties to enter the brain. NPs could be used as vectors to carry natural products across the BBB to treat AD. Among them, metal NPs can easily be synthesized, coated, or combined to carry these natural products. Metal NPs carrying natural products can be used for in vitro detection of Aβ using confocal microscopy and also to manipulate Aβ aggregation to treat neurodegenerative diseases [38].

2.3.3. Nanoparticle Technology for Treating AD

There are several routes in which nanocarriers carry therapeutic drugs across the BBB into the brain to treat degenerative neurological disease: (A) open the tight connections between BCECs or cause local toxic effects that make the BBB more permeable, allowing NPs to enter the brain; (B) through endocytosis through BCECs, NPs enter the BCECs cytoplasm and then are expelled into the brain by the BCECs lumen; (C) through transcellular action through BCECs into the brain. NPs' biocompatibility and biodegradability allow them to protect pharmaceuticals, increase their bioavailability, and enable active targeting through surface functionalization, making it easier to distribute drugs to specific places. NPs may be able to transport therapeutic medications directly to the brain due to these advantageous effects without endangering the BBB's neuroprotective qualities [8]. Therefore, NPs can be used to target amyloid Aβ aggregation, excessive *Tau* phosphorylation, neurotransmitter dysfunction, neuroinflammation, oxidative stress, and neurotrophic factors in the brain to restore degenerative nerves and thus achieve the therapeutic effect of AD. NPs carry fluorescent molecules for early diagnosis of brain diseases. In conclusion, application of NPs in treatment of AD across the BBB has shown great potential.

In the systemic delivery system, cell membrane biomimetic NPs have shown great advantages for brain drug delivery, with the features of high drug loading, good biocompatibility, long circulation time, instinctual targeting ability, and low immunogenicity. Cell membrane biomimetic NPs simultaneously combine the advantages of unique natural cell membranes and an artificial core and can disguise as autologous cells, providing a new idea for brain drug delivery.

3. Core NPs

With the introduction of the concept of nanotechnology, nanotechnology has become a field to ensure safety of human life, involving many aspects, such as medicine and bioscience, agriculture, the food industry, electronics, transportation, communication, energy, etc. [39]. NPs consisting of nanomaterials and therapeutic agents [40] have characteristics of tissue selectivity, long circulation time, protecting and encapsulating drugs, enhancing drug absorption, increasing the loading and bioavailability of poorly soluble drugs, etc. [41]. On this basis, a variety of drug nanocarriers have been developed, including polymeric NPs, lipid-based NPs, and inorganic NPs.

3.1. NPs

3.1.1. Polymeric NPs

Because of their flexible architecture (10–1000 nm), low toxicity, biocompatibility, and regulated drug release, polymeric NPs—both synthetic and natural—have been extensively exploited in an astounding variety of drug delivery systems [42]. Therapeutic medications can be transported across the BBB by passive or active delivery when they are enclosed in polymeric NPs, protecting them from enzymatic and hydrolytic destruction [43]. According to reports, pharmaceutically loaded polymeric NPs boost brain penetration, enabling much higher drug concentrations at the target region and increasing the medicine's overall effectiveness [44].

The most common biodegradable and biocompatible polymers used to create polymeric NPs include poly(D,L-lactide-*co*-glycolide) (PLGA), polyethylene glycol, polylactic acid, poly(caprolactone), poly(glutamic acid), *N*-(2-hydroxypropyl)-methacrylate copolymers, poly(*n*-butylcyanoacrylate), 4-(Hydroxymethyl) phenylboronic acid pinacol ester (PBAP), and poly(amino acids), etc. PLGA is a synthetic polymer that has received FDA approval and has excellent biocompatibility and biodegradability features. It has been utilized extensively in medicinal applications, including treatment of AD [45].

Gao et al. prepared Cur-encapsulated PLGA NPs and camouflaged them with a red blood cell membrane (RBCm) (RBC-NP-Cur). In aneuronal-like cells (HT22) and primary brain capillary endothelial cell Transwell co-culture test, RBC-NP-Cur was confirmed to show significantly better permeability than Cur. In addition, after injection of RBC-NP-Cur in AD model mice, more accumulation of Cur, reduced cognitive decline, suppressed nerve cell death, and decreased *p*-tau levels in the brain were observed compared to free Cur group [46]. Tang et al. used macrophage membrane (MA)-encapsulated rapamycin-loaded PBAP NPs to treat AD. Confocal laser scanning microscope images revealed that a significant number of MA/1,19-Dioctadecyl-3,3,39,39-tetramethylindo-dicarbocyanine perchlorate (DiD) NPs accumulated in inflammatory human umbilical vein endothelial cells (HUVECs) after NPs were modified with DiD for 2 h [47]. These results imply that modified polymer NPs can actively target the sick region and release medications, resulting in increased effectiveness of drug delivery.

Polymer nanomicelles (PM) carrying a wide range of proteins, such as mRNAs or antibodies, can specifically and efficiently penetrate the BBB by injection to reach the brain parenchyma to release active agents' fragments. In addition to preventing early degradation of mRNA, use of mRNA-loaded PM altered intracellular mRNA transport, increased mRNA detection and expression in neurons in vivo, and reduced amyloid load in mouse models of acute amyloidosis [48]. It was also shown that accumulation of 3D6 antibody fragments (3D6-Fab) in the brain using the PM system was 41 times greater than that of free 3D6-Fab and successfully inhibited $A\beta_{1\text{-}42}$ aggregation in AD mice [49]. According to the characteristics of high impermeability of BBB, biotin and PECAM-1 protein on BBB were combined to form biotin targets on BCECs and avidin-functionalized PM with biotin specific binding were prepared. The PM can only target the brain and reduce accumulation in other organs in the body, thus reducing clinically limited peripheral side effects and effectively treating AD [50].

3.1.2. Lipid-Based NPs

Liposomes [51], solid lipid NPs (SLNs) [52], nanostructured lipid carriers [53], and nanoemulsions [54], among others [32], are the most common lipid-based NPs. Phospholipids, fatty acids, or cholesterol are generally used to create lipid-based NPs. Lipid-based NPs have the ability to form both unilamellar and multilamellar vesicular structures with diameters between 80 nm and 100 μm. Lipid-based NPs can carry various kinds of therapeutic drugs (such as nucleic acids, enzymes, and proteins) for effective transportation. The unique phospholipid structure of lipid-based NPs (similar to physiological membranes) makes them more compatible with the cellular lipid layer of the BBB, facilitating drug entry into the brain. Controlled and exact release of the materials at the targets is also made possible by lipid-based NPs, which can limit the rate of material breakdown. Lipid-based NPs are widely used in brain-targeted drug delivery because of high safety, good economic performance, large drug loading, good biodegradability, and biocompatibility [55].

Song et al. encapsulated rapamycin in liposomes and coated with platelet membrane by extrusion (P-Lipo). After intravenous injection of P-Lipo, the extracted brain tissue was observed under a fluorescence microscope and it was found that accumulation of P-Lipo in atherosclerotic lesions increased by 5.91 times compared with control liposomes, indicating that P-Lipo-specific targets to atherosclerotic plaques [56]. Han et al. prepared MA-coated SLNs for delivery of genistein to neuronal mitochondria (MASLNs). Using the brain microvascular cell (bEnd.3)/HT22 in vitro co-culture model to study the permeability of the BBB, it was found that MASLNs had a more pronounced ability to cross the BBB than SLNs. In vivo imaging in mice following tail vein injection of 1,1′-dioctadecyl-3,3,3′,3′-tetramethylindotricarbocyanine iodide (DiR)-labeled MASLNs and fluorescence intensities identified in isolated brain homogenates revealed that MASLNs can cross the BBB [57].

3.1.3. Inorganic NPs

Inorganic NPs are usually based on metals and non-carbon sources. The shape and size of inorganic NPs, including gold (Au) [58], silica (Si) [59], silver (Ag) [60], and magnetic (Fe_3O_4) [61] NPs, can be precisely tuned according to the synthesis process. Inorganic NPs have large surface area, controllable structure, diverse surface chemical properties, unique optical and magnetic properties, etc. At the same time, inorganic NPs also have chemical and physical stability in treatment of brain diseases and diagnostic applications [62]. Additionally, use of particular external stimuli, such as magnetic materials and near-infrared light, can assist the BBB's on-demand drug release and improve imaging [63]. However, because of their inherent toxicity, inorganic NPs are not always simply removed from the body, can have long-lasting immunological reactions, and have low biocompatibility [63].

Plissonneau et al. prepared sub-5 nm gadolinium-based NPs (AGuIX) co-modified by two small peptides derived from the sequence of Aβ_{1-42}, KLVFF and LPFFD. KLVFF matches the short hydrophobic core Aβ segment and LPFFD binds the hydrophobic area in Aβ's center, respectively, for Aβ-amyloid-plaque-targeted treatment of AD. Both functionalized NPs attach specifically to the amyloid plaque made up of Aβ protein in vitro hippocampus of AD model mice, as shown by immunohistochemical labeling with Pittsburgh compound on brain slices of transgenic mice with AD [64]. Gao et al. prepared an Au NPs scaffold with both polyoxometalates with LPFFD and Wells–Dawson structure (POMD) (AuNPs@POMD-pep). Thioflavin T assay demonstrated that AuNPs@POMD-pep successfully promoted disintegration of Aβ fibrils after co-incubating Aβ monomers with the compound. This was demonstrated by the fact that the fluorescence intensity was reduced by roughly 37%. After injection of AuNPs@POMD-pep to mice intravenously, inductively coupled plasma mass spectrometry analysis was involved to verify the success penetration of AuNPs@POMD-pep across the BBB [58].

3.2. *Synthesis of Core NPs*

3.2.1. Single Emulsification–Solvent Evaporation Method

Single emulsion (W/O) of polymeric NPs for hydrophobic drugs can be synthesized by emulsification–solvent evaporation method. First, the nano carries and interested ingredients are dissolved in organic solvents as organic phase. The organic phase is dropped into water phase containing sodium cholate, poloxamer, etc. Then, the mixtures are stirred and phaco-emulsified to produce a stable nano-emulsion. The organic solvent is evaporated off to generate NPs [65] (Figure 4).

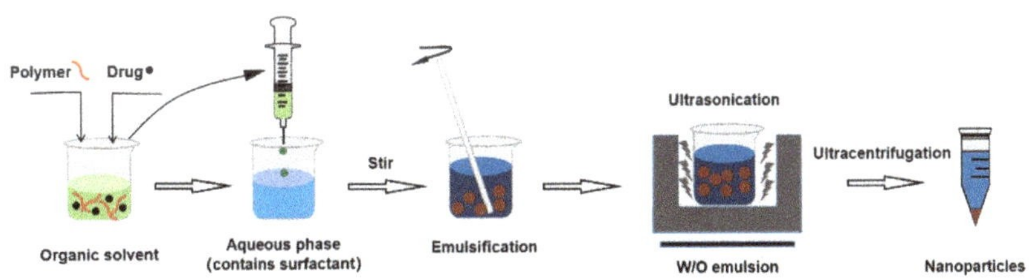

Figure 4. The procedure of single emulsification–solvent evaporation method.

3.2.2. Double Emulsion Method

Generally, hydrophilic drugs (such as proteins) can be prepared as polymeric NPs and lipid-based NPs by this double emulsion (W/O/W) method [66]. The hydrophilic drug and stabilizer are first dissolved in water and then dispersed in the organic solvent form colostrum. The colostrum is dispersed and dissolved in an aqueous phase containing an emulsifier, and the formulation is finally stirred to evaporate the organic solvent and obtain NPs [67]. The double emulsification method can prevent the decrease in encapsulation efficiency caused by the rapid dispersion of water-soluble drugs into the outer water phase during the emulsification process (Figure 5).

3.2.3. Nanoprecipitation Method

Nanoprecipitation method can be used to prepare hydrophobic polymers into NPs. Materials and drugs are dissolved and dispersed in organic solvents. The resulting organic solvent is added into an aqueous solution with surfactants magnetically stirred. Due to the difference in the solubility of hydrophobic polymers in the two solvents, the polymers that exist in stretched form in organic solvents will aggregate and form NPs once they enter the aqueous phase. By using lower pressure evaporation or nitrogen blowing, the solvent and water from the particle dispersions are eliminated. NPs are precipitated from the suspo-emulsion by centrifugation in a differential centrifuge [68] (Figure 6).

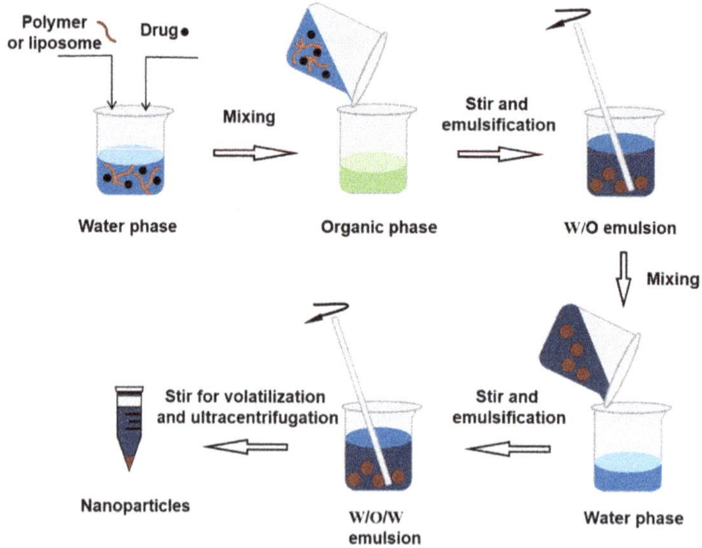

Figure 5. The procedure of double emulsion method.

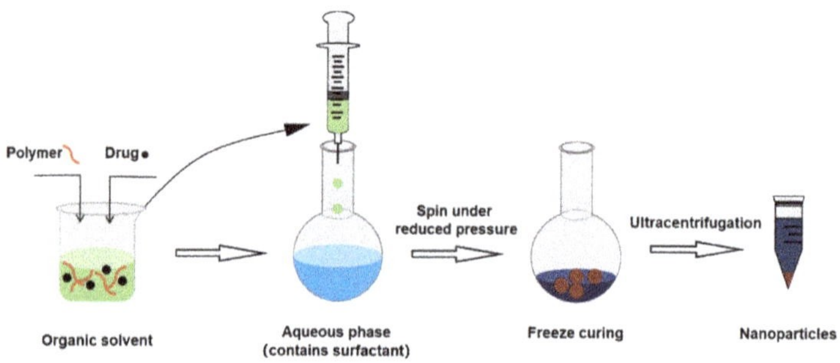

Figure 6. The procedure of nanoprecipitation method.

3.2.4. Salting out Emulsification–Diffusion Method

No toxic organic solvent is used in salting out emulsification–diffusion method. Natural polymer materials, such as albumin and gelatin, are used as carrier materials to prepare polymeric NPs. Dissolve nanocarriers and hydrophobic drugs in water with surfactant, and then add salt precipitating agent or change the pH value to precipitate the polymer while stirring. An emulsifier is added to emulsify the precipitate and an appropriate amount of curing agent is used to stabilize the NPs. Dialysis membrane or gel column chromatography can be used to purify the products [69] (Figure 7).

3.2.5. Supercritical Fluid Method

Supercritical fluid is a substance in a supercritical state that can improve solubility of poorly soluble drugs [70]. Polymers (or liposomes) and drugs are dissolved in a supercritical liquid. When the supercritical liquid is decompressed and atomized through a small-diameter nozzle, the NPs will be separated with rapid vaporization of the supercritical liquid [71]. Supercritical fluid technology is emerging as an attractive preparation method due to use of environmentally friendly solvents, high-purity processing of NPs, and absence of residual organic solvents [72] (Figure 8).

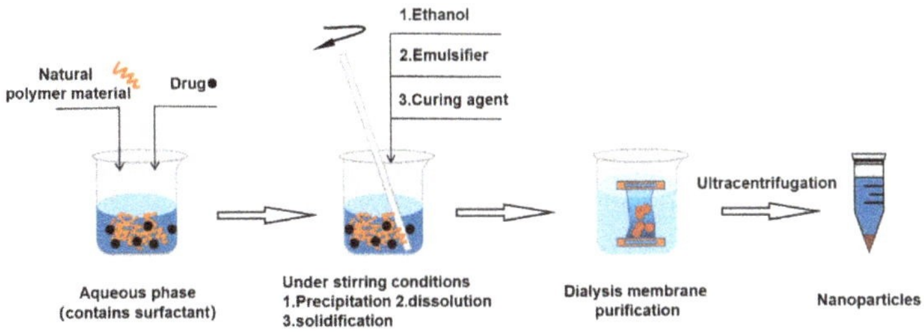

Figure 7. The procedure of salting out emulsification–diffusion method.

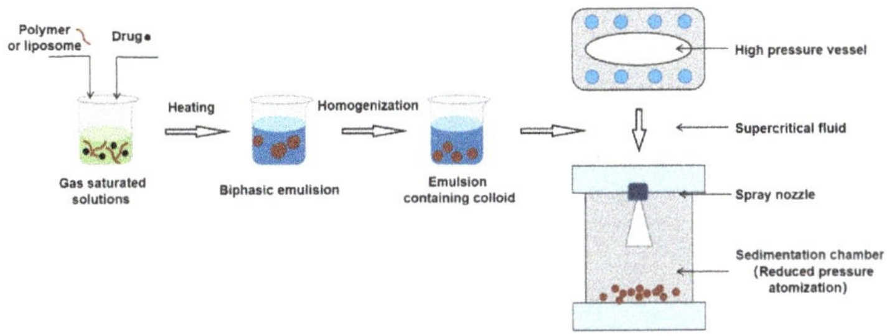

Figure 8. The procedure of supercritical fluid technology.

3.2.6. Spray Drying Method

Spray drying method has been shown to be an effective way for improving long-term stability of NPs and is suitable for industrial largescale preparation of NPs. With removal of water, NPs material turned from fluid state to powdered material. The atomizer atomizes a certain concentration of fluid, falls into a certain flow of dry gas for vaporization/drying, and finally separates NPs from the dry gas [73]. This method is further restricted to lipids with a melting point over 70 °C (Figure 9).

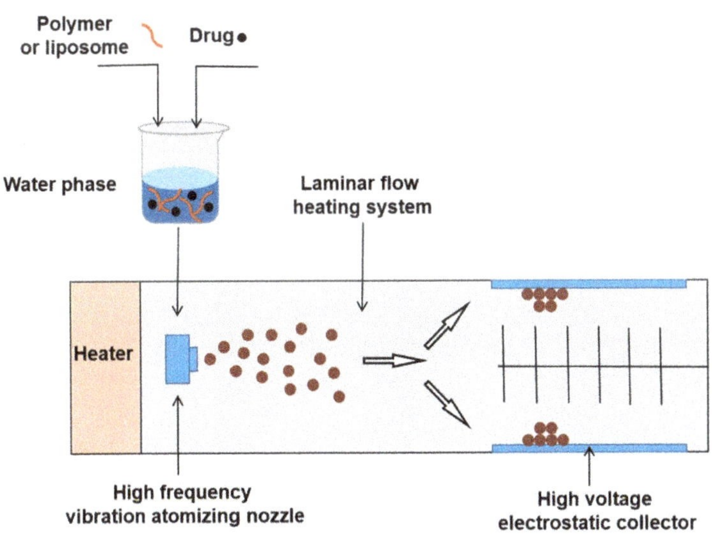

Figure 9. The procedure of spray drying method.

3.2.7. Solvothermal Method

In closed reactors (such as autoclave) with high temperatures and pressures, the solvothermal approach typically functioned and is suitable for preparation of inorganic NPs [74]. The raw material is dissolved in an organic solvent, stirred, sonicated, and then transferred to an autoclave for heat treatment. Then, the cores evolve into grains with a certain shape. The autoclave spontaneously cools down to ambient temperature in the presence of air following the solvothermal reaction [75]. The precipitate is then centrifuged separately, cleaned with deionized water, and finally dried [76]. The reaction process is relatively sluggish with this approach, taking between 18 and 36 h [77] (Figure 10).

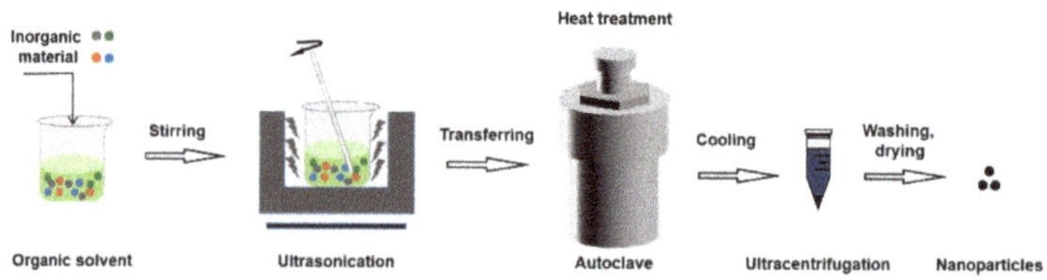

Figure 10. The procedure of solvothermal method.

3.2.8. Sol–Gel Method

When using the sol–gel process, the inorganic material is uniformly dissolved in the precursor solvent before being transferred to a container. Heat the container, store under vacuum for a period of time and cause its gelation, and then cool to room temperature. The product is washed with ethanol and subsequently dried under vacuum to obtain inorganic NPs with core–shell structure. By adjusting the reaction time and material ratio as well as the proportion of the reaction product, the sol–gel method can control the thickness of the shell, which in turn affects the overall particle size [78] (Figure 11).

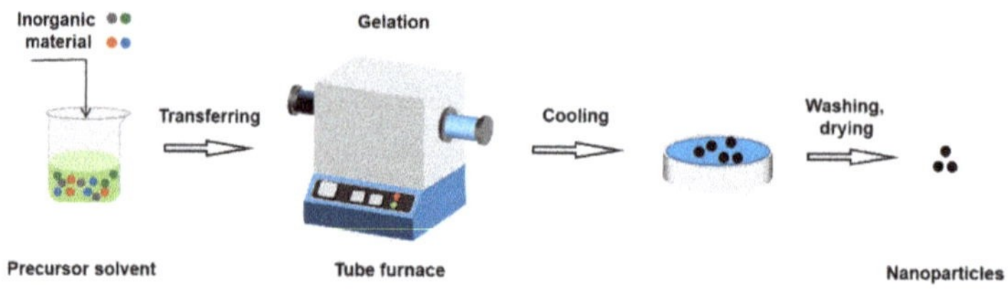

Figure 11. The procedure of sol–gel method.

3.2.9. Thermal Decomposition

The weighed precursor and inorganic material are added into an organic solvent. The mixture is stirred to dissolve during heating and then kept at a specific temperature in the reactor. The samples are allowed to cool down at room temperature. Products are collected by filtration, washed several times, and dried overnight [79]. Thermal decomposition has the benefit of allowing for efficient and speedy synthesis of functional NPs in accordance with experimental requirements (Figure 12).

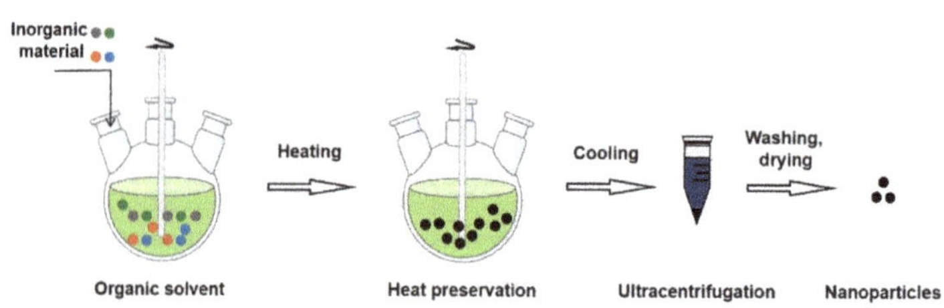

Figure 12. The procedure of thermal decomposition.

4. Cell Membrane

As the "shell" of the cell membrane biomimetic NPs, the cell membrane plays the role of modifying the NPs. Membrane proteins embedded in semipermeable phospholipid bilayers, such as integrins, peripherins, and lipid-anchored proteins, make up around one-third of all the proteins in an organism [80]. NPs, wrapped in membranes that embed endogenous proteins outwards, would have the properties of endogenous cells, enhancing immune escape and extending blood circulation [81]. This chapter summarized the cell extraction methods from blood or tissue and their corresponding membrane properties and limitations (as shown in Table 1).

Table 1. Extraction methods of different cell membranes and their characteristics and limitations.

Cell	Separation Methods	Properties	Limitations
Erythrocyte	Extrusion, ultrasound, freeze–thaw, and hypotonicity	Easy availability. Long circulatory lifespan (~120 days in humans and ~50 days in mice) and wide circulation range. Uniform in size and shape, with a good surface area to volume ratio, without organelles and any DNA. Good biocompatibility, biodegradability, and non-immunogenicity.	Poor targeting ability.
Platelet	Extrusion, freeze–thaw, and ultrasound	High targeting efficiency. Controlled drug release. Lower immunogenicity. Long systemic circulation (around 7–10 days). Targeting to plaque.	Small proportion of blood and undesirable activated.
Leukocyte	Extrusion and hypotonicity	Adhesion capacity. Migratory and chemotactic capacity in disease states. High loading capacity.	Organization residency restrictions.
Macrophage	Extrusion and hypotonicity	Good targeting ability to AD lesions. Innate immune evasion ability. Long circulation ability in vivo.	Organization residency restrictions.
Cancer cell	Extrusion and Dounce homogenizer	Strong homologous targeting ability.	Homologous tumor targeting.

4.1. Source Cell

Distinct types of cells in the human body perform several physiological tasks, such as lengthy blood circulation, migration to particular body areas, and traversing physical barriers. To deliver medications with retained cellular structure and function, it is crucial to choose particular cell types.

4.1.1. Erythrocyte

Erythrocytes, also known as red blood cells, lack organelles and nuclei and are biconcave blood cells, with a diameter of between 7 and 8 μm and a central thickness of about 1 μm. Erythrocytes are the most prevalent cell in blood, making up a quarter of the total number of cells in the body, and can be easily isolated from the blood [82]. In addition, because of a lifespan of more than 120 days and high surface area/volume ratio, the erythrocyte has long circulation time in the body for efficient transport. Erythrocytes can effectively avoid phagocytosis by the immune system because the surface of erythrocytes is rich in self-labeled proteins, such as CD47, polysaccharides, and acidic sialic acid moieties, which are essential for maintaining balance of erythrocytes [83]. Deactivation of myosin IIA, which is involved in contraction of macrophage actinomyosin, is brought about by binding of CD47 to SIRP-α and can prevent phagocytosis [84]. In addition to camouflaging their function and avoiding clearance by the immune system, NPs modified with RBCm can reduce toxic side effects, prolong circulation time, and enhance drug retention at the focal site [85]. In recent years, polymeric NPs encapsulated by RBCm have represented an emerging nano-drug delivery platform because of their properties of prolonging circulation in vivo [86].

Gao et al. coated Cur-loaded human serum albumin NPs with RBCm and then modified the RBCm surface with triphenylphosphine (TPP) molecules and AV-1451 (T807) (T807/TPP-RBC-Cur-NPs). In the in vitro co-culture model of BMECs, AS, and HT22 cells, significant fluorescence intensity was observed in the T807/TPP-RBC-NPs group, proving that RBCm-coated biomimetic NPs could effectively traverse the BBB and fully enhance the Cur cell uptake. Hematoxylin and eosin staining was used to check the survival of neurons in the hippocampus of AD model mice after injection of T807/TPP-RBC-Cur-NPs into the tail vein. The neuronal survival rate in the hippocampus of AD model mice treated with T807/TPP-RBC-Cur-NPs was greatly increased [87].

4.1.2. Platelet

Platelets are disc-shaped anucleate cellular fragments from bone marrow stem cell line megakaryocytes [88]. Platelets are less numerous (150,000-450,000/mL), shorter lifespan (7–10 days) [89], and smaller (average diameter 2–4 μm) compared to erythrocytes [88]. Platelets are commonly used for vascular injury, wound healing, inflammation, and hemostasis following thrombosis [90]. Due to the ability of platelets regarding immune evasion [91], subendothelial adhesion, and pathogen detection [92], platelet-membrane-coated NPs have gained great attention over the past few decades.

Xu et al. synthesized YGRKKRRQRRR-NH_2-modified platelet membranes coated with neuroprotectant (ZL006e) and recombinant-tissue-plasminogen-activator-loaded polymeric NPs of glucan derivatives (TP-NP-rtPA/ZL006e). It was found that the cell penetration rate of TP-NP-rtPA/ZL006e in BCECs cells was significantly higher than that of free ZL006e. The concentration of TP-NP-rtPA/ZL006e in the brain was 14.6% after injection of coumarin-6-labeled TP-NP-rtPA/ZL006e into a mouse model, which was higher than that in liver tissue at 2 h administration. TP-NP-rtPA/ZL006e was found to penetrate the BBB and accumulate in injured neural tissue [93].

4.1.3. Leukocyte

Leukocytes, commonly termed as white blood cells, are between 7 and 20 μm in diameter, larger than erythrocytes due to their nucleus. Leukocytes play an important function in protecting bodies from infection and injury and are widely distributed in blood arteries, lymphatics, and other organs. The CD11b protein on the surface of leukocyte membranes can target activated BCECs and evade uptake by the mononuclear phagocytosis system via CD45 protein [94]. Based on the characteristics of receptor proteins on the leukocytes membrane, the leukocytes membrane can be used as a general tool for therapeutic drug delivery [95]. Leukocytes come in five different subtypes: neutrophils (NCM), eosinophils, basophils, lymphocytes, and monocytes. Leukocytes are the guardians of the body, with unique physicochemical and biological properties. Therefore, NPs disguised with leukocyte membranes have the effect of evading opsonization and delaying uptake [96]. As the existence of nuclei, leukocytes are more difficult to be extracted and purified. Despite of their flaws, white blood cell membranes also are excellent candidates for NPs encapsulation due to their capacity to target and regulate tumors and inflammation.

Mesoporous Prussian blue nanozyme, which has a cell membrane coating of NCM (MPBzyme@NCM), was created by Feng et al. After co-culture with MPBzyme@NCM and Transwell system (bEnd.3 and mouse microglia cells), it was found that MPBzyme@NCM could not only cross BBB but also had strong reactive oxygen species scavenging ability. Fluorescence imaging of mice injected with fluorescein isothiocyanate labeled MPBzyme@NCM showed that NCM coating promoted continuous accumulation of MPBzyme@NCM in brain tissue compared with NCM or non-coating [97].

4.1.4. Macrophages

Macrophages are immune cells that recognize, engulf, and digest cellular debris and other foreign substances that lack biomarkers of their own [98]. Recently, macrophages have attracted much interest and have been developed to contain NPs [99]. As a kind of immune cell, macrophages have the function of immune evasion [98]. NPs that have been enclosed by the MA can easily move between macrophages, extravascular tissues, and blood vessels. Studies have shown that pathogeny of AD is related to damage of BCECs [100], which secrete adhesion molecules caused by immune cells. Thus, macrophages could be transferred to the lesion site and participate in various stages of AD [101].

Long et al. prepared Baicalin liposomes (BA-LP) modified with MA (MA-BA-LP). Intensity and duration of fluorescence in brains of mice injected with MA-DiR-LP in tail veins were substantially higher than those in the DiR-LP group. The findings demonstrated that MA-BA-LP had a greater brain targeting impact than BA-LP [102].

4.1.5. Cancer Cells

Cancer-cells-modified NPs can be easily bound to homologous tumor cells because of the homologous adhesion molecules on cell membranes, such as lectins, integrins, cadherins, selectors, and proteins [103]. Cancer-cell-membrane-modified NPs have strong homologous targeting capabilities without the need for laborious surface modifications, and they can be employed to deliver medications or contrast agents to specific tumors [104]. As a result, NPs coated with cancer cell membrane also can improve cellular uptake, tumor targeting, and accumulation in addition to enabling endogenous biomimetic "stealth" administration in vivo [105]. Furthermore, it has been established that one of the best strategies to improve NPs' ability to be biocompatible for treatment of homologous malignancies is through cancer cell membrane. Studies have shown that NPs disguised as glioma cell membranes have the ability to cross the BBB and long-term circulation [11], but, unfortunately, treatment of AD with cancer-cell-membrane-modified NPs is unclear [106].

4.1.6. Membrane Hybridization

Multi-membrane-modified NPs showed better performance compared with single-membrane-modified NPs [107]. Membrane hybridization can introduce membrane proteins specific to one cell type into another, giving the hybrid membrane greater targeting ability. Membrane hybridization can also enhance the immune escape of NPs by introducing another membrane with stronger stealth ability. Membrane hybridization is also used to introduce "homologous" characteristics that reduce unnecessary cells [108]. Mixed membranes exhibit superior biocompatibility, reduced immunogenicity, prolonged cyclicity, homologous targeting capability, and stimulation of the innate or adaptive immune system. For instance, modification of NPs by fusing of platelets and other functional membranes allows them to target damaged areas and treat diseases such as atherosclerosis and acute inflammation. Bionic neutral granulocytes and macroscopic cells with collaborative tumor micro-environment modify nano-particles to treat homologous tumors [109].

4.1.7. Other Cells

In a particular design found in the study, Niu et al. attached doxorubicin-loaded heparin NPs to the surface of native grapefruit extracellular vesicles, creating biomimetic grapefruit for drug delivery NPs; compared with traditional cell membrane encapsulation, the therapeutic effect of modified NPs can reach 4 times the drug loading. Biomimetic grapefruit NPs can bypass BBB and enter glioma tissue through receptor-mediated cell penetration and membrane fusion, which greatly promotes cellular internalization and anti-proliferation capabilities and extends the cycle time [110].

4.2. Isolation of Cell Membrane

Natural, intact, and functional cell membranes are separated from source cells by destroying or lysing cells to empty their intracellular components. Cell membranes can be separated from blood or tissues by ultrasound, freeze–thaw, extrusion, hypotonicity, and Dounce homogenizers (summarized in Figure 13).

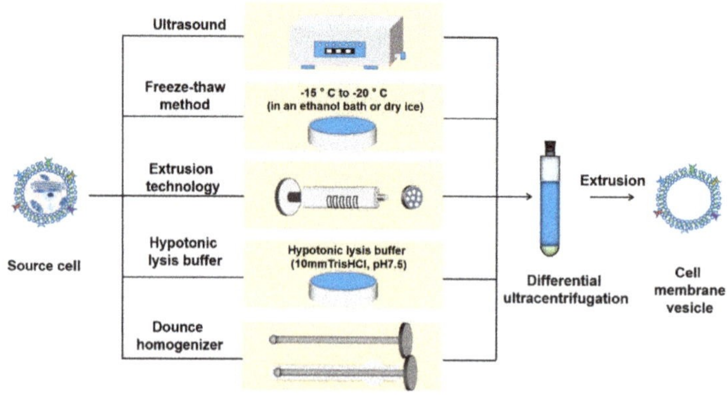

Figure 13. Schematic representation of different methods for isolating cell membranes from native cells.

4.2.1. Ultrasound

Ultrasound is a technique that agitates cells and their constituent parts with sound energy. The tube containing the cell suspension is placed in an ultrasonic bath [111]. The alternating process of compression and expansion through different acoustic frequencies produces intense shock waves (inertial cavitation) [112] and high-velocity microjets [113], known as cavitation. The cavitation leads to cell rupture and cell lysis, which makes it easier to separate the cell membranes. However, ultrasonic membrane separation technology still has some shortcomings. For example, free radicals generated in the process of ultrasound can affect the internal structure of cell membrane. The increasing temperature of the medium can change the properties of membrane proteins, resulting in unstable yield of cell membrane [80]. To prevent permanent harm to cell membranes, the power, frequency, time, and temperature parameters should be carefully optimized.

4.2.2. Freeze–Thaw

Freeze–thaw method is a gentle, simple, and convenient method of cell membrane isolation. The culture dish holding the cell suspension is quickly thawed at 40 °C or at ambient temperature after being instantly frozen at −15 °C to −20 °C (either dry ice or an ethanol bath). Cell destruction occurs after at least two cycles of freezing and thawing [114]. This is because cells grow larger by forming frozen ice crystals, which then contract as they melt. When the sizes of the ice crystals cells are periodically changed, the cells rupture and the membranes are separated. During freezing and thawing cycling, proteins embedded in the cell membrane are damaged and protein activity will be inhibited.

4.2.3. Extrusion

Cell membranes with large cross-sectional area are extruded through a die to obtain cell vesicles with smaller cross-section. After pretreatment of membranes with large cross-sectional areas, the cell membrane is mechanically pushed through a mold with a specified cross-section to obtain cell membrane vesicles of a certain desired shape and size [115]. The cell suspension is pushed through a membrane filter on the device using a liposome extruder to obtain cell vesicles in specified size range [116]. The main elements influencing the size distribution of the extruded material are pushing pressure, pushing timings, and pore size of the filter membrane. Extrusion can be conducted at room temperature or above the recrystallization temperature of the material.

4.2.4. Hypotonicity

When the hypotonic lysate is added to the culture dish containing the cells, the water molecules in the hypotonic lysate will diffuse into the cells and increase the volume of the cytoplasm, resulting in rupture of the cells to acquire the cell membrane [117]. Alternatively, cells are suspended in an ice bath in hypotonic lysis buffer for 15 min and then homogenized to obtain a supernatant containing cell membrane fragments and cytoplasmic extract. The pH and osmotic pressure of the lysate are regulated by buffer salts and ionic salts. The ready-to-use, detergent-free hypotonic lysis buffer (10 mm Tris HCl, pH 7.5) has a noticeable impact on cell lysis and cell membrane isolation; 0.25% PBS or 0.4% NaCl [80] is also recommended as a hypotonic lysis buffer for cell membrane isolation.

4.2.5. Dounce Homogenizer

Homogenization is a process of micronizing and homogenizing dispersion in a suspension (or emulsion) system. The Dounce homogenizer [118] is a cylindrical glass tube with two grinding rods of different sizes in each set. The smaller rod for preliminary tissue separation and the larger rod for finishing grinding are appropriate for cell suspension or soft tissue grinding, moderate homogenization of eukaryotic cells, and organelle separation [119]. The cells are placed in a Dounce homogenizer with the appropriate volume of lysis buffer. They are first tapped with a loose rod, and then a large and tight stick is tapped up and down in the glass bottle, usually five to ten times, to obtain the disrupted cell membranes. Previous studies showed that the combination of Dounce homogenizer and hypotonic lysis buffer can achieve better cell lysis effect [120]. Use of a hypotonic buffer caused the cytoplasm to swell, and then the cell membrane is obtained by gently breaking the cell by mechanical force using a Dounce homogenizer. Because the spherical design of the pestle head effectively reduces heat generation during friction, the Dounce homogenizer can avoid the effect of heat accumulation on the protein activity on the cell membrane surface.

4.3. *Fusion of Membrane Vesicles and NPs*

After the cell membrane is extracted, the extracted cell membrane vesicles need to be fused with NPs to form cell membrane biomimetic NPs. Several methods have been proposed to fuse cell membranes with NPs, including co-extrusion (by mechanical extrusion), ultrasound (endocytosis by ultrasonic energy), extrusion/microfluidic electroporation (by electrical pulses), etc. (Figure 14).

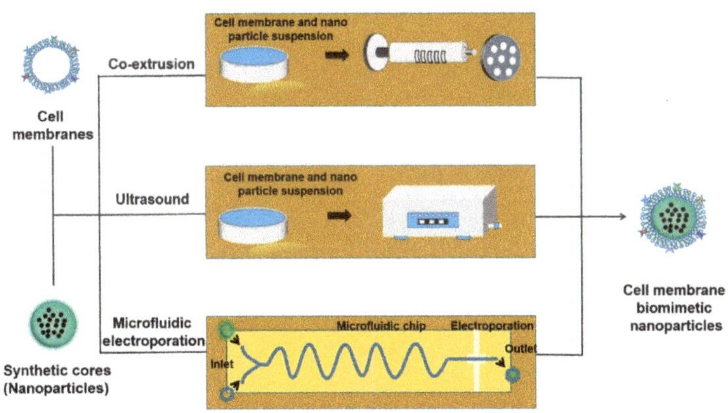

Figure 14. Schematic representation of different methods for fusing cell membranes with NPs.

4.3.1. Co-Extrusion

In the co-extrusion method, the cell membrane suspension and the NPs suspension are mixed in certain proportion. The mixed suspension is co-extruded multiple times through a porous filter membrane of the specified size of the extruder [102]. After extruder, NPs are wrapped by cell membrane vesicles to form cell membrane biomimetic NPs. The excess cell membrane vesicles and NPs are discarded by centrifugation. The lower residues after centrifugation are retained as cell membrane biomimetic NPs [116]. Co-extrusion method is easy and simple, and the desired size of cell membrane NPs can be obtained by adjusting the pore size of the filter membrane [121].

4.3.2. Ultrasound

The mixture of cell membranes and core NPs is incubated under the effect of ultrasound to obtain cell membrane biomimetic NPs [122]. The energy generated by the ultrasonic wave is destructive, which can make the cell membrane spontaneously remodel on the NPs to obtain cell membrane biomimetic NPs. Compared with the co-extrusion method, the ultrasonic method has less material loss and simple operation, which shows better application prospects. The ultrasonic method can also fuse multiple membranes to form membrane hybrids, giving the cell membrane more targeting capabilities. However, the film coating formed by ultrasonic method may not be uniform, and the long-term ultrasonic process will also break the NPs.

4.3.3. Microfluidic Electroporation

Microfluidic electroporation technology is a new technology developed in recent years that simultaneously solves the problems of destruction of NPs via ultrasonic/extrusion and time-consuming and labor-intensive nature of the co-extrusion method [123]. When the cell membrane suspension and the NPs suspension are separately injected into the instrument, the two components will first be combined in the first channel (Y shape), then mixed in the second channel (S shape). Under electrical impulses in the perforated area, NPs will penetrate into the cell membrane vesicles, and, finally, the cell membrane biomimetic NPs will be collected from the chip [124]. Even though the synthesis process is relatively complex, this method has high synthesis rate and good parallelism with great potential [125].

4.3.4. Other Coating Methods

In addition to the three methods summarized in Table 2, methods such as freeze–thaw/ultrasound, extrusion/ultrasound and stirring, extrusion/electroporation, and in situ packaging can also be used to prepare cell membrane biomimetic NPs.

Table 2. Methods of fusion of cell membrane and NPs and their advantages and disadvantages.

Method	Procedures	Advantages	Disadvantages
Co-extrusion	The mixed solution formed by mixing the cell membrane suspension and the NPs suspension is co-extruded through a porous filter membrane of specified size with an extruder for many times	The steps are simple and easy to use. The multi-layer target product can be prepared	Time-consuming and labor-intensive. Low synthesis rate
Ultrasound	The mixture formed by mixing the cell membrane suspension and the NPs suspension is sonicated at a certain frequency for a specified time	Less loss of raw materials; mass production is possible. The biomimetic NPs formed are highly stable. Membrane hybrids can be formed	Uneven coating, easy to form polydisperse particles. NPs are easily broken
Microfluidic electroporation	The cell membrane suspension and NPs suspension are mixed separately in the instrument, flow through the electroporation area, and finally the product is collected in the chip	High synthesis rate and good parallelism	Complex operation process

5. Targeting Peptides

Nowadays, application of membrane biomimetic NPs is becoming more and more common, and the multifunctional demand for membrane biomimetic NPs is also increasing. On this basis, peptides with additional functions can be used, which provide the particles with various additional functions beyond the natural functions of the cell membrane, greatly increasing application of NPs. The usual method includes (A) lipid insertion: ligand–joint–lipid junctions are first synthesized and then the lipid chains are inserted into the membrane depending on the fluidity of the bilayer lipid membrane [126]; (B) membrane hybridization: by fusing a variety of cell membranes, the combined hybrid membrane will have a variety of cell membrane functions [83]; (C) metabolic engineering: metabolic substrates are first bound to functional parts and then incubated with cells to participate in the absorption and metabolic processes, and metabolic engineering methods are expressed on cell membranes [127]; and (D) genetic modification: genetically modified membranes are created by selectively gene-editing cells, which are then coated with NPs [128]. The most widely used and easiest way to apply is to prepare dual-function joints Malayside-polyethylene glycol-active fat chemically modified living cells. Functional chains are attached to the ends of specific targeting peptides, giving the native cell membrane more function when the cell membrane is intact [129]. As shown in Table 3, a variety of targeting peptides have been applied to treat brain diseases through BBB.

Table 3. Targeting peptides related to BBB and their protein sequences and corresponding targets.

Target Receptor or Transport Pathway	Name	Peptide Sequence	Ref.
Low-density lipoprotein receptor	Angiopep-2	TFFYGGSRGKRNFKTEEY	[130]
	ApoB	SSVIDALQYKLEGTTRLTRKRGLKLATALSLSNKFVEGS	[131]
	ApoE	LRKLRKRLL	[132]
	mApoE	CWGLRKLRKRLLR	[133]
	Peptide-22	Ac-CMPRLRGC-NH_2	[134]
Transferrin receptor	B6	CGHKAKGPRK	[135]
	D-T7	D-HRPYIAH	[136]
	T7	HAIYPRH	[136]
	THR	THRPPMWSPVWP-NH_2	[137]
	THRre	pwvpswmpprht-NH_2	[138]
	CRT	CRTIGPSVC	[139]
Leptin receptor	Leptin30	YQQILTSMPSRNVIQISNDLENLRDLLHVL	[140]
Nicotinic acetylcholine receptor	RVG29	YTIWMPENPRPGTPCDIFTNSRGKRASNG-OH	[57]
	^{D}CDX	GreirtGraerwsekf-OH	[116]
	D8	^{D}RTG^{D}R^{D}A^{D}RE^{D}W	[141]
Potassium or calcium channel	Apamin	CNCKAPETALCARRCQQH-NH_2	[142]
	MiniAp-4	H-[Dap]KAPETAL D-NH_2	[135]
Glutathione transporter	GSH	γ-L-glutamyl-CG-OH	[143]
	G23	HLNILSTLWKYRC	[144]
Adsorption-mediated endocytosis	TAT(47-57)	YGRKKRRQRRR-NH_2	[145]
	SynB1	RGGRLSYSRRRFSTSTGR	[146]
Unknown receptor	CGN	D-GNHPLAKYNGT	[136]
	TGN	TGNYKALHPHNG	[147]
	TP10	AGYLLGKINLKALAALAKKIL-NH_2	[148]
Aβ aggregates	LVFFA	LVFFA	[149]
	KLVFF	KLVFF	[64]
	LPFFD	LPFFD	[147]
	QSH	QSHYRHISPAQV	[150]
Sphingomyelin and ganglioside GT1B on neurons	Tet1	HLNILSTLWKYR	[151]

Note: the amino acids are expressed in a single letter; the capital letter represents L-configured amino acids, and the lowercase letters indicate D-type amino acids.

On this basis, bi-functional ligands can also be used to modify the cell membrane surface (Figure 15).

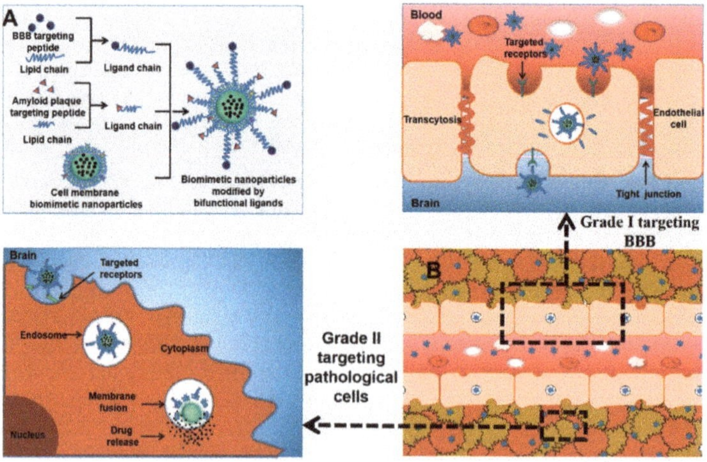

Figure 15. (**A**) Preparation of biomimetic NPs modified by targeting peptides. (**B**) Schematic illustration of the possible mechanism of stepwise targeting of cell membrane biomimetic NPs modified with targeting peptides to the affected area through the BBB for treatment.

6. Concluding Remarks and Future Perspectives

Nanomaterials have been developed to treat AD based on promotion of drug delivery across the BBB to achieve accumulation at desired sites. NPs carry therapeutic drugs by encapsulation or surface modification, which has the advantage of effectively delivering drugs to the target area and enhancing the therapeutic effect. Cell membrane biomimetic NPs, which fuse NPs with the membrane of the extracted cell, have the main biological traits and additional physiological functions of the source cell. Cell membrane biomimetic NPs are shielded from the body's immune system, which prevents immune cells from being absorbed. Surface-modified targeting peptides on cell membrane biomimetic NPs can improve the targeting capabilities and precision to a damaged location.

At present, biomimetic nanomedicine, represented by cell membrane biomimetic NPs used to treat AD, is still in its infancy and has many problems that need to be improved upon. First, maintaining stability of cell membrane biomimetic NPs is one of the issues that must be resolved for application, which requires certain stability of drugs for long-term effective preservation. Delivery efficiency of cell membrane biomimetic NPs is greatly influenced by their size, shape, elasticity, and other physical and chemical properties. Additionally, therapeutic and diagnostic nanomedicine products are currently administered via parenteral injection, typically intravenously. Oral administration is an ideal administration, with high patient compliance. Due to low absorption of solid NPs and biochemical barriers in the gastrointestinal tract, oral delivery of NPs has not proven feasible. Therefore, effective implementation of cell membrane biomimetic NPs administered orally will represent significant advancement in the field of nanomedicine.

Author Contributions: Conceptualization, X.Z. and F.G.; writing—original draft preparation, X.Z., Y.N., S.Y., C.Y., J.G. and N.Z.; writing—review and editing, X.Z., N.Z. and F.G. finalized the review. All authors have read and agreed to the published version of the manuscript.

Funding: This work was supported by the National Natural Science Foundation of China (82174007).

Institutional Review Board Statement: Not applicable.

Informed Consent Statement: Not applicable.

Data Availability Statement: Not applicable.

Conflicts of Interest: The authors declare no conflict of interest.

References

1. Bukhari, S.N.A. Nanotherapeutics for Alzheimer's disease with preclinical evaluation and clinical trials: Challenges, promises and limitations. *Curr. Drug Deliv.* **2022**, *19*, 17–31. [CrossRef] [PubMed]
2. Vermunt, L.; Sikkes, S.A.M.; Hout, A.V.D.; Handels, R.; Bos, I.; Flier, W.M.V.D.; Kern, S.; Ousset, P.J.; Maruff, P.; Skoog, I.; et al. Duration of preclinical, prodromal, and dementia stages of Alzheimer's disease in relation to age, sex, and APOE genotype. *Alzheimers Dement.* **2019**, *15*, 888–898. [CrossRef]
3. WHO. *Dementia*; World Health Organization: Geneva, Switzerland, 2022.
4. Todd, S.; Barr, S.; Roberts, M.; Passmore, A.P. Survival in dementia and predictors of mortality: A review. *Int. J. Geriatr. Psychiatry* **2013**, *28*, 1109–1124. [CrossRef] [PubMed]
5. Li, Y.X.; Leng, F.D.; Xiong, Q.; Zhou, J.; Du, A.L.; Zhu, F.Q.; Kou, X.W.; Sun, W.; Chen, L.Z.; Wang, H.L.; et al. Factors associated with Alzheimer's disease patients' caregiving status and family caregiving burden in China. *Front. Aging Neurosci.* **2022**, *14*, 865933. [CrossRef] [PubMed]
6. Gupta, G.L.; Samant, N.P. Current druggable targets for therapeutic control of Alzheimer's disease. *Contemp. Clin. Trials.* **2021**, *109*, 106549. [CrossRef] [PubMed]
7. Pardridge, W.M. BBB-genomics: Creating new openings for brain-drug targeting. *Drug Discov. Today* **2001**, *6*, 381–383. [CrossRef]
8. Tsou, Y.H.; Zhang, X.Q.; Zhu, H.; Syed, S.; Xu, X.Y. Drug delivery to the brain across the blood–brain barrier using nanomaterials. *Small* **2017**, *13*, 1701921. [CrossRef]
9. Tripathi, P.; Shukla, P.; Bieberich, E. Theranostic applications of nanomaterials in Alzheimer's disease: A multifunctional approach. *Curr. Pharm. Des.* **2022**, *28*, 116–132. [CrossRef]
10. Chai, Z.L.; Hu, X.F.; Lu, W.Y. Cell membrane-coated nanoparticles for tumor-targeted drug delivery. *Sci. China Mater.* **2017**, *60*, 504–510. [CrossRef]
11. Jia, Y.L.; Wang, X.B.; Hu, D.H.; Wang, P.; Liu, Q.H.; Zhang, X.J.; Jiang, J.Y.; Liu, X.; Sheng, Z.H.; Liu, B.; et al. Phototheranostics: Active targeting of orthotopic glioma using biomimetic proteolipid nanoparticles. *ACS Nano* **2018**, *13*, 386–398. [CrossRef]
12. Wang, H.J.; Liu, Y.; He, R.Q.; Xu, D.L.; Zang, J.; Weeranoppanant, N.; Dong, H.Q.; Li, Y.Y. Cell membrane biomimetic nanoparticles for inflammation and cancer targeting in drug delivery. *Biomater. Sci.* **2019**, *8*, 552–568. [CrossRef] [PubMed]
13. Zou, Y.; Liu, Y.J.; Yang, Z.P.; Zhang, D.Y.; Lu, Y.Q.; Zheng, M.; Xue, X.; Geng, J.; Chung, R.; Shi, B.Y. Effective and targeted human orthotopic glioblastoma xenograft therapy via a multifunctional biomimetic nanomedicine. *Adv. Mater.* **2018**, *30*, 1803717. [CrossRef] [PubMed]
14. Zhang, W.Y.; Zhao, M.; Gao, Y.L.; Cheng, X.; Liu, X.Y.; Tang, S.K.; Peng, Y.B.; Wang, N.; Hu, D.D.; Peng, H.S.; et al. Biomimetic erythrocytes engineered drug delivery for cancer therapy. *Chem. Eng. J.* **2021**, *433*, 133498. [CrossRef]
15. Cummings, J.; Lee, G.; Zhong, K.; Fonseca, J.; Taghva, K. Alzheimer's disease drug development pipeline. *Alzheimers Dement.* **2021**, *7*, e12179.
16. Melnikova, I. Therapies for Alzheimer's disease. *Nat. Rev. Drug Discov.* **2007**, *6*, 341–342. [CrossRef]
17. Matsunaga, S.; Kishi, T.; Nomura, I.; Sakuma, K.; Okuya, M.; Ikuta, T.; Iwata, N. The efficacy and safety of memantine for the treatment of Alzheimer's disease. *Expert Opin. Drug Saf.* **2018**, *17*, 1053–1061. [CrossRef]
18. McKeage, K. Memantine: A review of its use in moderate to severe Alzheimer's disease. *CNS Drugs* **2009**, *23*, 881–897. [CrossRef]
19. Atri, A.; Hendrix, S.B.; Pejović, V.; Hofbauer, R.K.; Edwards, J.; Molinuevo, J.L.; Graham, S.M. Cumulative, additive benefits of memantine-donepezil combination over component monotherapies in moderate to severe Alzheimer's dementia: A pooled area under the curve analysis. *Alzheimer's Res. Ther.* **2015**, *7*, 28. [CrossRef]
20. Dhillon, S. Aducanumab: First approval. *Drugs* **2021**, *81*, 1437–1443. [CrossRef]
21. Mahase, E. Aducanumab: European agency rejects Alzheimer's drug over efficacy and safety concerns. *The BMJ* **2021**, *375*, n3127. [CrossRef]
22. Cano, A.; Turowski, P.; Ettcheto, M.; Duskey, J.T.; Tosi, G.; Sánchez-López, E.; García, M.L.; Camins, A.; Souto, E.B.; Ruiz, A.; et al. Nanomedicine-based technologies and novel biomarkers for the diagnosis and treatment of Alzheimer's disease: From current to future challenges. *J. Nanobiotechnology* **2021**, *19*, 122. [CrossRef] [PubMed]
23. Benz, F.; Liebner, S. Structure and function of the blood-brain barrier (BBB). *Handb. Exp. Pharmacol.* **2020**, *273*, 3–31.
24. Abbott, N.J.; Rönnbäck, L.; Hansson, E. Astrocyte–endothelial interactions at the blood–brain barrier. *Nat. Rev. Neurosci.* **2006**, *7*, 41–53. [CrossRef] [PubMed]
25. Chowdhury, E.A.; Noorani, B.; Alqahtani, F.; Bhalerao, A.; Raut, S.; Sivandzade, F.; Cucullo, L. Understanding the brain uptake and permeability of small molecules through the BBB: A technical overview. *J. Cereb. Blood Flow Metab.* **2021**, *41*, 1797–1820. [CrossRef]
26. Pardridge, W.M. The blood-brain barrier: Bottleneck in brain drug development. *NeuroRx.* **2005**, *2*, 3–14. [CrossRef]
27. Zhao, J.J.; Ren, T.J.; Yang, M.B.; Zhang, Y.F.; Wang, Q.W.; Zuo, Z. Reduced systemic exposure and brain uptake of donepezil in rats with scopolamine-induced cognitive impairment. *Xenobiotica* **2019**, *50*, 389–400. [CrossRef]
28. Karasova, J.Z.; Soukup, O.; Korabecny, J.; Hroch, M.; Krejciova, M.; Hrabinova, M.; Misik, J.; Novotny, L.; Hepnarova, V.; Kuca, K. Tacrine and its 7-methoxy derivate; time-change concentration in plasma and brain tissue and basic toxicological profile in rats. *Drug Chem. Toxicol.* **2019**, *44*, 207–214. [CrossRef]
29. Ganipineni, L.P.; Danhier, F.; Préat, V. Drug delivery challenges and future of chemotherapeutic nanomedicine for glioblastoma treatment. *J. Control. Release* **2018**, *281*, 42–57. [CrossRef]

30. Chatterjee, B.; Gorain, B.; Mohananaidu, K.; Sengupta, P.; Mandal, U.K.; Choudhury, H. Targeted drug delivery to the brain via intranasal nanoemulsion: Available proof of concept and existing challenges. *Int. J. Pharm.* **2019**, *565*, 258–268. [CrossRef]
31. Lu, X.; Zhang, Y.; Wang, L.; Li, G.; Gao, J.; Wang, Y. Development of L-carnosine functionalized iron oxide nanoparticles loaded with dexamethasone for simultaneous therapeutic potential of blood brain barrier crossing and ischemic stroke treatment. *Drug Deliv.* **2021**, *28*, 380–389. [CrossRef]
32. Pinheiro, R.G.R.; Granja, A.; Loureiro, J.A.; Pereira, M.C.; Pinheiro, M.; Neves, A.R.; Reis, S. RVG29-functionalized lipid nanoparticles for quercetin brain delivery and Alzheimer's disease. *Pharm. Res.* **2020**, *37*, 139. [CrossRef] [PubMed]
33. Yusuf, M.; Khan, M.; Alrobaian, M.M.; Alghamdi, S.A.; Warsi, M.H.; Sultana, S.; Khan, R.A. Brain targeted polysorbate-80 coated PLGA thymoquinone nanoparticles for the treatment of Alzheimer's disease, with biomechanistic insights. *J. Drug Deliv. Sci. T echnol.* **2020**, *61*, 102214. [CrossRef]
34. Meng, Q.; Wang, A.; Hua, H.; Jiang, Y.; Wang, Y.; Mu, H.; Wu, Z.; Sun, K. Intranasal delivery of huperzine A to the brain using lactoferrin-conjugated N-trimethylated chitosan surface-modified PLGA nanoparticles for treatment of Alzheimer's disease. *Int. J. Nanomed* **2018**, *13*, 705–718. [CrossRef]
35. Xu, R.; Wang, J.; Xu, J.; Song, X.; Huang, H.; Feng, Y.; Fu, C. Rhynchophylline loaded-mPEG-PLGA nanoparticles coated with Tween-80 for preliminary study in Alzheimer's disease. *Int. J. Nanomed.* **2020**, *15*, 1149–1160. [CrossRef]
36. Barbalace, M.C.; Malaguti, M.; Giusti, L.; Lucacchini, A.; Hrelia, S.; Angeloni, C. Anti-inflammatory activities of marine algae in neurodegenerative diseases. *Int. J. Mol. Sci.* **2019**, *20*, 3061. [CrossRef] [PubMed]
37. Wang, C.; Du, W.; Lu, H.; Lan, J.; Liang, K.; Cao, S. A review: Halogenated compounds from marine actinomycetes. *Molecules* **2021**, *26*, 2754. [CrossRef]
38. Vio, V.; Marchant, M.J.; Araya, E.; Kogan, M.J. Metal nanoparticles for the treatment and diagnosis of neurodegenerative brain diseases. *Curr. Pharm. Des.* **2017**, *23*, 1916–1926. [CrossRef]
39. Bayda, S.; Adeel, M.; Tuccinardi, T.; Cordani, M.; Rizzolio, F. The history of nanoscience and nanotechnology: From chemical–physical applications to nanomedicine. *Molecules* **2019**, *25*, 112. [CrossRef]
40. Joy, R.; George, J.; John, F. Brief outlook on polymeric nanoparticles, micelles, niosomes, hydrogels and liposomes: Preparative methods and action. *ChemistrySelect* **2022**, *7*, e202104045. [CrossRef]
41. Tosi, G.; Duskey, J.T.; Kreuter, J. Nanoparticles as carriers for drug delivery of macromolecules across the blood-brain barrier. *Expert Opin. Drug. Deliv.* **2019**, *17*, 23–32. [CrossRef]
42. Danhier, F.; Ansorena, E.; Silva, J.M.; Coco, R.; Breton, A.L.; Préat, V. PLGA-based nanoparticles: An overview of biomedical applications. *J. Control. Release* **2012**, *161*, 505–522. [CrossRef] [PubMed]
43. Khan, A.R.; Yang, X.Y.; Fu, M.F.; Zhai, G.X. Recent progress of drug nanoformulations targeting to brain. *J. Control. Release* **2018**, *291*, 37–64. [CrossRef]
44. Rocha, C.V.; Gonçalves, V.; Silva, M.C.D.; Bañobre-López, M.; Gallo, J. PLGA-based composites for various biomedical applications. *Int. J. Mol. Sci.* **2022**, *23*, 2034. [CrossRef]
45. Khan, I.; Gothwal, A.; Sharma, A.K.; Kesharwani, P.; Gupta, L.; Lyer, A.K.; Gupta, U. PLGA nanoparticles and their versatile role in anticancer drug delivery. *Crit. Rev. Ther. Drug Carrier Syst.* **2016**, *33*, 159–193. [CrossRef] [PubMed]
46. Gao, C.; Chu, X.; Gong, W.; Zheng, J.; Xie, X.; Wang, Y.; Yang, M.; Li, Z.; Gao, C.; Yang, Y. Neuron tau-targeting biomimetic nanoparticles for curcumin delivery to delay progression of Alzheimer's disease. *J. Nanobiotechnology* **2020**, *18*, 71. [CrossRef] [PubMed]
47. Tang, D.; Wang, Y.; Wijaya, A.; Liu, B.Y.; Maruf, A.; Wang, J.X.; Xu, J.X.; Liao, X.L.; Wu, W.; Wang, G.X. ROS-responsive biomimetic nanoparticles for potential application in targeted anti-atherosclerosis. *Regen Biomater.* **2021**, *8*, rbab033. [CrossRef]
48. Perche, F.; Uchida, S.; Akiba, H.; Lin, C.Y.; Ikegami, M.; Dirisala, A.; Nakashima, T.; Itaka, K.; Tsumoto, K.; Kataoka, K. Improved brain expression of anti-amyloid β scFv by complexation of mRNA including a secretion sequence with PEG-based block catiomer. *Curr. Alzheimer Res.* **2016**, *14*, 295–302. [CrossRef]
49. Xie, J.; Gonzalez-Carter, D.; Tockary, T.A.; Nakamura, N.; Xue, Y.; Nakakido, M.; Akiba, H.; Dirisala, A.; Liu, X.; Toh, K.; et al. Dual-sensitive nanomicelles enhancing systemic delivery of therapeutically active antibodies specifically into the brain. *ACS Nano* **2020**, *14*, 6729–6742. [CrossRef]
50. Gonzalez-Carter, D.; Liu, X.; Tockary, T.A.; Dirisala, A.; Toh, K.; Anraku, Y.; Kataoka, K. Targeting nanoparticles to the brain by exploiting the blood-brain barrier impermeability to selectively label the brain endothelium. *Proc. Natl. Acad. Sci. USA* **2020**, *117*, 19141–19150. [CrossRef]
51. Akbarzadeh, A.; Rezaei-Sadabady, R.; Davaran, S.; Joo, S.W.; Zarghami, N.; Hanifehpour, Y.; Samiei, M.; Kouhi, M.; Nejati-Koshki, K. Liposome: Classification, preparation, and applications. *Nanoscale Res. Lett.* **2013**, *8*, 102. [CrossRef]
52. Tulbah, A.S.; Lee, W.H. Physicochemical characteristics and in vitro toxicity/anti-SARS-CoV-2 activity of favipiravir solid lipid nanoparticles (SLNs). *Pharmaceuticals* **2021**, *14*, 1059. [CrossRef]
53. Khosa, A.; Reddi, S.; Saha, R.N. Nanostructured lipid carriers for site-specific drug delivery. *Biomed. Pharmacother.* **2018**, *103*, 598–613. [CrossRef] [PubMed]
54. Wilson, R.J.; Li, Y.; Yang, G.Z.; Zhao, C.X. Nanoemulsions for drug delivery. *Particuology* **2021**, *64*, 85–97. [CrossRef]
55. Daraee, H.; Etemadi, A.; Kouhi, M.; Alimirzalu, S.; Akbarzadeh, A. Application of liposomes in medicine and drug delivery. *Artif. Cells Nanomed. Biotechnol.* **2014**, *44*, 381–391. [CrossRef] [PubMed]

56. Song, Y.N.; Zhang, N.; Li, Q.Y.; Chen, J.; Wang, Q.Z.; Yang, H.B.; Tan, H.P.; Gao, J.F.; Dong, Z.H.; Pang, Z.Q.; et al. Biomimetic liposomes hybrid with platelet membranes for targeted therapy of atherosclerosis. *Chem. Eng. J.* **2020**, *408*, 127296. [CrossRef]
57. Han, Y.; Gao, C.H.; Wang, H.; Sun, J.J.; Liang, M.; Feng, Y.; Liu, Q.Q.; Fu, S.Y.; Cui, L.; Gao, C.S.; et al. Macrophage membrane-coated nanocarriers Co-modified by RVG29 and TPP improve brain neuronal mitochondria-targeting and therapeutic efficacy in Alzheimer's disease mice. *Bioact. Mater.* **2021**, *6*, 529–542. [CrossRef]
58. Gao, N.; Sun, H.J.; Dong, K.; Ren, J.S.; Qu, X.G. Gold-nanoparticle-based multifunctional amyloid-β inhibitor against Alzheimer's disease. *Chem. Eur. J.* **2014**, *21*, 829–835. [CrossRef]
59. Tengjisi; Hui, Y.; Yang, G.Z.; Fu, C.K.; Liu, Y.; Zhao, C.X. Biomimetic core-shell silica nanoparticles using a dual-functional peptide. *J. Colloid Interface Sci.* **2020**, *581*, 185–194. [CrossRef]
60. Nakamura, S.; Sato, M.; Sato, Y.; Ando, N.; Takayama, T.; Fujita, M.; Ishihara, M. Synthesis and application of silver nanoparticles (Ag NPs) for the prevention of infection in healthcare workers. *Int. J. Mol. Sci.* **2019**, *20*, 3620. [CrossRef]
61. Liu, D.Z.; Cheng, Y.; Cai, R.Q.; Wang, W.W.; Cui, H.; Liu, M.; Zhang, B.L.; Mei, Q.B.; Zhou, S.Y. The enhancement of siPLK1 penetration across BBB and its anti glioblastoma activity in vivo by magnet and transferrin co-modified nanoparticle. *Nanomedicine* **2018**, *14*, 991–1003. [CrossRef]
62. Ehlerding, E.B.; Chen, F.; Cai, W.B. Biodegradable and renal clearable inorganic nanoparticles. *Adv. Sci.* **2015**, *3*, 1500223. [CrossRef] [PubMed]
63. Yang, G.B.; Phua, S.Z.F.; Lim, W.Q.; Zhang, R.; Feng, L.Z.; Liu, G.F.; Wu, H.W.; Bindra, A.K.; Jana, D.; Liu, Z.; et al. A hypoxia-responsive albumin-based nanosystem for deep tumor penetration and excellent therapeutic efficacy. *Adv. Mater.* **2019**, *31*, e1901513. [CrossRef] [PubMed]
64. Plissonneau, M.; Pansieri, J.; Heinrich-Balard, L.; Morfin, J.F.; Stransky-Heilkron, N.; Rivory, P.; Mowat, P.; Dumoulin, M.; Cohen, R.; Allémann, É.; et al. Gd-nanoparticles functionalization with specific peptides for ß-amyloid plaques targeting. *J. Nanobiotechnology* **2016**, *14*, 60. [CrossRef] [PubMed]
65. Pooja, D.; Tunki, L.; Kulhari, H.; Reddy, B.B.; Sistla, R. Optimization of solid lipid nanoparticles prepared by a single emulsification-solvent evaporation method. *Data Brief* **2016**, *6*, 15–19. [CrossRef] [PubMed]
66. Cortesi, R.; Esposjto, E.; Luca, G.; Nastruzzi, C. Production of lipospheres as carriers for bioactive compounds. *Biomaterials* **2002**, *23*, 2283–2294. [CrossRef]
67. Si, W.; Yang, Q.; Zong, Y.; Ren, G.; Zhao, L.; Hong, M.; Xin, Z. Toward understanding the effect of solvent evaporation on the morphology of PLGA microspheres by double emulsion method. *Ind. Eng. Chem. Res.* **2021**, *60*, 9196–9205. [CrossRef]
68. Almoustafa, H.A.; Alshawsh, M.A.; Chik, Z. Technical aspects of preparing PEG-PLGA nanoparticles as carrier for chemotherapeutic agents by nanoprecipitation method. *Int. J. Pharm.* **2017**, *533*, 275–284. [CrossRef]
69. Sheth, P.; Sandhu, H.; Singhal, D.; Malick, W.; Shah, N.; Kislalioglu, M.S. Nanoparticles in the pharmaceutical industry and the use of supercritical fluid technologies for nanoparticle production. *Curr. Drug Deliv.* **2012**, *9*, 269–284. [CrossRef]
70. Maqbool, F.; Moyle, P.M.; Thurecht, K.J.; Falconer, J.R. Dispersibility of phospholipids and their optimization for the efficient production of liposomes using supercritical fluid technology. *Int. J. Pharm.* **2019**, *563*, 174–183. [CrossRef]
71. Islam, T.; Ragib, A.A.; Ferdosh, S.; Uddin, A.B.M.H.; Akanda, M.J.H.; Mia, M.A.R.; M, R.P.D.; Kamaruzzaman, B.Y.; Sarker, M.Z.I. Development of nanoparticles for pharmaceutical preparations using supercritical techniques. *Chem. Eng. Commun.* **2022**, *209*, 1642–1663. [CrossRef]
72. Ali, M.E.; Lamprecht, A. Spray freeze drying as an alternative technique for lyophilization of polymeric and lipid-based nanoparticles. *Int. J. Pharm.* **2016**, *516*, 170–177. [CrossRef] [PubMed]
73. Lee, S.H.; Heng, D.; Ng, W.K.; Chan, H.-K.; Tan, R.B.H. Nano spray drying: A novel method for preparing protein nanoparticles for protein therapy. *Int. J. Pharm.* **2011**, *403*, 192–200. [CrossRef] [PubMed]
74. Li, R.X. Progress in preparation methods and applications of inorganic nanoparticles. *J. Phys. Conf. Ser.* **2020**, *1676*, 012093. [CrossRef]
75. Li, Y.; Han, Q.L.; Yao, Y.; Li, M.; Dong, P.; Han, L.; Zeng, X.Y.; Liu, J.; Liu, J.M.; Zhang, Y.J.; et al. Comparative study of yttria-stabilized zirconia synthesis by Co-precipitation and solvothermal methods. *JOM* **2019**, *71*, 3806–3813. [CrossRef]
76. Mousavi, S.H.; Müller, T.S.; Karos, R.; Oliveira, P.W.D. Faster synthesis of CIGS nanoparticles using a modified solvothermal method. *J. Alloys Compd.* **2016**, *659*, 178–183. [CrossRef]
77. Chun, Y.G.; Kim, K.H.; Yoon, K.H. Synthesis of CuLnGaSe2 nanoparticles by solvothermal route. *Thin Solid Films* **2005**, *480–481*, 46–49. [CrossRef]
78. Lismont, M.; Páez, C.A.; Dreesen, L. A one-step short-time synthesis of 2 core–shell nanoparticles. *J. Colloid Interface Sci.* **2015**, *15*, 2903–2911.
79. Sheng, S.; Jin, S.; Cui, K. Thermal decomposition of nanostructured bismuth subcarbonate. *Materials* **2020**, *13*, 4287. [CrossRef]
80. Oroojalian, F.; Beygi, M.; Baradaran, B.; Mokhtarzadeh, A.; Shahbazi, M.A. Immune cell membrane-coated biomimetic nanoparticles for targeted cancer therapy. *Small* **2021**, *17*, e2006484. [CrossRef]
81. Chen, L.; Hong, W.Q.; Ren, W.Y.; Xu, T.; Qian, Z.Y.; He, Z.Y. Recent progress in targeted delivery vectors based on biomimetic nanoparticles. *Signal Transduct. Target. Ther.* **2021**, *6*, 225. [CrossRef]
82. Huang, Y.X.; Tuo, W.W.; Wang, D.; Kang, L.L.; Chen, X.Y.; Luo, M. Restoring the youth of aged red blood cells and extending their lifespan in circulation by remodelling membrane sialic acid. *J. Cell. Mol. Med.* **2015**, *20*, 294–301. [CrossRef] [PubMed]

83. Dehaini, D.; Wei, X.L.; Fang, R.H.; Masson, S.; Angsantikul, P.; Luk, B.T.; Zhang, Y.; Ying, M.; Jiang, Y.; Kroll, A.V.; et al. Erythrocyte–platelet hybrid membrane coating for enhanced nanoparticle functionalization. *Adv. Mater.* **2017**, *29*, 1606209. [CrossRef] [PubMed]
84. Zhao, H.; Song, S.S.; Ma, J.W.; Yan, Z.Y.; Xie, H.W.; Feng, Y.; Che, S.S. CD47 as a promising therapeutic target in oncology. *Front. Immunol.* **2022**, *13*, 757480. [CrossRef] [PubMed]
85. Hu, C.M.J.; Fang, R.H.; Zhang, L. Erythrocyte-inspired delivery systems. *Adv. Healthc. Mater.* **2012**, *1*, 537–547. [CrossRef] [PubMed]
86. Liu, B.; Wang, W.M.; Fan, J.L.; Long, Y.; Xiao, F.; Daniyal, M.; Tong, C.Y.; Xie, Q.; Jian, Y.Q.; Li, B.; et al. RBC membrane camouflaged prussian blue nanoparticles for gamabutolin loading and combined chemo/photothermal therapy of breast cancer. *Biomaterials* **2019**, *217*, 119301. [CrossRef]
87. Gao, C.H.; Wang, Y.L.; Sun, J.J.; Han, Y.; Gong, W.; Li, Y.; Feng, Y.; Wang, H.; Yang, M.Y.; Li, Z.P.; et al. Neuronal mitochondria-targeted delivery of curcumin by biomimetic engineered nanosystems in Alzheimer's disease mice. *Acta Biomater.* **2020**, *108*, 285–299. [CrossRef] [PubMed]
88. Meijden, P.E.J.V.D.; Heemskerk, J.W.M. Platelet biology and functions: New concepts and clinical perspectives. *Nat. Rev. Cardiol.* **2019**, *16*, 166–179. [CrossRef]
89. Avecilla, S.T.; Hattori, K.; Heissig, B.; Tejada, R.; Liao, F.; Shido, K.; Jin, D.K.; Dias, S.; Zhang, F.; Hartman, T.E.; et al. Chemokine-mediated interaction of hematopoietic progenitors with the bone marrow vascular niche is required for thrombopoiesis. *Nat. Med.* **2004**, *10*, 64–71. [CrossRef]
90. Koupenova, M.; Clancy, L.; Corkrey, H.A.; Freedman, J.E. Circulating platelets as mediators of immunity, inflammation, and thrombosis. *Circ. Res.* **2018**, *122*, 337–351. [CrossRef]
91. Rayes, J.; Watson, S.P.; Nieswandt, B. Functional significance of the platelet immune receptors GPVI and CLEC-2. *J. Clin. Investig.* **2019**, *129*, 12–23. [CrossRef]
92. McDonald, B.; Dunbar, M. Platelets and intravascular immunity: Guardians of the vascular space during bloodstream infections and sepsis. *Front. Immunol.* **2019**, *10*, 2400. [CrossRef] [PubMed]
93. Xu, J.P.; Wang, X.Q.; Yin, H.Y.; Cao, X.; Hu, Q.Y.; Lv, W.; Xu, Q.W.; Gu, Z.; Xin, H.L. Sequentially site-specific delivery of thrombolytics and neuroprotectant for enhanced treatment of ischemic stroke. *ACS Nano* **2019**, *13*, 8577–8588. [CrossRef]
94. Zinger, A.; Soriano, S.; Baudo, G.; Rosa, E.D.; Taraballi, F.; Villapol, S. Biomimetic nanoparticles as a theranostic tool for traumatic brain injury. *Adv. Funct. Mater.* **2021**, *31*, 2100722. [CrossRef] [PubMed]
95. Martinez, J.O.; Molinaro, R.; Hartman, K.A.; Boada, C.; Sukhovershin, R.; Rosa, E.D.; Kuri, D.; Zhang, S.R.; Evangelopoulos, M.; Carter, A.M.; et al. Biomimetic nanoparticles with enhanced affinity towards activated endothelium as versatile tools for theranostic drug delivery. *Theranostics* **2018**, *8*, 1131–1145. [CrossRef]
96. Li, R.; He, Y.; Zhang, S.; Qin, J.; Wang, J. Cell membrane-based nanoparticles: A new biomimetic platform for tumor diagnosis and treatment. *Acta Pharm. Sin. B* **2017**, *8*, 14–22. [CrossRef] [PubMed]
97. Feng, L.S.; Dou, C.R.; Xia, Y.G.; Li, B.H.; Zhao, M.Y.; Yu, P.; Zheng, Y.Y.; El-Toni, A.M.; Atta, N.F.; Galal, A.; et al. Neutrophil-like cell-membrane-coated nanozyme therapy for ischemic brain damage and long-term neurological functional recovery. *ACS Nano* **2021**, *15*, 2263–2280. [CrossRef]
98. Liu, R.; An, Y.; Jia, W.F.; Wang, Y.S.; Wu, Y.; Zhen, Y.H.; Cao, J.; Gao, H.L. Macrophage-mimic shape changeable nanomedicine retained in tumor for multimodal therapy of breast cancer. *J. Control. Release* **2020**, *321*, 589–601. [CrossRef]
99. Pang, L.; Qin, J.; Han, L.; Zhao, W.; Liang, J.; Xie, Z.; Yang, P.; Wang, J. Exploiting macrophages as targeted carrier to guide nanoparticles into glioma. *Oncotarget* **2016**, *7*, 37081–37091. [CrossRef]
100. Yurdagul, A.; Finney, A.C.; Woolard, M.D.; Orr, A.W. The arterial microenvironment: The where and why of atherosclerosis. *Biochem. J.* **2016**, *473*, 1281–1295. [CrossRef]
101. Nagenborg, J.; Goossens, P.; Biessen, E.A.L.; Donners, M.M.P.C. Heterogeneity of atherosclerotic plaque macrophage origin, phenotype and functions: Implications for treatment. *Eur. J. Pharmacol.* **2017**, *816*, 14–24. [CrossRef]
102. Long, Y.; Xiang, Y.; Liu, S.Y.; Zhang, Y.L.; Wan, J.Y.; Ci, Z.M.; Cui, M.Q.; Shen, L.; Li, N.; Guan, Y.M. Macrophage membrane modified baicalin liposomes improve brain targeting for alleviating cerebral ischemia reperfusion injury. *Nanomedicine* **2022**, *43*, 102547. [CrossRef] [PubMed]
103. Sun, H.; Su, J.; Meng, Q.; Yin, Q.; Chen, L.; Gu, W.; Zhang, P.; Zhang, Z.; Yu, H.; Wang, S.; et al. Cancer-cell-biomimetic nanoparticles for targeted therapy of homotypic tumors. *Adv. Mater.* **2016**, *28*, 9581–9588. [CrossRef]
104. Li, J.; Wang, X.D.; Zheng, D.Y.; Lin, X.Y.; Wei, Z.W.; Zhang, D.; Li, Z.F.; Zhang, Y.; Wu, M.; Liu, X.L. Cancer cell membrane-coated magnetic nanoparticles for MR/NIR fluorescence dual-modal imaging and photodynamic therapy†. *Biomater. Sci.* **2018**, *6*, 1834–1845. [CrossRef] [PubMed]
105. Drolez, A.; Vandenhaute, E.; Julien, S.; Gosselet, F.; Burchell, J.; Cecchelli, R.; Delannoy, P.; Dehouck, M.-P.; Mysiorek, C. Selection of a relevant in vitro blood-brain barrier model to investigate pro-metastatic features of human breast cancer cell lines. *PLoS ONE* **2016**, *11*, e0151155. [CrossRef] [PubMed]
106. Wang, C.X.; Wu, B.; Wu, Y.T.; Song, X.Y.; Zhang, S.S.; Liu, Z.H. Camouflaging nanoparticles with brain metastatic tumor cell membranes: A new strategy to traverse blood–brain barrier for imaging and therapy of brain tumors. *Adv. Funct. Mater.* **2020**, *30*, 1909369. [CrossRef]

107. Zhao, Y.N.; Li, A.; Jiang, L.D.; Gu, Y.W.; Liu, J.Y. Hybrid membrane-coated biomimetic nanoparticles (HM@BNPs): A multifunctional nanomaterial for biomedical applications. *Biomacromolecules* **2021**, *22*, 3149–3167. [CrossRef]
108. Ai, X.Z.; Wang, S.Y.; Duan, Y.O.; Zhang, Q.Z.; Chen, M.S.; Gao, W.W.; Zhang, L.F. Emerging approaches to functionalizing cell membrane-coated nanoparticles. *Biochemistry* **2020**, *60*, 941–955. [CrossRef]
109. Yin, Y.; Tang, W.; Ma, X.Y.; Tang, L.; Zhang, Y.; Yang, M.; Hu, F.F.; Li, G.L.; Wang, Y.Z. Biomimetic neutrophil and macrophage dual membrane-coated nanoplatform with orchestrated tumor-microenvironment responsive capability promotes therapeutic efficacy against glioma. *Chem. Eng. J.* **2021**, *433*, 133848. [CrossRef]
110. Niu, W.B.; Xiao, Q.; Wang, X.J.; Zhu, J.Q.; Li, J.H.; Liang, X.M.; Peng, Y.M.; Wu, C.T.; Lu, R.J.; Pan, Y.; et al. A biomimetic drug delivery system by integrating grapefruit extracellular vesicles and doxorubicin-loaded heparin-based nanoparticles for glioma therapy. *Nano Lett.* **2021**, *21*, 1484–1492. [CrossRef]
111. Hao, Q.; Liu, Q.H.; Wang, X.B.; Wang, P.; Li, T.; Tong, W.Y. Membrane damage effect of therapeutic ultrasound on Ehrlich ascitic tumor cells. *Cancer Biother. Radiopharm.* **2009**, *24*, 41–48. [CrossRef]
112. Fabiilli, M.L.; Haworth, K.J.; Fakhri, N.H.; Kripfgans, O.D.; Carson, P.L.; Fowlkes, J.B. The role of inertial cavitation in acoustic droplet vaporization. *IEEE Trans. Ultrason. Ferroelectr. Freq. Control* **2009**, *56*, 1006–1117. [CrossRef] [PubMed]
113. Wang, W.J.; Chen, W.J.; Zou, M.M.; Lv, R.L.; Wang, D.L.; Hou, F.R.; Feng, H.; Ma, X.B.; Zhong, J.J.; Ding, T.; et al. Applications of power ultrasound in oriented modification and degradation of pectin: A review. *J. Food Eng.* **2018**, *234*, 98–107. [CrossRef]
114. Amini, M.; Niemi, E.; Hisdal, J.; Kalvøy, H.; Tronstad, C.; Scholz, H.; Rosales, A.; Martinsen, Ø.G. Monitoring the quality of frozen-thawed venous segments using bioimpedance spectroscopy. *Physiol. Meas.* **2020**, *41*, 044008. [CrossRef]
115. Fu, Q.; Lv, P.P.; Chen, Z.K.; Ni, D.Z.; Zhang, L.J.; Yue, H.; Yue, Z.G.; Wei, W.; Ma, G.H. Programmed co-delivery of paclitaxel and doxorubicin boosted by camouflaging with erythrocyte membrane†. *Nanoscale* **2015**, *7*, 4020–4030. [CrossRef]
116. Chai, Z.L.; Hu, X.F.; Wei, X.L.; Zhan, C.Y.; Lu, L.W.; Jiang, K.; Su, B.X.; Ruan, H.T.; Ran, D.N.; Fang, R.H.; et al. A facile approach to functionalizing cell membrane-coated nanoparticles with neurotoxin-derived peptide for brain-targeted drug delivery. *J. Control. Release* **2017**, *264*, 102–111. [CrossRef] [PubMed]
117. Klenk, C.; Heim, D.; Ugele, M.; Hayden, O. Impact of sample preparation on holographic imaging of leukocytes. *Opt. Eng.* **2019**, *59*, 102403. [CrossRef]
118. Kang, T.; Zhu, Q.Q.; Wei, D.; Feng, J.X.; Yao, J.H.; Jiang, T.Z.; Song, Q.X.; Wei, X.B.; Chen, H.Z.; Gao, X.L.; et al. Nanoparticles coated with neutrophil membranes can effectively treat cancer metastasis. *ACS Nano* **2017**, *11*, 1397–1411. [CrossRef] [PubMed]
119. Barua, P.; Ahn, S.B.; Mohamedali, A.; Liu, F. Improved sensitivity in cell surface protein detection by combining chemical labeling with mechanical lysis in a colorectal cancer cell model. *Biotechnol. Lett.* **2020**, *42*, 683–695. [CrossRef]
120. DeCaprio, J.; Kohl, T.O. Using Dounce homogenization to lyse cells for immunoprecipitation. *Cold Spring Harb. Protoc.* **2019**, *2019*, 551–554. [CrossRef]
121. Rahman, M.A.; Wang, J.; Zhang, C.; Olah, A.; Baer, E. Novel micro-/nano- porous cellular membranes by forced assembly co-extrusion technology. *Eur. Polym. J.* **2016**, *83*, 99–113. [CrossRef]
122. He, W.P.; Frueh, J.; Wu, Z.W.; He, Q. Leucocyte membrane-coated janus microcapsules for enhanced photothermal cancer treatment. *Langmuir* **2016**, *32*, 3637–3644. [CrossRef] [PubMed]
123. Movahed, S.; Li, D.Q. Microfluidics cell electroporation. *Microfluid Nanofluidics* **2010**, *10*, 703–734. [CrossRef]
124. Rao, L.; Cai, B.; Bu, L.L.; Liao, Q.Q.; Guo, S.S.; Zhao, X.Z.; Dong, W.F.; Liu, W. Microfluidic electroporation-facilitated synthesis of erythrocyte membrane-coated magnetic nanoparticles for enhanced imaging-guided cancer therapy. *ACS Nano* **2017**, *11*, 3496–3505. [CrossRef] [PubMed]
125. Huang, D.; Zhao, D.Y.; Li, J.H.; Wu, Y.T.; Zhou, W.B.; Wang, W.; Liang, Z.C.; Li, Z.H. High cell viability microfluidic electroporation in a curved channel. *Sens. Actuators B Chem.* **2017**, *250*, 703–711. [CrossRef]
126. Marqués-Gallego, P.; Kroon, A.I.P.M.d. Ligation strategies for targeting liposomal nanocarriers. *BioMed. Res. Int.* **2014**, *2014*, 129458. [CrossRef]
127. García-Granados, R.; Lerma-Escalera, J.A.; Morones-Ramírez, J.R. Metabolic engineering and synthetic biology: Synergies, future, and challenges. *Front. Bioeng. Biotechnol.* **2019**, *7*, 36. [CrossRef]
128. Stephan, M.T.; Irvine, D.J. Enhancing cell therapies from the outside in: Cell surface engineering using synthetic nanomaterials. *Nano Today* **2011**, *6*, 309–325. [CrossRef]
129. Zhou, H.; Fan, Z.Y.; Lemons, P.K.; Cheng, H. A facile approach to functionalize cell membrane-coated nanoparticles. *Theranostics* **2016**, *6*, 1012–1022. [CrossRef]
130. Wang, R.R.; Wang, C.W.; Dai, Z.Z.; Chen, Y.Z.; Shen, Z.W.; Xiao, G.; Chen, Y.F.; Zhou, J.N.; Zhuang, Z.R.; Wu, R.H. An amyloid-β targeting chemical exchange saturation transfer probe for in vivo detection of Alzheimer's disease. *ACS Chem. Neurosci.* **2019**, *10*, 3859–3867. [CrossRef]
131. Spencer, B.; Trinh, L.; Rockenstein, E.; Mante, M.; Florio, J.; Adame, A.; El-Agnaf, O.M.A.; Kim, C.; Masliah, E.; Rissman, R.A. Systemic peptide mediated delivery of an siRNA targeting α-syn in the CNS ameliorates the neurodegenerative process in a transgenic model of Lewy body disease. *Neurobiol. Dis.* **2019**, *127*, 163–177. [CrossRef]
132. Topal, G.R.; Mészáros, M.; Porkoláb, G.; Szecskó, A.; Polgár, T.F.; Siklós, L.; Deli, M.A.; Veszelka, S.; Bozkir, A. ApoE-targeting increases the transfer of solid lipid nanoparticles with donepezil cargo across a culture model of the blood–brain barrier. *Pharmaceutics* **2020**, *13*, 38. [CrossRef] [PubMed]

133. Corti, R.; Cox, A.; Cassina, V.; Nardo, L.; Salerno, D.; Marrano, C.A.; Missana, N.; Andreozzi, P.; Silva, P.J.; Stellacci, F.; et al. The clustering of mApoE anti-amyloidogenic peptide on nanoparticle surface does not alter its performance in controlling beta-amyloid aggregation. *Int. J. Mol. Sci.* **2020**, *21*, 1066. [CrossRef] [PubMed]
134. Séguy, L.; Guyon, L.; Maurel, M.; Verdié, P.; Davis, A.; Corvaisier, S.; Lisowski, V.; Dallemagne, P.; Groo, A.C.; Malzert-Fréon, A. Active targeted nanoemulsions for repurposing of tegaserod in Alzheimer's disease treatment. *Pharmaceutics* **2021**, *13*, 1626. [CrossRef] [PubMed]
135. Israel, L.L.; Galstyan, A.; Cox, A.; Shatalova, E.S.; Sun, T.; Rashid, M.-H.; Grodzinski, Z.; Chiechi, A.; Fuchs, D.-T.; Patil, R.; et al. Signature effects of vector-guided systemic nano bioconjugate delivery across blood-brain barrier of normal, Alzheimer's, and tumor mouse models. *ACS Nano* **2022**, *16*, 11815–11832. [CrossRef] [PubMed]
136. Hou, Q.H.; Zhu, L.N.; Wang, L.; Liu, X.Y.; Xiao, F.; Xie, Y.Z.X.; Zheng, W.F.; Jiang, X.Y. Screening on-chip fabricated nanoparticles for penetrating the blood–brain barrier. *Nanoscale* **2022**, *14*, 3234–3241. [CrossRef] [PubMed]
137. Zhang, X.T.; He, T.; Chai, Z.; Samulski, R.J.; Li, C.W. Blood-brain barrier shuttle peptides enhance AAV transduction in the brain after systemic administration. *Biomaterials* **2018**, *176*, 71–83. [CrossRef]
138. Díaz-Perlas, C.; Oller-Salvia, B.; Sánchez-Navarro, M.; Teixidó, M.; Giralt, E. Branched BBB-shuttle peptides: Chemoselective modification of proteins to enhance blood–brain barrier transport†. *Chem. Sci.* **2018**, *9*, 8409–8415. [CrossRef]
139. Falanga, A.; Melone, P.; Cagliani, R.; Borbone, N.; D'Errico, S.; Piccialli, G.; Netti, P.; Guarnieri, D. Design, synthesis and characterization of novel co-polymers decorated with peptides for the selective nanoparticle transport across the cerebral endothelium. *Molecules* **2018**, *23*, 1655. [CrossRef]
140. Liu, Y.; Li, J.F.; Shao, K.; Huang, R.Q.; Ye, L.Y.; Lou, J.N.; Jiang, C. A leptin derived 30-amino-acid peptide modified pegylated poly-L-lysine dendrigraft for brain targeted gene delivery. *Biomaterials* **2010**, *31*, 5246–5257. [CrossRef]
141. Farshbaf, M.; Mojarad-Jabali, S.; Hemmati, S.; Khosroushahi, A.Y.; Motasadizadeh, H.; Zarebkohan, A.; Valizadeh, H. Enhanced BBB and BBTB penetration and improved anti-glioma behavior of bortezomib through dual-targeting nanostructured lipid carriers. *J. Control. Release* **2022**, *345*, 371–384. [CrossRef]
142. Fattahi, H.; Esmaeil, N.; Aliomrani, M. Apamin as a BBB shuttle and its effects on T cell population during the experimental autoimmune encephalomyelitis-induced model of multiple sclerosis. *Neurotox. Res.* **2021**, *39*, 1880–1891. [CrossRef] [PubMed]
143. Najmi, A.; Wang, S.G.; Huang, Y.; Seefeldt, T.; Alqahtani, Y.; Guan, X.M. 2-(2-Cholesteroxyethoxyl)ethyl 3′-S-glutathionylpropionate and its self-assembled micelles for brain delivery: Design, synthesis and evaluation. *Int. J. Pharm.* **2021**, *600*, 120520. [CrossRef] [PubMed]
144. Zhang, H.Y.; Os, W.L.v.; Tian, X.B.; Zu, G.Y.; Ribovski, L.; Bron, R.; Bussmann, J.; Kros, A.; Liu, Y.; Zuhorn, I.S. Development of curcumin-loaded zein nanoparticles for transport across the blood–brain barrier and inhibition of glioblastoma cell growth. *Biomater. Sci.* **2021**, *35*, 456–465. [CrossRef]
145. Maderna, E.; Colombo, L.; Cagnotto, A.; Fede, G.D.; Indaco, A.; Tagliavini, F.; Salmona, M.; Giaccone, G. In situ tissue labeling of cerebral amyloid using HIV-related Tat peptide. *Mol. Neurobiol.* **2018**, *55*, 6834–6840. [CrossRef]
146. Rousselle, C.; Clair, P.; Temsamani, J.; Scherrmann, J.-M. Improved brain delivery of benzylpenicillin with a peptide-vector-mediated strategy. *J. Drug Target.* **2002**, *10*, 309–315. [CrossRef]
147. Yang, L.C.; Sun, J.; Xie, W.J.; Liu, Y.N.; Liu, J. Dual-functional selenium nanoparticles bind to and inhibit amyloid β fiber formation in Alzheimer's disease. *J. Mater. Chem. B* **2017**, *5*, 5954–5967. [CrossRef] [PubMed]
148. Rusiecka, I.; Ruczyński, J.; Kozłowska, A.; Backtrog, E.; Mucha, P.; Kocić, I.; Rekowski, P. TP10-dopamine conjugate as a potential therapeutic agent in the treatment of Parkinson's disease. *Bioconjug. Chem.* **2019**, *30*, 760–774. [CrossRef]
149. Loureiro, J.A.; Gomes, B.; Fricker, G.; Coelho, M.A.N.; Rocha, S.; Pereira, M.C. Cellular uptake of PLGA nanoparticles targeted with anti-amyloid and anti-transferrin receptor antibodies for Alzheimer's disease treatment. *Colloids Surf. B* **2016**, *145*, 8–13. [CrossRef] [PubMed]
150. Zhang, C.; Wan, X.; Zheng, X.Y.; Shao, X.Y.; Liu, Q.F.; Zhang, Q.Z.; Qian, Y. Dual-functional nanoparticles targeting amyloid plaques in the brains of Alzheimer's disease mice. *Biomaterials* **2014**, *35*, 456–465. [CrossRef]
151. Guo, Q.; Xu, S.T.; Yang, P.; Wang, P.Z.; Lu, S.; Sheng, D.Y.; Qian, K.; Cao, J.X.; Lu, W.; Zhang, Q.Z. A dual-ligand fusion peptide improves the brain-neuron targeting of nanocarriers in Alzheimer's disease mice. *J. Control. Release* **2020**, *320*, 347–362. [CrossRef]

MDPI AG
Grosspeteranlage 5
4052 Basel
Switzerland
Tel.: +41 61 683 77 34

Molecules Editorial Office
E-mail: molecules@mdpi.com
www.mdpi.com/journal/molecules

www.ingramcontent.com/pod-product-compliance
Lightning Source LLC
Chambersburg PA
CBHW040807250926
51850CB00007BA/1106
* 9 7 8 3 7 2 5 8 8 0 4 5 4 *